T0198431

AI Doctor

AI Doctor: The Rise of Artificial Intelligence in Healthcare

A Guide for Users, Buyers, Builders, and Investors

RONALD M. RAZMI, MD

WILEY

Published by John Wiley & Sons, Inc., Hoboken, New Jersey.
Published simultaneously in Canada.

For general information on our other products and services or for technical support, please contact our Customer Care Department within the United States at (800) 762-2974, outside the United States at (317) 572-3993 or fax (317) 572-4002.

Wiley also publishes its books in a variety of electronic formats. Some content that appears in print may not be available in electronic formats. For more information about Wiley products, visit our web site at www.wiley.com.

Library of Congress Cataloging-in-Publication Data applied for
9781394240166 (paperback); 9781394240180 (ePDF); 9781394240173 (ePUB); 9781394240197 (oBook)

Cover Design: Wiley
Cover Images: © Kittipong Jirasukhanont/Alamy Stock Photo; Sandipkumar Patel/Getty Images

Set in 10/12pt STIX Two Text by Straive, Pondicherry, India
SKY10082230_081724

This work is dedicated to my amazing parents and brothers, whose love and support have always been the foundation upon which I've built. To friends and mentors whom I've learned from and who have always helped me pursue my goals.

Contents

Part III   The Business Case for AI in Healthcare   275

About the Author

DR. RONALD M. RAZMI IS A CARDIOLOGIST who's occupied many roles in healthcare and has a 360-degree view of the practice and business of healthcare. He completed his medical training at the Mayo Clinic and was one of the pioneers in studying the applications of emerging digital technologies in managing cardiac patients. During his training, he was involved in research and published several peer-reviewed articles in scientific journals. He is a co-author of the *Handbook of Cardiovascular Magnetic Resonance Imaging* (CRC Press 2006) and launched one of the first training centers in the world for cardiologists to learn emerging technologies for managing their patients.

Ron earned his MBA from Northwestern University's Kellogg School of Management and joined McKinsey & Company in their healthcare group, where he advised large and small companies in corporate strategy, M&A, buyout deals, and investments in emerging health technologies. In 2011, he founded Acupera, a software company that uses healthcare data and analytics to improve the management of patients with chronic diseases. Ron was the CEO of Acupera for six years and saw the challenges of bringing innovation into healthcare organizations or achieving patient adoption. Much of what he learned is covered in this book to educate innovators, buyers, and investors about the roadmap for technology adoption in healthcare. Ron has been one of the prominent voices in the digital revolution in healthcare and has written many articles and bylines, participated in interviews, and spoken at conferences.

Ron is the co-founder and managing director of Zoi Capital, a venture capital firm that invests in digital health technologies with a focus on the applications of AI in healthcare. In 2021, he launched AI Doctor, one of the only blogs focused solely on the applications of AI in healthcare. He's a frequent speaker at conferences, a guest on podcasts, and the author of medical and business articles.

Foreword

FROM THE EARLIEST DAYS of Alan Turing's 1950s speculations about the possibility of computers developing some general form of intelligence, scholars have thought that healthcare would be an ideal application area for such capabilities. After all, everyone desires more effective health care, medical practice has never approached perfection, and computers and their applications have increased by nearly a billion-fold in computational abilities over these years. So, it is not beyond the realm of imagination to think that the computer and its sophisticated machine learning abilities can form an ideal technology to help revolutionize the practice of medicine and public health. After all, if we can capture all the healthcare situations in which patients have found themselves, record the decisions their clinicians have made in their care, and evaluate the outcomes in those myriad trials, we (and our tools) should be able to learn what works best for which kinds of patients in what conditions, and perhaps even why, based on a growing understanding of the biology that underlies medicine. That knowledge should then form the basis of clinical decision support, which should help doctors, nurses, technicians, and patients themselves make optimal choices and thus lead to an era of precision medicine, achieving the best possible outcomes for each individual patient.

Despite the optimism embedded in such projections, this vision has largely not been fulfilled. Of course, the practice of medicine has improved greatly over the past seventy years, but mostly because we have developed better tools to examine the operations of the human body, a much-improved understanding of the biological and environmental processes and genetic influences that cause disease, and highly targeted medications and procedures that can interfere with disease processes. Yet most of the traditional tasks of medicine—diagnosis, prognosis, and treatment—are still rife with uncertainty.

The vast increases in computer power have enabled widespread application of imaging tools such as CT and MRI, have contributed to sequencing and analyzing the human genome, and have made it possible to create electronic health records for billions of patients around the world, whose data had previously largely remained in inaccessible paper collections of handwritten notes. Nevertheless, despite tremendous advances in what we now call artificial intelligence (AI), we see surprisingly few successful applications of those technologies in healthcare. The ones that are successful tend to focus on very specific clinical problems, such as interpreting retinal fundus images to identify patients developing diabetic retinopathy or examining mammograms to estimate the risk of a patient developing breast cancer. And even in such narrow domains, success is often elusive.

Ron Razmi has spent the past three years wrestling with this conundrum, and in this book reviews what he has learned from that struggle. Ron is a Renaissance man of healthcare, who trained and practiced as a cardiologist, then was a consultant for one of the world's largest consulting companies, became a digital health entrepreneur, and now serves as a venture capitalist, helping others to realize the above dreams.

My own interest in medical AI began in 1974 when I joined the computer science faculty at MIT and quickly found myself attracted to the problems of how one could represent medical knowledge in a formal way in computer programs and how those programs could use that knowledge to apply diagnostic reasoning, therapy planning, and prognoses to individual patient cases. I began to work with a cohort of brilliant doctors who were excited to formalize these ideas for a very different reason: they taught the next generation of medical students and wanted to know how to teach the best ways to reason about clinical decision-making. They thought that capturing what they knew and how they reasoned would crystalize what they wanted to pass on to their students. My motivation was to build decision support systems that could improve the practice of most doctors by providing a built-in "second opinion" on their challenging cases. Replacing doctors' decision-making was never the goal, as we realized that our systems were unlikely to be perfect, so a man-machine team was likely to make better decisions than either alone.

At that time, most medical records were still kept as handwritten paper notes and the machine learning methods we today take for granted had not yet been developed, so our approach was to ask experienced doctors how they thought through difficult problems and then to write computer programs to simulate that thinking. Those programs, based on symbolic pattern matching or on chaining of symbolic inference rules, did a good job of handling the "textbook" cases but broke down on more complex cases where, for example, a patient suffered from an unusual combination of disorders. We tried to fix this problem by developing methods that reasoned about the pathophysiology of multiple diseases, but unfortunately, even today, with our much better understanding of biology and genetics, variations among patients and their responses to treatments are often unexplainable.

Fortunately, by the mid-1990s, many academic medical centers had implemented electronic medical/health/patient records, so it became possible to learn relationships among symptoms, lab data, drug prescriptions, procedures, and their outcomes from such empirical data. By the end of the 2000s, government subsidy for EHR adoption had made such systems ubiquitous, today implemented in about 98% of all US hospitals. At the same time, research on machine learning, starting with the tried-and-true methods of statistics, had been extended to model much more complex relationships among data.

In the 2010s, a new method was developed to represent concepts as vectors in a high-dimensional space—i.e. as long lists of numbers—derived from the frequency and nearness of co-occurrence of the concepts in papers, medical notes, etc. Concepts whose meanings are similar to each other are often found in similar contexts, so their representations wind up near each other in that space. Furthermore, relations also take on a numerical relationship. For example, the vector of the distance and direction of the difference between the embeddings of "bone marrow" and "red blood cells" is similar to that between "adrenal gland" and "cortisol". So, that vector is approximately a representation of "produces". At the same time, an older idea, to build learning systems inspired by neuroscience, became practical because of the enormous improvements in computer power. To learn a model that can, say, predict the outcome of a medical intervention on a patient in a certain clinical state, we can start with a random neural network and train it on a large body of known cases of the state of a patient, the treatment, and the outcome. Initially, the network will predict randomly, but each time it makes an error, we can assign blame for that error proportionally to the parts of the network that computed the wrong outcome and adjust their influence to reduce the error. As we keep doing so, often repeatedly for thousands or even millions of cases, the error is reduced and the model becomes more accurate. The numerical representation of concepts makes this possible, so those two insightful methods now account for most machine learning approaches. Indeed, the Large Language Models that are so much in the news today are trained very much as just described, where their task is simply to predict the next word from previous ones in a vast number of human-written (or spoken) texts.

In the past dozen or so years, therefore, many projects have succeeded in using repositories of clinical data to learn predictive models that could estimate the likelihood that a patient would develop some disease within a certain period of time, whether particular interventions were likely to cure them, how long they might live with an incurable disease, etc.

Nevertheless, much technical work remains to be done. We learned that systems built from data at one hospital might not work nearly as well at another because the patient populations differed in genetics, socioeconomic status, attitudes toward complying with medical advice, the prevalence of environmental influences in their neighborhood, etc. Medical records were often incomplete: a patient treated at multiple institutions might have records at only some of them, clerical errors dropped some data, heterogeneous vendors could have incompatible data formats that prevented their matching, etc. Clinical practice, often based on local traditions, might differ, so the tests and treatments used in different hospitals may not be the same. Most significantly, medical records do not typically record why some action was taken, yet that reasoning may be the most useful predictor of how well a patient eventually thrives. Finally, faced with a clinical situation in which two alternative therapies seem reasonable, in each case only one of them is chosen, so we have no way to know what would have happened had the other—the counterfactual therapy—been chosen.

Clinical trials address this problem by randomizing the choice of intervention, so we can know that nothing about the case has influenced the treatment choice, so its success or failure must depend only on the patient's condition and treatment, and not on confounders that in a non-trial context probably influenced the choice of treatment. However, most clinical decisions have not been studied by clinical trials. Also, the trials that have been done are typically done with a limited number of patients and for a limited period of time, so they may easily miss phenomena that arise rarely or only in the long term. They also tend to recruit subjects without comorbidities unrelated to the trial; thus, most of the patients whose care is ultimately determined by the outcome of the trial may not have been eligible to participate in it. Thus, clinical trials are also an imperfect method to determine the right interventions, so, despite methodological difficulties, analyzing the vast amount of non-trial clinical data must have great value to improve healthcare.

Focusing on the technical problems of how to build the best possible models makes researchers such as me myopic. Only with decades of experience have I come to realize that a working predictive model will not necessarily be adopted and used. Institutions' choices are driven by their own perceptions of what they need most, what they can afford to do, what they have the energy to take on, and what is consistent with their culture. These are not computational questions but fall more into areas such as management and sociology. Thus, improvement of healthcare through machine learning is a socio-technical problem that requires insights and collaboration among many specialists.

This book is organized into three major sections. The first section ("Roadmap") introduces the development of AI technologies over many decades and indicates the current state of the art, especially how it might be applied in healthcare. It then asks the question of how we can build robust applications and enters a very detailed discussion of what data are needed to train AI models, how these may be obtained (with difficulty), how they are processed, and how their availability and nature influence the quality of the models we can build from them. The need for robustness also raises critical questions about whether a model can be used on different populations and related issues of bias and fairness. This section then presents a bad news/good news pair of chapters, first summarizing the impediments to the vision the book outlines, followed by a more optimistic chapter describing the forces that are likely to make the vision come to fruition.

Section II ("Applications of AI in Healthcare") examines in great detail the opportunities for AI health care applications in diagnostics, therapeutics, decision support, population health, clinical workflows, administration, and the related basic life sciences. Each subsection delves into Ron's insights about specific clinical areas of opportunity, e.g. radiology, ophthalmology, cardiology, neurology, etc. It also details examples of particular projects and companies that are currently pursuing these opportunities, thus painting a vivid picture of where the field stands. Although the tone is overall optimistic, these discussions also cover potential problems and places where we don't yet know how things will turn out.

The third section ("The Business Case for AI in Healthcare") is Ron's assessment of the business case for the possibilities described in the earlier chapters. Doctors, patients, hospitals, clinics, insurers, etc., each have a limited attention span and many competing potential projects vying for their attention. Thus, even applications that technically work are often not adopted if they are not seen as solving critical problems, doing so rapidly, while offering significant financial returns on investment. Ron uses his experience as an entrepreneur to discuss the myriad problems encountered in taking an application to successful adoption and then his experience as an investor to show the constraints on developing new applications placed by financial considerations. This section serves as a cautionary tale on what one might expect from new ventures but also includes suggestions on the kinds of applications that are ripe for contemporary exploitation, those expected to become practical in the medium term, and those whose potential is in the more distant future.

The value of this book is in explaining the technical background that makes sophisticated healthcare applications possible, surveying the field of such applications currently being fielded or developed, and describing the landscape into which any such efforts must fit. The specific projects will, of course, change rapidly as the trends outlined here make more data available to learn from in a more standardized way, as the field figures out how to conduct trials of these technologies that can convincingly pave the way for their adoption, and as the priorities of providers and payers adjust to the growing capabilities of the systems.

The underlying technologies will also change rapidly. The convolutional neural networks that underlie most machine vision and image interpretation algorithms only became practical a little over a decade ago. The large language models that drive generative AI applications have only become capable in the past two or three years and continue to develop rapidly. Pioneers of these technologies anticipate that newer methods will arise that can much more accurately identify subtle image features and generate answers to queries that are free of the "hallucinations" that sometimes plague current methods. Such technical advances, if realized, will open up new avenues of application in healthcare and will change the ROI calculations that influence adoption. Despite the consequent changes that I would expect in an edition of this book five years from now, the principles identified by Ron and the way of thinking exemplified by the analyses in this book are going to continue to be of great value.

Peter Szolovits, PhD
Professor of Computer Science and Engineering
Massachusetts Institute of Technology
Cambridge, MA
January 15, 2024

Preface

OVER THE COURSE OF my career as a cardiologist, consultant, CEO, and investor, I've always been astonished at the pace of medical innovation and how we're making rapid progress in maintaining health and treating diseases. Only 100 years ago, we didn't have anesthesia for surgeries, antibiotics for infections, cancer treatments, or the knowledge of what caused heart disease (or much else, for that matter). How did we get this far in 100 years or so when for 300,000 years, progress was negligible? Well, the industrial revolution that started about 250 years ago set in motion the kind of technological progress and wealth creation that paved the way for the medical breakthroughs we've seen over the last few decades. You need resources and know-how to do good medical research.

Much of the progress in healthcare stems from the creation of institutions that established standards for research, private sector incentives such as patents for discoveries and inventions, and robust public sector funding. Life expectancy is way up and the pace of progress is accelerating every day. This has a ripple effect throughout the rest of the economy. When people are healthier and live longer, they're happier and more productive. This results in economic growth, which means more employment and better standards of living. It also means higher tax revenues for the government, the entity that funds most of the basic research that leads to new industries, creating future employment opportunities and improving our lives. Examples of this include the internet, the pharmaceutical industry, and now artificial intelligence (AI). According to the McKinsey Global Institute, about a third of all economic growth in advanced economies in the past 100 years can be attributed to health improvements among the global population.[1]

Although AI has been discussed for decades, it's only in the last decade that breakthroughs in its core methodologies have pushed it to the forefront. In healthcare, we've only recently accepted its potential to become a breakthrough technology. It was only after it started to be used in other sectors and people noticed its power to solve complex problems that innovators in healthcare realized how well-suited it is for medical research and care delivery. After all, AI is at its most powerful when it has access to a large amount of data with many dimensions. Perhaps there's no industry with more of that than healthcare, from genetics and proteomics to epigenetics, clinical data, social data, and more!

But that's not always been the case, and until a few decades ago, we had limited data to work with. Gradually, as the number of labs we could order increased, we carried out more sophisticated radiological imaging and tissue analysis with pathology, while genetics was introduced into certain specialties. However, reviewing all of this information and putting it all together has remained a clinician's job. It will most likely *remain* their job, but the amount of data has exploded and keeps growing. Molecular data (and the insights it provides) introduces a whole new dimension to the practice of medicine. When you add this to data from smartphones, smartwatches and wearables, and environmental and socioeconomic data, you have a lot to analyze. Figuring out patterns in all of this data to predict, diagnose, or manage disease is beyond the capabilities of the human mind and the traditional analytical methods we've relied on.

Since this explosion of health data only started in the last couple of decades, AI is arriving at just the right moment. It's the technology of the moment and can help us to take advantage of all of this data. It can help us to make the data usable, to figure out key relationships, to make predictions, and to do things that aren't even on our radar today. There's a wealth of insights inside existing medical research that we're yet to uncover. AI will eventually help us to arrive at those insights. It will also allow us to sift through genomics and other 'omics data and uncover new insights to come up with the treatments of the future. It can transform how medicine is practiced in terms of risk analysis, decision support, better workflows, automated administration, and many other areas.

You'll notice that throughout this book, I try to separate fact from fiction. Many of these promising areas are works-in-progress and will take years to materialize. That shouldn't lead to disillusionment or disappointment, though. We need to accept a less-than-perfect start and use AI in all of these areas to figure out where it's falling short and to focus on the next round of AI research. A prime example of that is natural language processing (NLP), which will be critical for AI in healthcare because so much of the data is unstructured. However, it's currently not as advanced as machine learning algorithms for structured data. This means more manual work in the near future to abstract key concepts and data from unstructured healthcare data. It's not ideal, but that's what we have to work with for now, until NLP methodologies improve. Recent advances in large language models that underpin self-supervised learning and generative AI (e.g. ChatGPT) are a pleasant surprise that also holds great promise in healthcare, but those applications are not yet commonplace in everyday practice of medicine.

This book is separated into three parts. In the first part, I focus on defining AI and examining its history, its promise in healthcare, the drivers and barriers of its applications in healthcare, and the data issues that will ultimately be the key factor in fulfilling its promise. The next part is about its applications to date and where it's poised to make the biggest impact. The last part is about the business of AI in healthcare. It will examine which applications are ready today from a methodological point of view to solve mission-critical issues for the buyers, as well as which use cases can see short- and medium-term demand from those same buyers: health systems, life science companies, long-term care facilities, telemedicine companies, etc. Lastly, we examine the key issues that every entrepreneur and investor needs to analyze before embarking on building or investing in a health AI company. Ultimately, the business case for the innovators and buyers needs to be established before adoption accelerates. Having been both a physician and a digital technology entrepreneur and investor in healthcare, I've experienced how issues like workflow implications, data ownership, and reimbursement impact the bottom line and can make or break new innovations.

I'm optimistic about what lies ahead in healthcare. I see great progress ahead but make no unrealistic or wildly optimistic predictions. The state of data in healthcare is chaotic and there are powerful technical and business barriers to the adoption of these technologies. As such, my focus is to lay out the promise, discuss the drivers and barriers, and examine how innovators can successfully navigate them to fulfill that promise.

I deliberately wrote this book to cover technical, clinical, and business issues that will be critical for this technology to fulfill its immense promise in healthcare. It is meant to be technical and clinical enough for those who are involved in the field and want to better understand the current state of affairs, what's holding back faster adoption, which technologies or use cases are ready now, and how they can create or invest in a successful business model on either side of the commercial transaction. On the other hand, I've tried to use plain language and to avoid getting too technical so that those who are trying to familiarize themselves with this field can follow along.

I hope you find it useful during your journey in this exciting field.

Ronald M. Razmi, MD
New York
January 15, 2024

Reference

1. Remes, J., Linzer, K., Singhal, S. et al. (2022, August 4). *Prioritizing Health: A Prescription for Prosperity*. McKinsey & Company https://www.mckinsey.com/industries/healthcare-systems-and-services/our-insights/prioritizing-health-a-prescription-for-prosperity.

Acknowledgments

MANY PEOPLE HELPED IMPROVE this book. They reviewed and edited each chapter. I'm extremely grateful to each one of them for their contributions. Special thanks to Pete Szolovits, PhD, Seymour Dunker, Matthew Kittay, JD, Eli Khedouri, Kang Zhang, MD, Justin Graham, MD, Greg Wolff, Gerasimos Petratos, MD, and Alex Fair.

PART I

Roadmap of AI in Healthcare

CHAPTER 1

History of AI and Its Promise in Healthcare

ARTIFICIAL INTELLIGENCE TECHNOLOGY has been "around" for some 80 years. Although it's gained significant traction recently and its applications are transforming almost every industry, its foundations date back to the Second World War. Alan Turing is considered one of the pioneers in computing and artificial intelligence (AI), and his papers from the time reveal some of the earliest mentions of machines that could mimic the human mind and its ability to reason. Back then, scientists were beginning to build computer systems that were meant to process information in the same way as the human brain. A paper by Warren McCulloch and Walter Pitts, who proposed an artificial neuron as early as 1943, refers to a computational model of the "nerve net" in the brain and is one of the first mentions of the topic in scientific literature.[1] This laid the foundation for the first wave of research into the topic.

In the 1950s, in his paper *Computing Machinery and Intelligence*, Turing offered a framework for building intelligent machines and methods for testing their intelligence. Bernard Widrow and Ted Hoff at Stanford University developed a neural network application for reducing noise in phone lines in the late 1950s.[2] Around the same time, Frank Rosenblatt built the Perceptron while working as an academic and with the US government.[3] The Perceptron was based on the concept of a neural network and was meant to be able to perform tasks that humans usually performed, such as recognizing images and even walking and talking. However, the Perceptron only had a single layer of

AI Doctor: The Rise of Artificial Intelligence in Healthcare: A Guide for Users, Buyers, Builders, and Investors, First Edition. Ronald M. Razmi.
© 2024 Ronald M. Razmi. Published 2024 by John Wiley & Sons, Inc.

neurons and was limited in how much it could do. Marvin Minsky, a colleague of Rosenblatt's and an old high school classmate of his, and Seymour Papert wrote a book called *Perceptrons: An Introduction to Computational Geometry* in which he detailed the limitations of the Perceptron and neural networks. This led to an AI winter that lasted until the mid-1980s.[4]

By 1986, there was renewed interest in neural networks by physicists who were coming up with novel mathematical techniques. There was also a landmark paper by Geoffrey Hinton about the applications of back propagation in neural networks as a way to overcome some of their limitations, although some practitioners point to a Finnish mathematician, Seppo Linnainmaa, as having invented back propagation in the 1960s.[5, 6] This led to a revival of the field and the creation of some of the first practical applications, such as detecting fraud in credit card transactions.

The 1986 paper by Geoffrey Hinton and few others in Canada highlighted the potential of multi-layered neural networks.[5] This, along with the potential it subsequently showed in speech recognition, re-ignited interest in neural networks and was enough to start attracting interest and research dollars. At Carnegie Melon in the late 1980s, Dean Pomerleau built a self-driving car using neural networks. NYU's Yann LeCun started using neural networks for image recognition and released a paper in 1998 that introduced convolutional neural networks (CNNs) as a way to mimic the human visual cortex.[7] In parallel, John Hopfield popularized the Hopfield network, which was the first recurrent neural network (RNN).[8] This was expanded upon by Jurgen Schmidhuber and Sepp Hochreiter in 1997 with the introduction of long short-term memory, which greatly improved the efficiency and practicality of RNNs.[9] Although these applications in the 1980s and 1990s created momentum for the field, they soon reached their limits due to a lack of data and insufficient computing power. There was another AI winter—fortunately, a shorter one—for about a decade or so.

As computing power and the amount of data increased, over the next few years, companies like Microsoft and Google ramped up their research in the field dramatically. In 2012, Hinton and two of his students highlighted the power of deep learning (DL) when they obtained significant results in the well-known ImageNet competition, based on a dataset collated by Fei-Fei Li and others.[10]

Seymour Duncker, CEO of Mindscale.ai, who's developed many AI-based products in healthcare and other sectors, told me, "Fei-Fei's work that led to ImageNet was a watershed moment that changed how the field of AI came to view data and its key role for making progress in the field of AI. Before ImageNet, the predominant thinking was that a better algorithm would make better decisions, regardless of the data. Fei-Fei had the key insight that even the best algorithms wouldn't be able to perform if the data they operated on wasn't representative of the world. That's why she went out and curated a large dataset representing visual objects found in the world and then made it open source. The ImageNet competition spawned a range of vision models that took the accuracy of classifying objects from 71.8% to 97.3%, beating human abilities. Essentially, Fei-Fei showed that big data leads to better decisions."

At the same time as Hinton's work in 2012, Jeffrey Dean and Andrew Ng were doing breakthrough work on large-scale image recognition at Google Brain.[11] DL also enhanced the existing field of reinforcement learning, thanks largely to researchers like Richard Sutton, leading to the game-playing successes of systems developed by DeepMind.[12] Given the impressive results that this algorithm showed the world, everyone woke up to the potential of DL and neural networks. In 2014, Ian Goodfellow published his paper on generative adversarial networks (GANs), which along with reinforcement learning has become the focus of much of the recent research in the field.[13]

This led to an initiative at Stanford University called the One Hundred Year Study on Artificial Intelligence. The study was founded by Eric Horvitz and aimed to build on the existing research that Horvitz and his team had carried out at Microsoft. The rest, as they say, is history! Progress came fast and in various sectors thanks to large amounts of digitized data and significantly stronger computers. Figure 1.1 summarizes some of the key milestones in the evolution of AI.

Today, we're at the dawn of AI's true potential. Most of the applications to date use supervised learning, which teaches algorithms by giving them annotated data (thousands or millions of records) and allowing the algorithm to learn from that data to identify patterns and make predictions. The long-term power of neural nets will reside in unsupervised learning, where the algorithms can learn without being trained on annotated data but by just being given the data. Generative AI is surprising everyone with its rapid progress and the level of sophistication it's showing in generating text, images, voice, art, etc. Reinforcement learning, which mimics human learning mechanisms, will also lead the charge toward AI's full potential.[15]

1.1   What is AI?

AI isn't magic, and nor is it going to spark a robot uprising or replace your doctor entirely. Mathematical terms like machine learning (ML) and DL are used as easy ways to explain statistical computer algorithms that use data to identify patterns and make accurate predictions. The term AI is used to refer to a range of technologies that can be combined in different ways to sense, comprehend, and act, as well as to learn from experience and to adapt over time (Figure 1.2).[16]

As an umbrella term, AI can refer to both natural language processing (NLP) and ML. NLP powers translations, understanding meaning in written

History of Artificial Intelligence

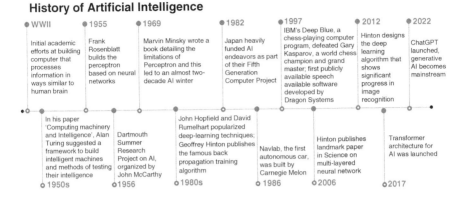

● WWII	● 1955	● 1969	● 1982	● 1997	● 2012	● 2022
Initial academic efforts at building computer that processes information in ways similar to human brain	Frank Rosenblatt builds the perceptron based on neural networks	Marvin Minsky wrote a book detailing the limitations of Perceptron and this led to an almost two-decade AI winter	Japan heavily funded AI endeavors as part of their Fifth Generation Computer Project	IBM's Deep Blue, a chess-playing computer program, defeated Gary Kasparov, a world chess champion and grand master; first publicly available speech available software developed by Dragon Systems	Hinton designs the deep learning algorithm that shows significant progress in image recognition	ChatGPT launched, generative AI becomes mainstream

In his paper 'Computing machinery and Intelligence', Alan Turing suggested a framework to build intelligent machines and methods of testing their intelligence	Dartmouth Summer Research Project on AI, organized by John McCarthy	John Hopfield and David Rumelhart popularized deep-learning techniques; Geoffrey Hinton publishes the famous back propagation training algorithm	Navlab, the first autonomous car, was built by Carnegie Melon	Hinton publishes landmark paper in Science on multi-layered neural network	Transformer architecture for AI was launched
○ 1950s	○ 1956	○ 1980s	○ 1986	○ 2006	○ 2017

FIGURE 1.1 *(source: original research[14])*: *1936–1969: Early progress, 1969–1986: AI winter, 1986: Hinton's paper on back propagation in neural networks, 1997–2012: Progress in AI methodologies: 1997 IBM beat Kasperov, 2007 ImageNet, 2011 IBM beat Jeopardy, 2012–Present: Rapid progress in deep-learning applications*

or spoken language, pattern recognition, as well as smart assistants like Google Assistant, Siri, and Alexa. ML is one of the most exciting areas of AI and uses computational approaches to make sense of data and to provide insights into what that data shows. It's a dynamic, iterative process that uses examples and experiences as opposed to predefined rules (Figure 1.3). With ML, instead of providing a set of rules that define what a cat looks like, the operator provides

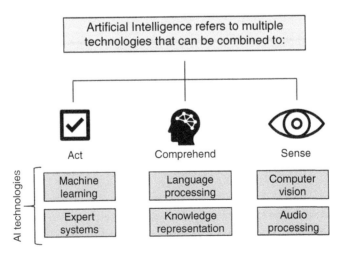

FIGURE 1.2 *(source: Accenture)[16]*

Artificial intelligence encompasses machine learning and neural networks. NLP cuts through the three

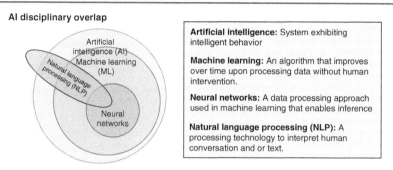

AI disciplinary overlap

Artificial intelligence: System exhibiting intelligent behavior

Machine learning: An algorithm that improves over time upon processing data without human intervention.

Neural networks: A data processing approach used in machine learning that enables inference

Natural language processing (NLP): A processing technology to interpret human conversation and or text.

FIGURE 1.3   *(source: HIMSS 2019)[17]*

the algorithm with a bunch of cat photos and leaves the software to arrive at its own conclusions. ML allows computers to retain information and to get smarter over time, just like human beings. But unlike human beings, these algorithms aren't susceptible to sleep deprivation, distractions, information overload, and short-term memory loss. That's why this powerful technology is so exciting.[18]

Then there's cognitive computing, an approach that uses computers to simulate human understanding, reasoning, and thought-processing.

The thing to remember is that AI isn't like other software and you can't just install it and get going. Instead, it's a sophisticated combination of inter-related technologies that needs to be customized for each application. Done properly, it can process data and come to its own conclusions about what that data means, and it can then carry out a set of actions based on what it's learned. It's true that AI can mimic the human brain, but it can also outperform us mere humans by discovering complex patterns that no human being could ever process and identify.

And not all AI applications are created equally. Some of the simpler use cases for AI include chatbots and automated phone screeners, which are able to provide basic responses to voice or text inputs. More complex AI algorithms can process unfathomably large sets of data to discover underlying trends and to answer questions ranging from which film a Netflix subscriber is most likely to enjoy to which treatment option is best for any given patient. They work by making predictions on how to interpret what's happening and how best to respond (Figure 1.4).

ML is a subcategory of AI in which algorithms and statistical models are used to allow computers to perform tasks. The interesting thing about ML is

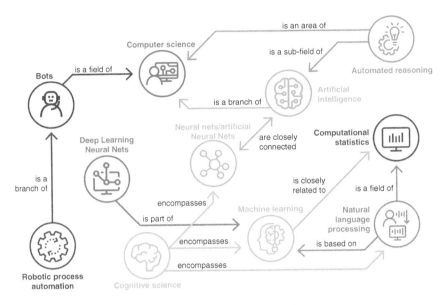

FIGURE 1.4 *(source: IQVIA)*[19]

that it goes above and beyond classic rules-based approaches and instead taps into inference and patterns to address sophisticated challenges. It's able to tap into DL and other complex mathematical techniques to parse large datasets and make predictions. As time goes on, the algorithm figures out which patterns and approaches will deliver the best results and uses that to adapt itself for the future.

In general, the more data that they have access to, the more ML algorithms can improve themselves. Recent technological advances in big data have made it more practical to apply ML to massive datasets to derive insights that were previously impossible to detect.

We typically use ML to build inference tools where we find patterns in existing data that allow us—when presented with new data—to infer something interesting about that data, such as recognizing abnormalities in an MRI image.[20] The great thing about ML is that it doesn't require interference or human intuition because it's driven entirely by data.

Neural networks are a subcategory of ML that simulates connected artificial neurons. This allows them to model themselves on the natural neurons and the way that they interact in the human brain. Computational models that are inspired by neural connections have been studied since the 1950s and are more relevant than ever before because processing power has continued to increase and we have access to even larger training datasets that can allow algorithms to analyze input data such as images, video, and speech.

AI practitioners refer to these techniques as DL, since neural networks have many ("deep") layers of simulated, interconnected neurons.[19] DL is a branch of ML that's emerged in the last decade as a breakthrough technology and its applications hold significant promise in the coming decades. DL is possible due to the architecture and design of neural networks, which mimic the neural connections in the human brain.

Artificial neural networks (ANNs) are clusters of interconnected nodes, like brain neurons. ANNs with multiple layers of connected nodes are able to take advantage of DL. They typically also use convolutional layers, which take the input data and group it together into blocks. These blocks are then fed into multiple deep processing layers, which filter them and then feed that filtered data into further layers with more filters. They identify features that are inherent to the original data and combine those features to produce a hierarchic estimation of patterns, called concepts.

Seymour Duncker explains, "These hierarchic estimations are represented by numerical weights, each of which represents the relative importance of two nodes in the network. A trained AI model is represented by a matrix of these numerical weights which gets combined with live data to produce a prediction." That might sound complicated, but that's what we humans do every day. When machines do this, it's called AI.

Neural networks run datasets through what the ML community calls a black box. This black box represents a series of mathematical calculations and statistical computations that are far beyond our understanding. Learning typically happens by feeding back an error signal from incorrect predictions, to alter the myriad weights the network uses to compute an answer from the inputs. The actual decision-making process can't usually be traced from beginning to end in a way that can be easily understood.

Neural networks and DL can and should be used as tools to aid the medical community. But these algorithms and this technology won't replace the expertise of medical professionals. Human experts will always be needed to train these algorithms and to identify the unique situations that exceed the scope of what can easily be defined.

Here are the four different types of neural networks and their benefits (Figure 1.5):

- **Feed-forward neural networks:** This is the simplest type of ANN in which information moves in only one direction (forward) with no loops in the network. Information typically starts out from the input layer and moves through the hidden layers to the output layer. The first single-neuron network was proposed by AI pioneer Frank Rosenblatt back in 1958.

- **Recurrent neural networks (RNNs):** These are ANNs with connections between the neurons, which are perfectly suited for processing sequential data like speech and language. RNNs are composed of an additional hidden state vector that contains "memory" about the data

We examined artificial intelligence (AI), machine learning, and other analytics techniques.

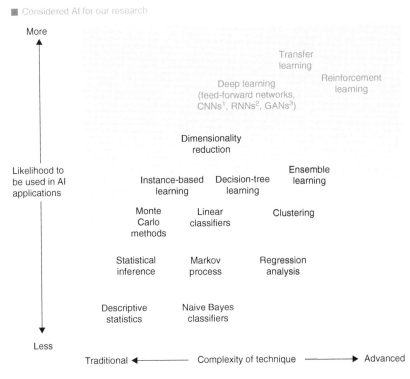

■ Considered AI for our research

¹Convolutional neural networks.
²Recurrent neural networks.
³Generative adversarial netwerks.

FIGURE 1.5 *(source: McKinsey Global Institute analysis/https://www.mckinsey.com/ featured-insights/artificial-intelligence/notes-from-the-ai-frontier-applications-and-value-of-deep-learning)*

that it's observed over time. As Seymour Duncker told me, "Recurrent neural networks have largely been replaced by the transformer architecture, which provides a more effective way of representing patterns in sequences and enables parallel processing, allowing algorithms to process extremely large volumes of data more efficiently than the original RNNs."

- **Convolutional neural networks (CNNs):** CNNs are ANNs where the connections between neural layers are inspired by biological visual cortexes, the portion of the brain that processes images. This makes them ideal for perceptual tasks.

- **Generative adversarial networks (GANs)**: This approach uses two neural networks that compete against one other in a zero-sum game framework (which is why we call them "adversarial"). GANs can learn to mimic various distributions of data (such as text, speech, and images), which makes them useful for generating test datasets when they're not readily available. This is where we're seeing the exciting new developments with ChatGPT and other generative AI and possibly the foundation for the next breakthroughs in AI capabilities.

I mentioned earlier about the astounding results that generative AI is showing. You could say that generative AI is a branch of AI that involves creating new content. This new content can be in the form of audio, code, images (art!), text, and videos. Recent advancements in the field mean that AI is on its way to being one step ahead of interpreting data and to start creating the types of content that have previously been only the domain of human beings.

Generative AI is a form of ML algorithm that uses self-supervised learning to train on large amounts of historic data. For example, with ChatGPT, which generates text, the training involved feeding the model a massive amount of text from the internet so that it was able to generate predictions. It's a breakthrough in that rather than simply perceiving and classifying data, ML is now able to create content on demand. Given their ability to do self-supervised learning and not require labeled training data (as in supervised learning), the models can be trained on large datasets much faster. For example, a large language model can be trained on historic medical literature and be ready to answer medical questions in short order. Up until recently, our thinking has been that the medical literature needs to be annotated and key concepts abstracted in order to use ML models to extract insights.

Generative AI outputs are carefully calibrated combinations of the data used to train the algorithms. Because the amount of data used to train these algorithms is so large, the models can appear to be "creative" when producing outputs. What's more, the models usually have random elements, which means they can produce a variety of outputs from one input request—making them seem even more lifelike.[21]

In healthcare, the initial applications of generative AI could include generating images for training radiology models, creating clinical content for educating patients about their conditions, answering general questions about various conditions, carrying out administrative tasks such as medical coding and documentation, supporting mental health services, and helping with research.

Now, you may be wondering how AI, ML, DL, and other related technologies are different from statistics or analytics. The short answer is that the new methods are better suited for large volumes of data and high-dimensional data like pictures, video, and audio files. Also, AI is better suited for data where we're not aware of all of the complex relationships within the dataset and so we can't provide specific instructions to the model. AI is particularly effective at uncovering hidden relationships in the datasets, uncovering patterns, and making predictions.

Classical statistics methods require more input from humans about the variables, the relationship between the variables, and the desired outcome. Traditional statistical analyses aim to find inferences about sample or population parameters, while ML aims to algorithmically represent the data structure and to make predictions or classifications. ML typically starts out with fewer assumptions about the underlying data than traditional statistical analysis and results in algorithms that are much more accurate when it comes to prediction and classification (Figure 1.5).

Healthcare analytics have traditionally been rooted in understanding a given set of data by using business intelligence-focused tools.[22] The people using those tools are typically analysts, statisticians, and business users as opposed to engineers. The problem with traditional enterprise data analytics is that you don't learn from the data, you only understand what's in it. To learn from it, you need to use ML and effective feedback loops from all of the relevant stakeholders. This will help you to uncover hidden patterns in the data, especially when there are non-linear relationships that aren't easily identifiable to humans.

For DL models to get good at classification and to perform at the same level as humans, they require thousands—or in some cases, millions—of data records. One estimate found that supervised DL algorithms generally achieve acceptable performance with around 5000 labeled examples per category and match or exceed human performance when trained with at least 10 million.[23] In some cases, so much data is available (often millions or billions of rows per dataset) that AI is the most appropriate technique. However, if a threshold of data volume isn't reached, AI might not add value to traditional analytics techniques.

It can be difficult to source these massive datasets, and labeling remains a challenge. Most current AI models are trained with supervised learning, which requires humans to label and categorize the underlying data. However, promising new techniques are emerging to overcome these data bottlenecks, such as large language models, reinforcement learning, transfer learning, and "one-shot learning," which allows a trained AI model to learn about a subject based on a small number of real-world demonstrations or examples—and sometimes just one.

Neural AI techniques are particularly good at analyzing images, videos, and audio data because they're complex and multidimensional. AI practitioners often call this "high dimensionality." Neural networks are well suited to high dimensionality because multiple layers in a network can learn to represent the many different features that are present in the data.

For example, with facial recognition, the first layer in the network could focus on raw pixels, the next on edges and lines, another on generic facial features, and the final layer on identifying the face (Figure 1.6). Unlike previous generations of AI, which often required human expertise to do "feature engineering," these neural network techniques are often able to learn to represent these features in their simulated neural networks as part of the training process (Figure 1.7).

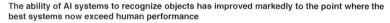

The ability of AI systems to recognize objects has improved markedly to the point where the best systems now exceed human performance

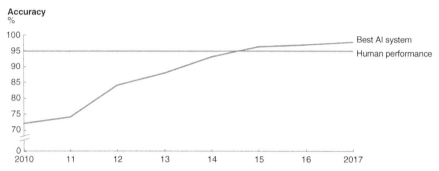

FIGURE 1.6 *(source: McKinsey Global Institute analysis/https://www.mckinsey.com/~/media/ mckinsey/featured%20insights/artificial%20intelligence/notes%20from%20the%20ai%20frontier%20 applications%20and%20value%20of%20deep%20learning/notes-from-the-ai-frontier-insights-from-hundreds-of-use-cases-discussion-paper.ashx)[23]*

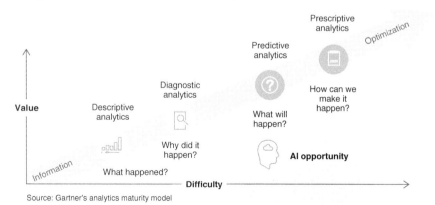

FIGURE 1.7 *(source: Gartner/McKinsey & Company)[24]*

1.2   A Classification System for Underlying AI/ML Algorithms

There are different levels of AI systems, with plenty of different algorithms being capable of consuming and classifying data or using it to make predictions. Some systems operate strictly on hard-wired rules, while more recent systems are far more autonomous and require very little human input other than the data and the desired output (Figures 1.8 and 1.9).[25]

Within the industry, we often classify algorithms into three main categories—expert systems, traditional ML, and frontier ML. Algorithms can be sorted into these categories according to two main attributes:

- Their autonomy (measured by how much human guidance they need).

- Their explainability (measured by how easily humans can understand how the algorithm makes its predictions or arrives at its outputs).[26]

One of the interesting things about these attributes is that they're inversely related. This means that if the explainability is high, the autonomy is low—and vice versa.

When it comes to ML, there are four different classifications to think about—supervised learning, unsupervised learning (including self-supervised learning used in large language models), semi-supervised learning, and reinforcement learning (Figure 1.10).

John Guttag, head of the Data Driven Inference Group at MIT's Computer Science and Artificial Intelligence Laboratory, explains, "In supervised machine learning, we're given the data and some outcome associated

Spectrum of algorithms underpinning AI (excerpt)

ROCK
HEAL+H

	Expert systems	Traditional machine learning	Frontier machine learning
Summary	Human-programmed, static program to perform a single, deterministic task	Algorithms mathematically proven to make an optimum or best prediction based on data they are trained with	Algorithms with the same characteristics as traditional machine learning (learn from and improve predictions through data) but with greater autonomy and less explainability
Period of major breakthroughs	1980s–1990s	2000s	2010s–present
Autonomy	Low, program is entirely dependent on human-provided information	Medium, generally humans guide the model to take into account certain features and to remove "noisy" outlier data	High, generally the model decides on feature selection and weighting and has to account for outlier data independently
Explainability	High	Medium	Low, "black box"

FIGURE 1.8   *(source: Rock Health[25])*

History of AI in medicine

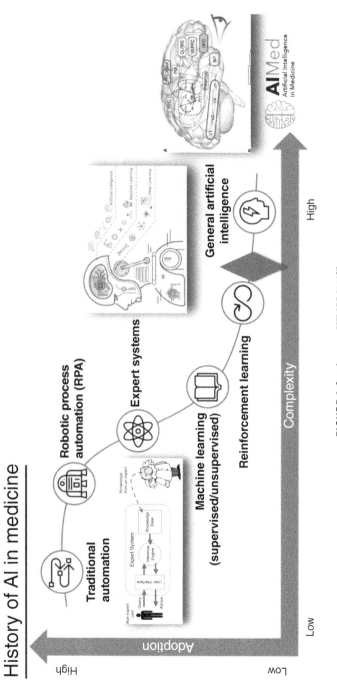

FIGURE 1.9 *(source: HIMSS 2019[26])*

AI in medicine:

Artificial Intelligence (AI) is computer science that uses algorithms, heuristics, pattern matching, rules, deep learning and cognitive computing to approximate conclusions without direct human input.

The application of AI in medicine has two main branches: virtual and physical.
* The virtual component includes machine learning (ML) and algorithms,
* physical AI includes medical devices and robots for delivering care.

 VIRTUAL

* There are three main types of machine learning algorithm:
1. **Unsupervised:** finding patterns): involves a system looking for patterns in the unlabelled input data and further classifying the input data depending on these patterns identified
2. **Supervised:** classifying and predicting algorithms based on past learning. In supervised learning, Ml provides the system with labelled data, which helps the system categories the various inputs depending on what has been learnt with the labelled data.
3. **Reinforcement learning:** using rewards and punishments for forming a strategy to operate in a designed problem space.

 PHYSICAL

* The physical branch of AI in medicine encompasses medical devices and advanced, sophisticated robots responsible for care delivery ('carebots') that can even help during surgery
* Nanobots have been designed to overcome problems associated with the permeation and diffusion of the therapeutic agent at the site of application for targeted delivery. An example of such use is targeting a tumour that is deficit in vascularity but shows active proliferation.

FIGURE 1.10   *(source: Original Research)*

with the data. We're given all the people who have Zika infections and then we know which of the women have children with birth defects and which don't. And maybe from that we could build a model saying that if the woman is pregnant and has Zika, what's the probability that her baby has a birth defect? And it might be different for 30-year-old women than for 40-year-old women. Who knows what the factors would be? But there we have a label – all sorts of details about the woman, and was the baby healthy or not? So that would be supervised learning: We have a label about the outcome of interest."[27]

The upshot of all of this is that supervised ML tries to model how independent variables relate to a dependent variable. In ML, you need to choose a strategy (by picking a particular algorithm) to discover those relationships. For example, by annotating a lot of images of patients with stroke findings on a CT scan, you can train an algorithm to find that abnormality on future CT scans.

Ninety Percent of the value of AI in healthcare so far is coming from supervised learning.[28]

Unsupervised ML means we wouldn't have a label.[29] By using an unsupervised algorithm on a lot of data, we try to identify hidden structures within that data. For example, you can use an unsupervised algorithm on clinical data from patients with heart failure and try to discern which of the many clinical factors are related to the deterioration of those patients. The great thing about unsupervised learning is that you can discover things that you didn't think to look for, and it can also help when the data is impossible to label. This helps with cohort analysis and anomaly detection.

You can also often take features that you discover with unsupervised learning and incorporate them into your supervised learning models. For

Box 1| Key terms in artificial intelligence

- Artificial intelligence: A branch of applied computer science wherein computer algorithms are trained to perform tasks typically associated wiht human intelligence.
- Machine learning: Providing knowledge to computers through data without explicit programming. Attempts to optimize a 'mapping' between inputs and outputs.
- Represntation learnings: Learning effective representations of a data source algorithmically, as opposed to hand-crafting combinations of data features.
- Deep learning: Multiple processing layers are used to learn representations of data with multiple layers of abstraction.
- Supervised learning: Training is conducted with specific labels or annotations.
- Unsupervised learning: Training is conducted without any specific labels, and the algorithm clusters data to reveal underlying patterns.
- Natural language processing: The organization of unstructured narrative text into a structured form that can be interpreted by a machine and allows for automated information extraction.

FIGURE 1.11   *(source: McKinsey Global Institute)*

example, if your unsupervised learning shows that a previously undetected subtle abnormality on radiological images correlates with a disease (e.g. dementia), you can then label those abnormalities on a large number of scans and train a new algorithm using supervised learning to detect that abnormality in future patients.

There's also semi-supervised learning, where some data may be labeled with outcomes while other data is unlabeled. In this case, the labeled data can help the algorithm to understand the unlabeled data.

Reinforcement learning involves being able to sequentially interact, learn, and improve your models. It's a subcategory of ML where systems are given virtual rewards or punishments, allowing us to train them through trial and error. This is the technique that Google DeepMind used to develop systems that could play video games and board games like chess and Go better than human champions (Figure 1.11).

1.3   AI and Deep Learning in Medicine

Although medicine has been notoriously slow to adopt innovations—and digital innovations in particular—the massive applications of AI in medicine are gaining significant momentum. This is mostly because everyone is starting to realize that AI can be a big part of the solution for making the practice of medicine more effective and efficient. This includes everything from screening and diagnosis to decision support, therapeutics, and administration. Also, in the life sciences industry, AI has the potential to be a game changer for drug discovery, development, manufacturing, and the supply chain.

Given the increasing amounts of data being generated by the practice of medicine, the increasing complexity of clinical literature, and older and sicker patients, AI won't be a luxury but a necessity in the practice of medicine. AI can process large amounts of data and identify relationships and patterns, predict risks and outcomes, and recommend the best courses of action. It can help with processing the large and growing knowledge base and make it available at the point of care, and it can certainly improve the efficiency of doctors and nurses, as well as improving the efficiency of the administrative part of healthcare.

Physicians need to identify, quantify, and interpret relationships between variables to improve patient care, and this isn't a new phenomenon. We can think of AI and ML as offering a variety of methods that allow us to use computers to do just that by analyzing the vast amount of data, finding patterns, and making predictions. In healthcare, AI has the potential to provide new tools to make physicians more efficient. We need this for a number of reasons. The increasing amount of data—from sources like whole-genome-sequencing, remote monitoring, social media, and community databases—requires physicians to interpret and synthesize information from many more sources than they're traditionally used to.[30–33]

Simultaneously, the increasing number and complexity of patients and the ever-increasing administrative burden are placing additional demands on physicians and healthcare systems.[34] Finally, there's an opportunity to drastically improve care by increasing personalization and immediacy.[35, 36] In short, physicians are getting more and more data, which requires more sophisticated interpretation and which takes more time. AI is the solution, enhancing every stage of patient care from research and discovery to diagnosis and therapy selection. As a result, clinical practice will become more efficient, convenient, personalized, and effective.

AI can be transformative in medicine. It can find new relationships and causes and effect—such as biomarkers for disease—teaching us what causes diseases and how to understand and predict them. It can help with everything from disease diagnosis and management to administrative and operational tasks and better management of patient populations.[37] AI can generate value through enhanced physician decision-making, reduced waste and fraud, and improved administrative efficiency.[38]

ML can help to identify complex relationships between different clinical variables and patient outcomes. Johnson et al. provide the example of a cardiologist who wanted to predict readmission in a heart failure patient and how the current statistical models have limitations.[39] They explain, "This is a difficult problem where machine learning techniques have been shown to improve on traditional statistical methods. Our hypothetical clinician possesses a large but 'messy' electronic health record (EHR) dataset (Figure 1.12). Typically, EHRs include variables such as International Classification of Diseases ninth revision and tenth revision billing codes, medication prescriptions, laboratory values, physiological measurements, imaging studies and encounter notes. It's difficult to decide a priori which variables should be included in a predictive model. Fitting a logistic regression model is algebraically impossible when there are more independent variables than observations. Techniques such as univariate significance screening (i.e. including independent variables only if each is associated with the outcome in univariate analyses) or forward step-wise regression are commonly used. Unfortunately, these methods lead to models that don't tend to validate in other datasets and are poorly generalizable to patients. Furthermore, there are often complex interactions between variables. For example, one drug may significantly interact with another drug only if other conditions are present. The quantity and quality of such interactions are difficult to describe using traditional methods. With machine learning, we can capture and use these complex relationships. Features

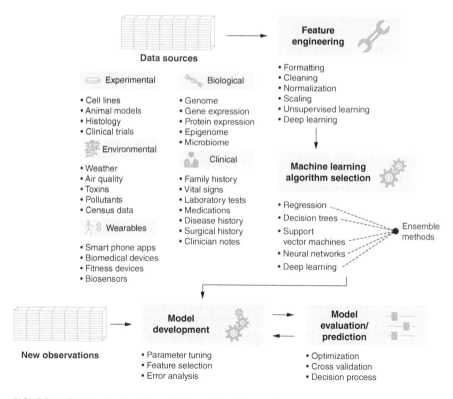

FIGURE 1.12   Developing AI medical models using variety of data sources *(source: Johnson et al.[39]/Elsevier/CC BY 4.0)*

engineered by unsupervised learning are also often incorporated into supervised learning models and new models that are far more predictive of patient outcomes and the drivers of those outcomes emerge."

In a multi-center observational study that compared traditional statistical models such as logistics regression with ML models, the ML models more accurately predicted clinical deterioration—defined as cardiac arrest, ICU transfer, or death—than traditional logistic regression models.[40]

1.4 The Emergence of Multimodal and Multipurpose Models in Healthcare

Given the emergence of large language models and generative AI, there's great excitement about the possibilities they represent in healthcare. Their ability to ingest large amounts of unlabeled data (such as medical literature or clinical notes) means that new models can be rapidly trained to perform key functions such as assisting in medical research or clinical decision support. Unlike medical models that are mostly developed using supervised learning and labeled data for narrow tasks, these new models can be trained using unlabeled data and perform multiple tasks.

Foundation models—the latest generation of AI models—are trained on massive, diverse datasets and can be applied to numerous downstream tasks.[41] Individual models can now achieve state-of-the-art performance on a wide variety of problems, ranging from answering questions about texts to labeling abnormalities on images and assisting with documentation. This versatility represents a stark change from the previous generation of AI models, which were designed to solve specific tasks, one at a time. This is made possible by growing datasets, increases in model size, and advances in model architectures.

Applying foundation models to healthcare introduces tougher barriers, mainly because of the difficulty to access large, diverse medical datasets, the complexity of the medical domain, and the recency of these developments. As data issues are resolved and there's more access to large and diverse datasets, the medical models promise to have multimodal architectures, self-supervised learning without explicit data labels, and the ability to perform a variety of tasks, rather than just one or two.[42, 43]

Moor et al. have described a new generation of medical models that they refer to as Generalist Medical AI (GMAI) that have three key capabilities that distinguish them from conventional medical AI models.[44] First, adapting a GMAI model to a new task will be as easy as describing the task in plain

English (or another language). Models will be able to solve previously unseen problems simply by having new tasks explained to them (dynamic task specification), without needing to be retrained. Second, GMAI models can accept inputs and produce outputs using varying combinations of data modalities (e.g. they can take in images, text, laboratory results, or any combination thereof). This flexible interactivity contrasts with the constraints of more rigid multimodal models, which always use predefined sets of modalities as input and output (such as by requiring images, text, and laboratory results together). Third, GMAI models will formally represent medical knowledge, allowing them to reason through previously unseen tasks and use medically accurate language to explain their outputs (Figure 1.13).

These AI models, including the medical versions of them, can introduce capabilities well beyond what we've experienced to date. We'll examine some of their potential applications throughout this book, but the bottom line is that decision support, extracting insights from existing medical literature, and researching and developing new treatments all seem ripe for this type of model. The issues with task-specific medical models to date have been that their development often depends on the creation of labeled datasets and that they perform best when trained on structured data. As such, applications in areas of medicine that depend on structured data for diagnosis and decision support—such as radiology, pathology, ophthalmology, and dermatology—have been at the forefront of AI in healthcare. However, with large language models that can be trained on unlabeled and unstructured data, which comprises more than 80% of the data in healthcare, a new world of possibilities opens up.

The advantages of large language models include their adaptability to changing contexts, their ability to learn in-context through new examples, the ability to perform multiple tasks (such as identifying multiple abnormalities on an x-ray without being explicitly trained on labeled data), and the fact that their output can be used downstream for specialist models.[45] The main disadvantage is that they'll need large and diverse datasets to be trained on.

As we'll discuss in the coming chapters, it isn't easy to obtain these kinds of datasets in medicine. If you have in-context learning through a few examples provided by the user, who will validate that the answers are correct? These models have been shown to fabricate answers and to present them in a convincing manner. As such, the regulatory issues for the launch and use of these models will be complex.

Given the difficulty in obtaining large and diverse datasets in healthcare, the issues of bias in the models' output will be even more pronounced. Also, given the size of these models, privacy issues will become more salient since it's more likely that patient information will be exposed.[46] Developing them will require collecting massive datasets and could incur high computational costs, and their size means that it will be difficult to implement them in the healthcare industry using existing infrastructure.

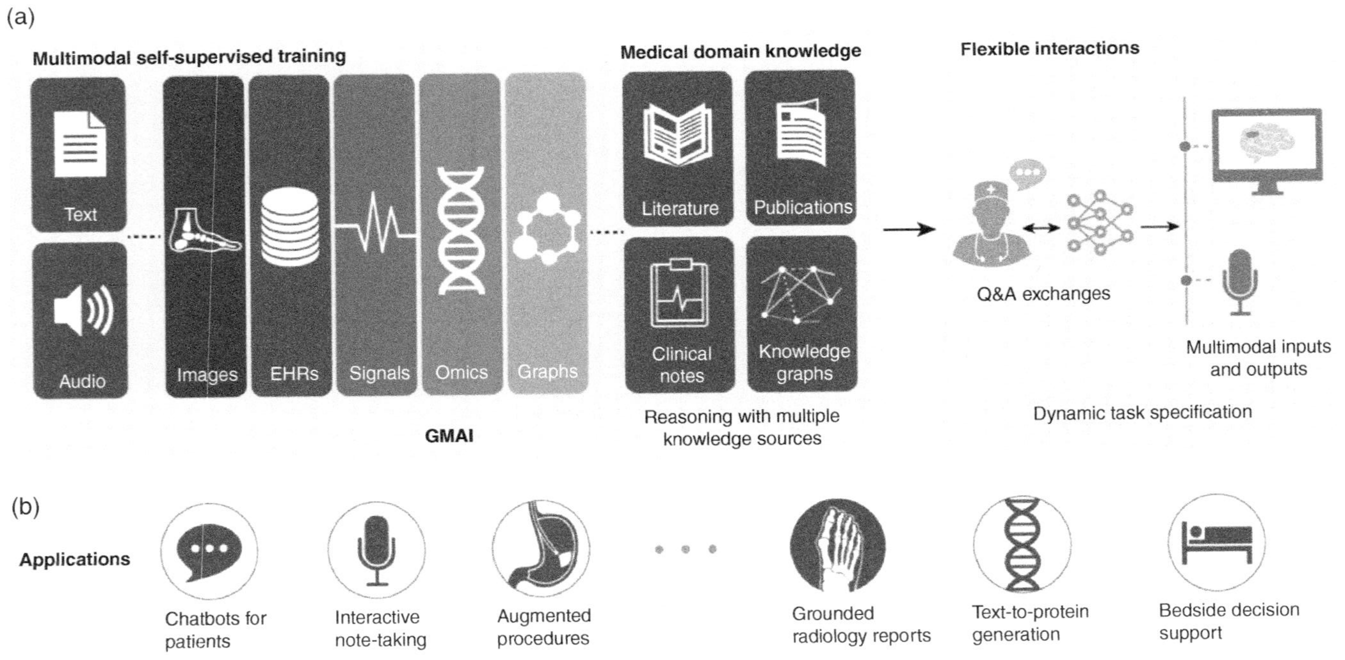

FIGURE 1.13 Foundation Models for Generalist Medical Artificial Intelligence (*source: Moore et al.[43]/Springer Nature*)

Pilots used to fly planes manually, but now they operate a dashboard with the help of computers. This has made flying safer and improved the industry. Healthcare can benefit from the same type of approach, with physicians practicing medicine with the help of data, dashboards, and AI. This will improve the quality of care they provide and make their jobs easier and more efficient.

References

1. McCulloch, W. S., & Pitts, W. (1943). A logical calculus of the ideas immanent in nervous activity. The Bulletin of Mathematical Biophysics, 5(4), 115–133. https://doi.org/10.1007/bf02478259
2. ETHW. (2021, January 26). Oral-History:Bernard Widrow. Engineering and Technology History Wiki. Retrieved August 4, 2022, from https://ethw.org/Oral-History:Bernard_Widrow
3. Rosenblatt, F. (1958). The perceptron: a probabilistic model for information storage and organization in the brain. Psychological Review, 65(6), 386–408. https://doi.org/10.1037/h0042519
4. Nievergelt, J. (1969). R69-13 perceptrons: an introduction to computational geometry. IEEE Transactions on Computers, C–18(6), 572. https://doi.org/10.1109/t-c.1969.222718
5. Rumelhart, D. E., Hinton, G. E., & Williams, R. J. (1986). Learning representations by back-propagating errors. Nature, 323(6088), 533–536. https://doi.org/10.1038/323533a0
6. Schmidhuber, J. (2014). Who Invented Backpropagation?Retrieved August 8, 2022, from https://people.idsia.ch/~juergen/who-invented-backpropagation.html
7. LeCun, Y., Bottou, L., Bengio, Y., & Haffner, P. (1998). Gradient-based learning applied to document recognition. Proceedings of the IEEE, 86(11), 2278–2324. https://doi.org/10.1109/5.726791
8. Hopfield, J. J. (1982). Neural networks and physical systems with emergent collective computational abilities. Proceedings of the National Academy of Sciences, 79(8), 2554–2558. https://doi.org/10.1073/pnas.79.8.2554
9. Hochreiter, S., & Schmidhuber, J. (1997). Long short-term memory. Neural Computation, 9(8), 1735–1780. https://doi.org/10.1162/neco.1997.9.8.1735
10. Krizhevsky, A., Sutskever, I., & Hinton, G. E. (2017). ImageNet classification with deep convolutional neural networks. Communications of the ACM, 60(6), 84–90. https://doi.org/10.1145/3065386
11. Dean, J., Corrado, G., Monga, R., Chen, K., Devin, M., Mao, M., Ranzato, M., Senior, A., Tucker, P., Yang, K., Le, Q., & Ng, A. (2012). Large scale distributed deep networks. Proceedings of a meeting held December 3-6, 2012, Lake Tahoe, Nevada, United States. https://papers.nips.cc/paper/2012/hash/6aca97005c68f1206823815f66102863-Abstract.html
12. Sutton, R. S., & Barto, A. G. (1998). Reinforcement Learning: An Introduction (Adaptive Computation and Machine Learning) (Adaptive Computation and Machine Learning series) (second edition). A Bradford Book.

13. Goodfellow, I., Pouget-Abadie, J., Mirza, M., Xu, B., Warde-Farley, D., Ozair, S., Courville, A., & Bengio, Y. (2020). Generative adversarial networks. Communications of the ACM, 63(11), 139–144. https://doi.org/10.1145/3422622

14. Razmi, R. M. (2021). History of AI. https://zoicap.com/ai_in_healthcare_blo/history-of-ai/

15. Vance, A. (2018, May 21). How We Got Here. Bloomberg Businessweek, 64–67.

16. The Next Generation of Medicine: Artificial Intelligence and Machine Learning. (2017). TM Capital. https://www.tmcapital.com/wp-content/uploads/2017/11/TMCC20AI20Spotlight20-202017.10.2420vF.PDF

17. Martin, A. (2019). Using AI and NLP to alleviate physician burnout. Machine Learning and AI for Healthcare. A HIMSS Event.

18. SysML 18: Michael Jordan, Perspectives and Challenges. (2018, March 4). [Video]. YouTube. https://www.youtube.com/watch?v=4inIBmY8dQI

19. IQVIA. (2019). AI in clinical development: improving safety and accelerating results. https://www.iqvia.com/-/media/iqvia/pdfs/library/white-papers/ai-in-clinical-development.pdf

20. Dreyer, K. J., & Geis, J. R. (2017). When machines think: radiology's next frontier. Radiology, 285(3), 713–718. https://doi.org/10.1148/radiol.2017171183

21. What is Generative AI? (2023). McKinsey and Company. Retrieved March 11, 2023, from https://www.mckinsey.com/~/media/mckinsey/featured%20insights/mckinsey%20explainers/what%20is%20generative%20ai/what%20is%20generative%20ai.pdf

22. Siwicki, B. (2021, June 9). What you need to know about data fluency and federated AI. Healthcare IT News. https://www.healthcareitnews.com/news/what-you-need-know-about-data-fluency-and-federated-ai

23. Goodfellow, I., Bengio, Y., & Courville, A. (2016). Deep Learning (Adaptive Computation and Machine Learning series) (Illustrated ed.). The MIT Press.

24. Chui, M., Manyika, J., Miremadi, M., Henke, N., Chung, R., Nel, P., & Malhotra, S. (2019, November 20). Notes from the AI Frontier: Applications and Value of Deep Learning. McKinsey & Company. https://www.mckinsey.com/featured-insights/artificial-intelligence/notes-from-the-ai-frontier-applications-and-value-of-deep-learning

25. Rock Health. (2018). Demystifying AI and Machine Learning in Healthcare. https://rockhealth.gumroad.com/l/uXbeg

26. Chang, A. (2019, February 11). Artificial intelligence in medicine, synergies between man and machine [Presentation]. AI in Medicine Symposium, Orlando, Florida.

27. Miliard, M. (2017, March 16). MIT professor's quick primer on two types of machine learning for. Healthcare IT News. https://www.healthcareitnews.com/news/mit-professors-quick-primer-two-types-machine-learning-healthcare

28. Artificial Intelligence in Healthcare Market. (2020). Markets and Markets. https://www.marketsandmarkets.com/Market-Reports/artificial-intelligence-healthcare-market-54679303.html

29. Rock Health. (2017, November 29). Podcast: Uncovering the real value of AI in healthcare with Andrew Ng | Rock Health.

30. Kuo, F. C., Mar, B. G., Lindsley, R. C., & Lindeman, N. I. (2017). The relative utilities of genome-wide, gene panel, and individual gene sequencing in clinical practice. Blood, 130(4), 433–439. https://doi.org/10.1182/blood-2017-03-734533

31. Muse, E. D., Barrett, P. M., Steinhubl, S. R., & Topol, E. J. (2017). Towards a smart medical home. The Lancet, 389(10067), 358. https://doi.org/10.1016/s0140-6736(17)30154-x

32. Steinhubl, S. R., Muse, E. D., & Topol, E. J. (2015). The emerging field of mobile health. Science Translational Medicine, 7(283). https://doi.org/10.1126/scitranslmed.aaa3487

33. Shameer, K., Badgeley, M. A., Miotto, R., Glicksberg, B. S., Morgan, J. W., & Dudley, J. T. (2016). Translational bioinformatics in the era of real-time biomedical, health care and wellness data streams. Briefings in Bioinformatics, 18(1), 105–124. https://doi.org/10.1093/bib/bbv118

34. Konstam, M. A., Hill, J. A., Kovacs, R. J., Harrington, R. A., Arrighi, J. A., & Khera, A. (2017). The academic medical system: reinvention to survive the revolution in health care. Journal of the American College of Cardiology, 69(10), 1305–1312. https://www.sciencedirect.com/science/article/pii/S0735109717301249

35. Steinhubl, S. R., & Topol, E. J. (2015). Moving from digitalization to digitization in cardiovascular care. Journal of the American College of Cardiology, 66(13), 1489–1496. https://doi.org/10.1016/j.jacc.2015.08.006

36. Boeldt, D. L., Wineinger, N. E., Waalen, J., Gollamudi, S., Grossberg, A., Steinhubl, S. R., McCollister-Slipp, A., Rogers, M. A., Silvers, C., & Topol, E. J. (2015). How consumers and physicians view new medical technology: comparative survey. Journal of Medical Internet Research, 17(9), e215. https://doi.org/10.2196/jmir.4456

37. Miliard, M. (2018, November 6). Use your words! Sorting through the confusing terminology of artificial intelligence. Healthcare IT News. https://www.healthcareitnews.com/news/use-your-words-sorting-through-confusing-terminology-artificial-intelligence

38. Using machine learning to unlock value across the healthcare value chain. (2018). [Infographic]. McKinsey. https://www.mckinsey.com/~/media/McKinsey/Industries/Healthcare%20Systems%20and%20Services/Our%20Insights/Using%20machine%20learning/2018_Using-machine-learning_Infographic.pdf

39. Johnson, K. W., Torres Soto, J., Glicksberg, B. S., Shameer, K., Miotto, R., Ali, M., Ashley, E., & Dudley, J. T. (2018). Artificial intelligence in cardiology. Journal of the American College of Cardiology, 71(23), 2668–2679. https://doi.org/10.1016/j.jacc.2018.03.521

40. Churpek, M. M., Yuen, T. C., Winslow, C., Meltzer, D. O., Kattan, M. W., & Edelson, D. P. (2016). Multicenter comparison of machine learning methods and conventional regression for predicting clinical deterioration on the wards. Critical Care Medicine, 44(2), 368–374. https://doi.org/10.1097/ccm.0000000000001571

41. Bommasani, R. (2021, August 16). On the opportunities and risks of foundation models. arXiv.org. https://arxiv.org/abs/2108.07258

42. Acosta, J. N., Falcone, G. J., Rajpurkar, P., & Topol, E. J. (2022). Multimodal biomedical AI. Nature Medicine, 28(9), 1773–1784. https://doi.org/10.1038/s41591-022-01981-2

43. Krishnan, R., Rajpurkar, P., & Topol, E. J. (2022). Self-supervised learning in medicine and healthcare. Nature Biomedical Engineering, 6(12), 1346–1352. https://doi.org/10.1038/s41551-022-00914-1

44. Moor, M., Banerjee, O., Abad, Z. S. H., Krumholz, H. M., Leskovec, J., Topol, E. J., & Rajpurkar, P. (2023). Foundation models for generalist medical artificial intelligence. Nature, 616(7956), 259–265. https://doi.org/10.1038/s41586-023-05881-4

45. Tiu, E., Talius, E., Patel, P., Langlotz, C. P., Ng, A. Y., & Rajpurkar, P. (2022). Expert-level detection of pathologies from unannotated chest X-ray images via self-supervised learning. Nature Biomedical Engineering, 6(12), 1399–1406. https://doi.org/10.1038/s41551-022-00936-9

46. Carlini, N., Tramèr, F., Wallace, E. S., Jagielski, M., Herbert-Voss, A., Lee, K. J., Roberts, A., Brown, T., Song, D., Erlingsson, Ú., Oprea, A., & Raffel, C. (2020). Extracting training data from large language models. In USENIX Security Symposium (pp. 2633–2650). https://www.usenix.org/system/files/sec21-carlini-extracting.pdf

CHAPTER 2

Building Robust Medical Algorithms

IF THERE'S ONE ISSUE that needs to be front and center in artificial intelligence (AI), it's the issue of data: getting enough of it to train the algorithms, having a steady flow of it when you implement the algorithms in the real world, ensuring that it's representative of the patient population and protecting it effectively. MIT Computer Science and Artificial Intelligence Laboratory Clinical Decision-Making Group head Peter Szolovits told me a few years ago, "A bad algorithm trained with lots of data will perform better than a good algorithm trained with little data." As such, the process of using AI to transform healthcare will only reach completion if the myriad issues with healthcare data are addressed over time. Fortunately, the quantity of digitized data in healthcare is exploding. From electronic health records (EHRs) to wearables and apps, this trend is expected to continue to increase exponentially (Figure 2.1).

But there are some serious issues. We'll delve into many of them in this and the next chapter, but those that come straight to mind include fragmented data that resides in different information systems (for the same patient!), unstructured data, data gaps, and errors, exchanging healthcare data between different providers, changing data, and so on. In the early days of digital health, I started a population health management software company., Acupera. Our platform used data from different sources such as EHRs, claim data, sociobehavioral data, and more to create care plans for patients with chronic diseases. For all of the years that we were selling and implementing care management software, we spent most of our time pulling out the data and cleaning it up, rather than just plugging our software into the EHR and immediately starting to manage chronically ill patients. Although there's been some progress since then, the overall state of affairs hasn't changed

AI Doctor: The Rise of Artificial Intelligence in Healthcare: A Guide for Users, Buyers, Builders, and Investors, First Edition. Ronald M. Razmi.
© 2024 Ronald M. Razmi. Published 2024 by John Wiley & Sons, Inc.

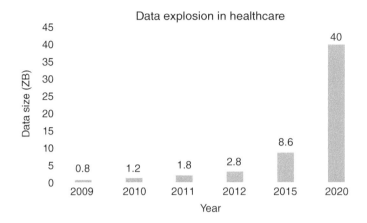

FIGURE 2.1   Big data in health care: Applications and challenges
(source: Hang et al.[1])

dramatically, so the data issues are the first problems that innovators in this space have to solve.

If the food for a robust algorithm is data, then in medicine we're often starved. Applications of AI in medicine often require expert annotation, which comes at a cost. As Eli-Shaoul Khedouri, CEO of Intuition Machines, told me, "Many of the most successful AI/ML systems today rely on a massive amount of labeled data. While most image recognition problems can be crowd-sourced or labeled by anyone with a few hours of training, medical AI applications are often bottlenecked by the cost and limited supply of experts required to build a new dataset in areas like radiology."

Will this change with the new language models we have access to? Well, it's certainly possible that we won't need to label all of the historic medical literature to extract insights, answer research questions, and receive point-of-care clinical decision support. There's early evidence that a new generation of large language models can be trained through self-supervision on large, unstructured, unlabeled datasets. These models will flexibly interpret different combinations of medical modalities, including data from imaging, EHRs, laboratory results, genomics, graphs, and medical text. They'll then produce expressive outputs, such as free-text explanations, spoken recommendations, or image annotations that demonstrate advanced medical reasoning abilities.[2]

Most medical models approved to date are for narrow tasks and are developed using supervised learning through labeled data. An example is a medical model that's trained using CT scans of patients presenting with acute stroke. Using labeled, historic scans, an algorithm can be trained to recognize an acute ischemic or hemorrhagic stroke on a CT scan. This requires a few thousand images, hopefully from patients of different demographics that represent a heterogeneous dataset. The promise of large language models is that they can be trained using different types of data (e.g. images, text, labs, and genetics) and will be able to perform many different tasks, ranging from answering questions about texts to describing images and more. However, these models will still require massive amounts of diverse data.

All of this points to the fact that solving data issues will be a prerequisite for developing and incorporating fancy algorithms into the practice of medicine. It's not that we don't know what needs to be done, but rather that there are serious political, business, and technical challenges to implementing the changes that need to be made. Let's dive into some of these data issues and assess their impact on AI in healthcare. Whether it's the use of labeled and structured data to train a model to perform a single task or using large amounts of unlabeled and unstructured data to train multi-purpose models, we'll need large datasets that are diverse and representative of the population that the model will be used for.

The success (or failure) of AI in healthcare will be determined based on its ability to deal with less glamorous issues like interoperability, data sourcing and labeling, the normalization of data, clinical workflow integration, and change management. Today, we have more digital data than ever and that's good news for the future of AI (Figure 2.2), but to take advantage of all this data, we need to solve many issues.

The data issue is so salient that many of the experts I spoke with mentioned that it will keep some of the key applications of AI in healthcare, such as clinical decision support, at bay for a long time. Decision support may

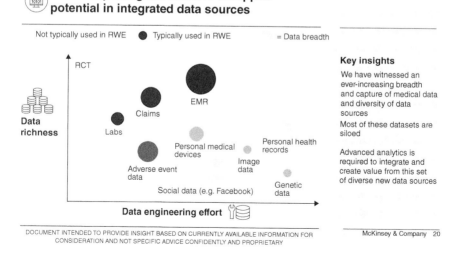

FIGURE 2.2   *(source: McKinsey & Company)*

end up being one of the last applications to gain widespread adoption due to the fragmented and unstructured nature of the data that needs to be used to develop and launch such applications. The challenge is even greater when you launch such an algorithm and the data needs to be fed into the algorithm in real time. Then there's structured or unstructured data that remain fragmented and which might not be easily available for the algorithm to provide the right output. These aren't trivial issues for the development and deployment of algorithms in the real world.

For example, when clinical algorithms were launched at Mount Sinai Hospital, a number of issues were encountered, including data quality, managing different data sources, and a lack of standardization. This can be particularly difficult to deal with when integrating into a medical industry where patients are the priority while the documentation and data collection are considered secondary.[3]

Let's discuss some of the data issues that are relevant for the successful use of AI in healthcare.

2.1   Obtaining Datasets That are Big Enough and Detailed Enough for Training

It's a huge challenge for businesses to create or obtain these kinds of datasets. The best datasets have the perfect combination of quantity and quality, as well as enough diversity to be fully representative of the different types of patients that the algorithm will be used for. This data will need to be generated and shared by medical providers while caring for patients and will need to be de-identified before use. There'll be a real need to tackle issues like data standardization and interoperability if we want to pull together solid datasets and to operationalize the resulting algorithms in clinical settings. This issue becomes even more relevant with the foundation models that promise to be the cornerstone of future medical algorithms. Large language model development will require massive datasets that specifically focus on the medical domain and its modalities. These datasets must be diverse, anonymized, and organized in compatible formats.

Today, most modern AI algorithms use input-output pairs. For example, they'll be provided with thousands of MRI scans and told, "Here are 10,000 MRI scans, and for each scan, there's a specification that says 'there isn't a tumor' or 'here's where the tumors are'." Or at the very least, "This scan contains one or more tumors." This means that the algorithm can only do one thing, which in this case is to identify tumors in MRI scans. It might not be versatile,

Initial clinical AI solutions approved by the FDA

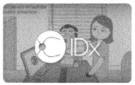 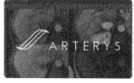 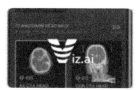

Diabetic retinopathy   Liver and lung AI lesion   CT scans analysis for strokes

FIGURE 2.3   *(source: CB Information Services, Inc.)*

but it will get very, very good at doing that one particular task accurately and at scale (Figure 2.3).

We need to remember that our patient data is siloed, messy, and super-sensitive. This leads us to the following basic questions:

- Where are we going to source the data for the problem we're trying to solve?
- Is the data accurately annotated?
- How will we obtain training data for rare diseases?
- How will we protect patient privacy while still training AI models?

We'll need data from multiple institutions if we want to create large and diverse datasets to train algorithms that will perform as planned in clinical practice. This will minimize the chance of using data that's too skewed toward a certain population and introducing algorithmic bias. It's important to remember that as well as needing data for the initial training, we'll also need a continual supply of data for training, validation, and the improvement of the AI algorithms. There will be secular changes in diseases, diagnoses, treatments, and practice patterns. The data might also need to be shared between multiple healthcare institutions and even across nations. This is usually very difficult as providers are concerned about sharing their data (and for good reason!).

Real-world data is often fragmented, and that can limit key applications such as decision support algorithms that rely on complete patient data from a variety of different sources. This isn't nearly as critical of an issue if the scope of decision support is narrow, such as in algorithms that help with the reading of radiological studies. In this instance, the data is limited to the radiology file and it's all structured. As such, AI applications that need limited data from a single file will be much easier to launch in the real world than those that rely on data from multiple sources.

For providers to meet their privacy obligations to patients, the data will need to be anonymized and de-identified. They'll also need to ensure that they're using informed consent processes which make it clear that there may be a need for wide distribution. With this scale of dissemination, the notions of patient confidentiality and privacy may need to be entirely reimagined.[4] Some IRBs will permit the distribution of de-identified data without consent for large patient populations where it's considered impractical to obtain (retrospective) consent and when they believe there's "minimal risk." Cybersecurity measures will also be increasingly important for addressing the inappropriate use of datasets, inaccurate or inappropriate disclosures, and limitations in de-identification techniques.[5] For example, it could come into play with data that's de-identified before it's used for research or data that's shared between institutions that are caring for the same patients. Modern de-identification techniques are good, but they're not perfect.

You can remove patients' identifying information from structured fields, but it can also be included in unstructured data such as physician notes or radiology reports. If we're not able to remove that, the data won't be fully de-identified and patients' identities could be exposed. There are worthwhile efforts that are showing promising results in removing patient identifying information from the unstructured data, but it's not yet been established whether they're 100% fool-proof. Dr. Szolovits of MIT also commented on the intersection between patient privacy and large language models. LLMs like GPT have such large capacities that they can effectively memorize notes, so the model itself contains much of the text. Although OpenAI doesn't disclose the model, there are clever ways to extract some of that information.

As you can see, these aren't isolated issues and overcoming them requires big-picture thinking, country-wide regulations and laws, and new approaches to the collection, storage, and sharing of data. This could threaten the business models of many current incumbents in health IT, and unless there are laws and regulations pushing them along, many of these incumbents will drag their feet in changing their approach. Worse still, some of the latest laws and regulations (such as General Data Protection Regulation [GDPR] in Europe) are making access to data and data sharing between institutions more difficult.

Even if you obtain a great dataset and do a good job of training a model, retrospective datasets used to train AI models are usually better than data that's fed into a model when it's in use in a live clinical environment, because the training datasets are cleaned up and more complete. Thus there will likely be gaps between how models perform on that data (or the data used in their validation, which is also retrospective![6]) and how they perform in the real world.

All of this means that even though many algorithms have been approved by the FDA based on their performance with limited retrospective data, they might not be trained for the optimal, real-world performance that their users will expect. This can happen when their developers are unable to access the large and diverse datasets that are needed to train their models.

2.2   Data Access Laws and Regulatory Issues

Obtaining high-quality (or any) data for the training and validation of AI models is challenging. High-profile cases in this area have been corrosive to public trust.[7, 8] There are excellent initial attempts at public policies to protect patient data and increase public confidence, like the European Union's GDPR[9] and the Consumer Privacy Act in California,[10] which show that the government is establishing standards on who can access data and what they can do with it. There are new proposals from the Center for Medicare and Medicaid Services which are designed to give patients access to and ownership of their healthcare data.[11] It's long been argued that patients themselves should be the owners and guardians of their health data, which is why their consent is being used to develop AI solutions.[12] However, this could present challenges as the creators of AI solutions would need to contact each patient individually to use their data. Given the amount of data needed to create good models, this doesn't seem realistic.

GDPR will have a huge impact on AI in healthcare. Perhaps the biggest impact will be because personal data can only be collected with individuals' "explicit and informed" consent. Informed consent is nothing new to the healthcare industry (in contrast to digital marketing), but obtaining informed consent for data collection is more difficult than it is to obtain consent for specific tasks, such as procedures or surgical interventions.

The new regulations also give more power to consumers, who now have the power to track which data is being collected and to file a request for its deletion. This will shift the power balance closer to the patient and is an important reminder of how healthcare professionals have a duty of care to protect patient privacy and to carry out appropriate governance.

Historically, China has been an easier place to get this data due to its lax data privacy laws. That, combined with its large population, made China an attractive place for building AI models. However, China has also passed some strict data privacy laws that took effect on November 2021. The Personal Information Protection Law is inspired by GDPR and means that moving forward, it will be more difficult to access data to train AI models. When combined with the data and security laws in Western countries, we can clearly see that it will be increasingly difficult for the developers of these technologies to get the necessary data.

In the United States, the current healthcare environment holds little incentive for data sharing.[13] The good news is that we can hope for change thanks to ongoing healthcare reforms that aim to prioritize outcome-based reimbursement over the old fee-for-service model. If this encouraging trend continues, there'll be more of an incentive for companies to compile and exchange information. We can also hope that the government will actively promote a move toward data sharing. The National Science and Technology Council Committee on Technology recommended that open data standards for AI should be a key priority for federal agencies.[14]

2.3   Data Standardization and Its Integration into Clinical Workflows

If we want to aggregate data from different sources so that we can train and use AI algorithms in healthcare, data standardization will be critical. The term refers to the act of taking data and transforming it so that it adheres to a common format, and when it's done well, it results in data that can be processed and understood by a variety of different tools. This is vital because data is collected in different ways and for different purposes, and it can also be stored in a variety of different formats. The same data (e.g. biomarkers like blood glucose levels) can be represented in different ways by different systems. Healthcare data is more heterogeneous and variable than the research data that other fields use.[15] Because of that, it needs to be standardized and ported to a common format if we want to use AI effectively in the healthcare industry.

The biggest (and arguably most valuable) healthcare data store can be found in our EMRs. The problem is that clinicians are dissatisfied with EMRs due to poor interfaces and workflows. This leads to poor documentation, variable completeness, and inconsistent data quality.

Seymour Duncker adds, "Additionally, imaging and labs data hold a lot of potential. There are over 100 trained algorithms on imaging data. Training algorithms on imaging data is more straightforward than using EMR-based data due to the standardized DICOM format and directly associated radiology reports that contain relevant findings and can be used in supervised training."

There are serious challenges when it comes to combining data from different sources, ranging from application programming interface (API) limitations to complex dependencies which lead to failure cascades, pipeline plus data engineering issues, and more. Over the last decade, we've seen a number of public and private attempts to address these challenges, but progress so far has been minimal at best. In spite of the widely-touted benefits of "data liberation," a sufficiently compelling business case hasn't been presented to overcome the vested interests maintaining the status quo and to justify the significant upfront investment that's necessary to build data infrastructure.[7]

Duncker says, "Another interesting development is the multi-modal approach, where individual models are pre-trained separately on siloed data sets (e.g. imaging, labs, EMRs) and then integrated into a multi-modal model that's designed for designated tasks. This potentially avoids the need to integrate data at the source, which is prohibitively expensive."[16]

We also discussed the initial promise shown by foundation models, the latest generation of AI models, which are trained on massive, diverse datasets and can be applied to numerous downstream tasks. Driven by growing datasets, increases in model size, and advances in architecture, foundation models offer previously unseen abilities. We'll still need to create large training datasets, but given their ability to train on unlabeled and unstructured data, we can tap into historical medical literature and other available medical data. This is a massive step forward and may mean that challenging applications such as clinical decision support could be closer than we thought.

All data that will or could be integrated with machine learning (ML) algorithms (administrative, clinical, claims, genomic, patient-generated, social determinants, or surveillance) need to be normalized, de-duplicated, tested, and, ultimately, integrated into workflows. Of course, the first step in all of this is to link all of the data about any specific patient. Here's what that looks like:

- **Normalization:** Data from disparate sources (such as EHRs, lab results, or claims) need to be organized into a standardized definition or vocabulary so that algorithms can understand it uniformly, regardless of the source.
- **De-duplication:** Data is often rendered differently across different sources. Information as simple as a name could be stored as Jeff Smith in the EHR, Jeffrey Smith in lab results and Jeffrey C. Smith in claims data. Such inconsistencies need to be corrected.
- **Testing:** Once the data has been normalized and de-duplicated, it needs to be tested for quality assurance to find and correct additional inconsistencies. Because duplicate datasets are unavoidable, organizations will need to conduct routine rounds of testing.
- **Workflow integration:** Determining the optimal point at which clinicians or administrative employees interface with the AI requires input from an interdisciplinary team. IT should work with clinicians to understand when it will be most effective for radiologists to receive information about suspicious legions in an image, for example.

Given the multiple components of clinical workflows, interoperability will be essential. For example, for an AI-assisted radiology workflow, algorithms developed for protocoling, study prioritization, feature analysis and extraction, and automated report generation could each conceivably be a product of individual specialized vendors, such as a radiology AI startup or a larger vendor like GE or Siemens.[17] We'll require a set of standards that are designed to allow different algorithms to be integrated together and for those algorithms to run on different equipment. Without a concerted, early effort to work toward interoperability, the efficacy of AI in healthcare will be severely limited.

It all comes down to interoperability, which is a super important topic even if it's not the most glamorous thing to talk about. The industry needs to go out of its way to prioritize interoperability, which itself is a loaded term. It can mean that the different data sources are connected to each other and can send and receive data. It can also mean that the different systems can talk to each other in the same language and that when they share data, the receiving systems can understand the data they're receiving.

One of the most promising solutions for the problem of interoperability in healthcare is the Fast Healthcare Interoperability Resources (FHIR). FHIR uses a set of modular components, known as "resources," which can be assembled into working systems that will facilitate data sharing within EHRs and mobile-based apps as well as cloud-based communications.[18] This is the most promising approach to ensuring that healthcare data, coded with different standards, can be exchanged between different systems with a unified language. This means that if the same concepts are coded differently in different EHRs or lab reporting systems, when those systems connect with each other, they'll be able to speak the same language. This is critical for making healthcare information more interoperable and to facilitate the ideal workflows we all need for providing better healthcare. Looking to the future, it'll be critical to have FHIR frameworks if we hope to implement AI-based technologies in the healthcare sector. It's similar to how Digital Imaging and Communications in Medicine (DICOM) and picture archiving and communications system (PACS) are vital to exchanging digital medical images (Figures 2.4 and 2.5).

By spending today focusing on the interoperability of information and systems, we can make sure that tomorrow, we're in a much better place than we are now. Because of that, interoperability, security, identity management, and differential privacy will all be important aspects of the future.

2.4 Federated AI as a Possible Solution

Federated learning is an up-and-coming approach to AI training that aims to protect the privacy of sensitive user data by ensuring that it never leaves their device. The applications that run specific programs on the edge of the network will still be able to learn how to process the data and build better, more efficient models by sharing a mathematical representation of key clinical features—but not the data.[20]

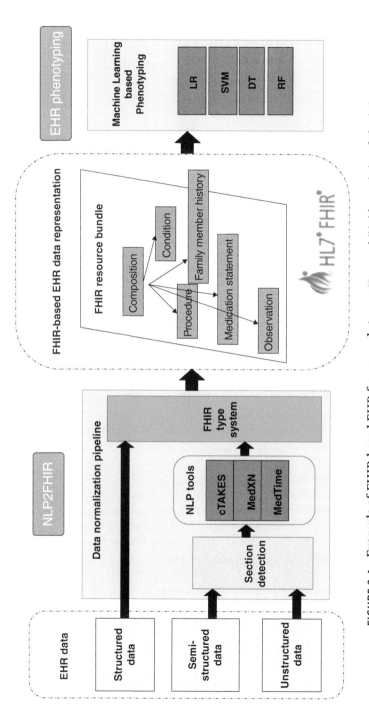

FIGURE 2.4 Example of FHIR-based EHR framework *(source: Hong et al.* [19]*/with permission of Elsevier)*

Mapping the ODM Data Model to FHIR Resources

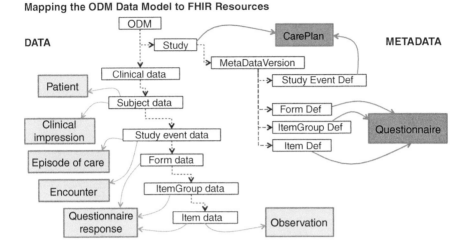

FIGURE 2.5   *(source: Ref. [18]/Springer Nature/CCB 4.0/Public domain)*

Federated learning gained prominence when Google started using it for Android keyboards (with Gboard). Now, a Google Ventures-backed company called OWKIN is applying the same techniques to patient data.[21] The idea is to create a system in which patient data never leaves the hospital and where it isn't uploaded to a centralized cloud server. Models will be updated at the hospital using local data, and only those updates will be uploaded to the cloud.

Traditional ML requires centralized data if we want to train and build models. Federated learning doesn't have the same drawback, and it could be combined with other privacy-preserving and zero-trust techniques to create models that use distributed data while reducing potential entry points for attacks or data leaks. It can also be used within the cloud, where the data won't have to leave the systems on which it exists for the algorithm to learn. This is called federated cloud learning, and it's notable for allowing collaboration between companies while simultaneously keeping data private.

The good news is that we can expect to see a federated learning platform for pharma called MELLODDY (Machine Learning Ledger Orchestration for Drug Discovery). MELLODDY is being built in collaboration between a number of major pharmaceutical companies, including Novartis, Merck, Janssen, Servier, Institut De Recherches Servier, GSK, Ingelheim, Boehringer, Bayer, AstraZeneca, Astellas, and Amgen.[22] The shared interest of reducing the cost and time it takes to bring a new drug to market has brought these competing players together on the project, which "aims to enhance predictive machine learning models on decentralized data from 10 pharmaceutical companies, without exposing proprietary information."

Data fluency is a framework and set of tools which aims to rapidly unlock the value within clinical data by ensuring that every stakeholder is simultaneously participating in a collaborative environment. An ML environment with a data fluency framework engages clinicians, actuaries, data engineers, data scientists, managers, infrastructure engineers, and all other business stakeholders to explore the data, ask questions, quickly build analytics, and even model the data.[22] This new and exciting approach to enterprise data analytics is set to help the healthcare industry streamline workflows, improve collaboration, and rapidly prototype ideas before resources are invested into building models.

Traditional healthcare systems work in siloes, and many companies in the industry are struggling to unlock the actionable trends and clinical insights that lie dormant in their data. This modern healthcare stack facilitates the collaboration of cross-functional teams from a single, data-driven point of view with a UI for non-engineering partners.[22]

Data fluency aims to provide an environment for key stakeholders to discover insights in a real-time, agile, and iterative way. The feedback from non-engineering teams can help to immediately improve the underlying model. Each domain expert can be provided with multiple data views that enable deep collaboration and data insight discovery. This will ensure that there's a continuous learning environment providing a feedback loop between care and research.

Federated AI and the concept of data fluency could also address the barriers to data acquisition, which usually revolve around privacy, trust, regulatory compliance, and intellectual property as opposed to being a technological challenge. This is especially the case in healthcare, where patients and consumers expect privacy when it comes to personal information and where organizations want to protect the value of their data while simultaneously following regulatory laws such as HIPAA in the United States and GDPR in Europe.[22]

It's difficult for companies to access healthcare data, and it's often hidden behind compliance walls. At best, access is usually only granted to de-identified data, and even then there are security measures in place. Federated AI and data fluency could enable the healthcare industry to create and share models without sharing the data that was used to train it, which could help to address those concerns. We can expect it to play a critical role in helping us to understand the insights that are hidden within distributed data silos without falling foul of non-compliance.

This approach to unlocking the value of healthcare data could help us to preserve privacy and thus prove vital in the future. As with everything else, it's all about driving actionable insights and better health outcomes, in this case by boosting ML adoption. Federated AI could allow us to create an ML environment that facilitates data fluency, leading to the creation of models that take data from multiple sources and run in parallel.

2.5   Synthetic Data

We have seen the ability of ChatGPT to generate text that is identical to human writings. Art generated by generative AI can be impossible to distinguish from a painting by humans. If you've spent any amount of time on Twitter and have been participating in discussions about AI, you might have seen people playing with generative AI to create fake images of everything from cats to pizzas and trees. Generative AI taps into AI's ability to create more realistic-looking synthetic images to train AI, and this has huge implications for the healthcare industry. NVIDIA, for instance, used generative adversarial networks (GANs) to create fake MRI images with brain tumors.[23] The company's research paper concluded that by augmenting real-world data with synthetic MRIs, they were able to improve tumor segmentation (Figure 2.6).

Synthetic data is one way of dealing with the issue of creating datasets for algorithm training. This approach is gaining traction, and just like Federated AI, it can offer a path to developing good models without having to go door-to-door from one medical center to another to create a heterogeneous dataset. Basically, you can use ML to create more data from the dataset you already have and then use that to train a better model.

The term synthetic data is used to refer to any data that doesn't come from direct measurement. Healthcare data comes from people seeking healthcare, which means that it's already biased toward those who have access to healthcare and those with certain mindsets and approaches. For rare conditions where there isn't enough data to develop good models, synthetic data could provide us with a solution. It is postulated that moving forward, synthetic data can be a major source of data for training AI models or for augmenting clinical trial data (Figure 2.7).

Michigan Medicine used this approach in a recent project to develop a decision support tool to improve pathologists' ability to accurately diagnose brain tumors in the operating room, allowing them to diagnose more quickly and more accurately.[23] They were trying to develop a computer vision model that could identify diagnostic regions and provide tentative diagnoses for pathologists to consider when making their final interpretations.

However, they were limited to using data that they'd collected themselves. They took slides that had been warehoused and then digitized them to create a set of training data for the network. That represented around 300 patients with five different brain tumor diagnoses. They then tried to validate the algorithm using a dataset from multiple institutions with the goal of ensuring high performance across different medical centers. Unfortunately, they observed an unexpected drop in accuracy once they started testing their model on images from other medical centers. It dropped as low as 50% when used on data from patients from Ohio State Medical Center.

By using synthetic data that was generated from large pathology datasets, the model improved its diagnostic accuracy significantly because the

"Together, these results offer a potential solution to two of the largest challenges facing machine learning in medical imaging, namely the small incidence of pathological findings, and the restrictions around sharing of patient data."

— NVIDIA RESEARCH PAPER

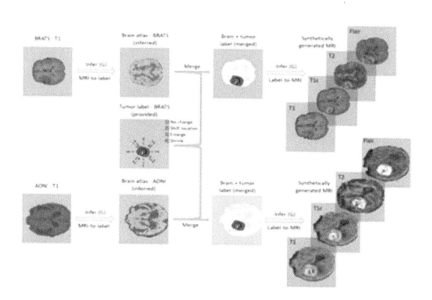

FIGURE 2.6   *(source: CB Information Services, Inc.[21] https://www.cbinsights.com/research/report/ai-trends-healthcare/last accessed 21 August, 2023)*

synthetic data meant there was more data available for training. In particular, the team needed more data for brain tumor types that were uncommon or that had disproportionately high diagnostic error rates.

The issue of not having enough data is a major challenge when training computer vision models for clinical decision support, but synthetic data can help to reduce the problem by creating more data. This will result in better algorithm training and diagnostic accuracy. The Michigan Medicine team

By 2030, synthetic data will completely overshadow real data in AI models

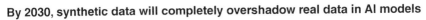

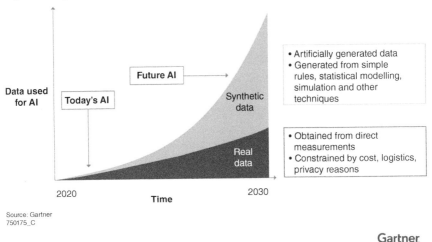

FIGURE 2.7   *(source: Gartner/https://www.gartner.com/en/newsroom/press-releases/2022-05-09-gartner-data-and-analytics-summit-london-2022-day-1-highlights)*

saw a huge improvement in diagnostic accuracy on both its own data and on pathology datasets from other medical centers. The team was also able to correctly classify challenging tumors that had been incorrectly classified by clinical pathologists at the time of surgery.

This synthetic data was generated using GANs by the synthetic data company, Synthetaic, to augment the existing data in an attempt to improve computer-aided diagnostic systems. We referred to GANs earlier as a novel AI approach that could help with some key issues in the development of good models.

The new algorithm trained with the additional synthetic data achieved 96% accuracy across major brain tumor types. This was a massive jump in performance when compared to the 68% accuracy it achieved without the synthetic data. They were also able to correctly diagnose 90% of the most challenging brain tumor types—primary central nervous system lymphomas—compared to a rate of 70% without the synthetic data.

Gretel provides another example, using real genotype and phenotype data to teach algorithms to generate artificial data. Also, MDClone creates synthetic data as a viable alternative to data de-identification (i.e. removing personally identifiable information from patient records) where patients could potentially be re-identified through cross-referencing.[24]

With the use of such trained datasets, even existing algorithmic bias could be overruled. There's an ongoing issue in AI-based programming due to the limited access to data focusing on race and skin color. An MIT Media

Lab study found that facial recognition systems from companies like IBM and Microsoft were 11–19% more accurate on lighter-skinned individuals.[25]

Synthetic data could help us to overcome this challenge as the training could focus on these kinds of variables, making use of real-world environments. For example, it could allow us to diagnose melanoma on darker-skinned patients—as previous algorithms have often failed to do.[26]

2.6   Data Labeling and Transparency

Labeling training data often requires a large amount of manual work. Most early applications in radiology and pathology use supervised learning, which means that human input is needed to label and categorize the data that's being used. This is time and labor intensive. However, promising new techniques are emerging to overcome these data bottlenecks, such as large language models that don't require labeled data, reinforcement learning, GANs, transfer learning, and "one-shot learning," which allows a trained AI model to learn about a subject based on a small number of real-world demonstrations or examples—and sometimes just one.

The transparency of data and AI algorithms is a major concern that's relevant at multiple levels.[15] Most applications rely on supervised learning, where accurate predictions are only possible if the underlying annotations are also accurate. Poorly labeled data will yield poor results, so transparent labeling is paramount to ensure that others can critically evaluate the training processes of supervised learning algorithms and therefore ensure their accuracy.[27]

Another challenge is that AI companies need experts from the healthcare industry to annotate images so that they can teach algorithms to pick up on anomalies. That's why both governments and tech giants are investing heavily in annotation and ensuring that the datasets are publicly available to other researchers (Figure 2.8).

For example, Google DeepMind recently partnered with Moorfield's Eye Hospital to use AI to detect eye diseases. The neural networks had a 94% accuracy rate when it came to recommending the right referral decisions for 50 sight-threatening eye diseases.[29] Even though this was just phase one of the study, DeepMind invested significant amounts of time into labeling and cleaning up the database of OCT (optical coherence tomography) scans and making it "AI ready." They needed trained ophthalmologists and optometrists to review the OCT scans and clinically label the 14,884 scans in the dataset to ensure that it was accurate and in the right format. Around 1000 scans were graded by junior ophthalmologists, and any disagreements in labeling were resolved by a certified senior specialist with over 10 years of experience.[21]

Yitu Technology—a Chinese "unicorn" company worth over $1 billion and owned by private investors—has a team of 400 doctors working part-time

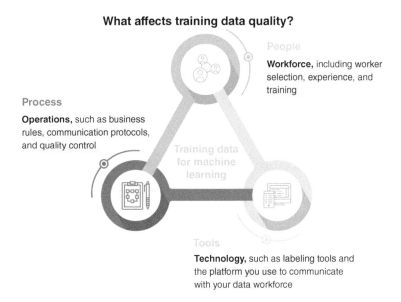

What affects training data quality?

People

Workforce, including worker selection, experience, and training

Process

Operations, such as business rules, communication protocols, and quality control

Training data for machine learning

Tools

Technology, such as labeling tools and the platform you use to communicate with your data workforce

FIGURE 2.8 *(source: Ref.[28]/Cloudfactory)*

purely on the labeling of data. However, higher salaries in the United States mean that it would be an expensive option for startups in the States.[21] It was a similar case for Alibaba when it moved into the field of AI for diagnostics back in 2016.[29] And the National Institutes of Health (NIH) released a dataset of 32,000 lesions annotated and identified in CT images anonymized from 4400 patients.[21]

Fortunately, there are emerging techniques to address this challenge, including reinforcement learning and in-stream supervision, which allow data to be labeled in the course of natural usage. In fact, models that have been trained to support healthcare and life sciences can give us the ability to automatically normalize, index, and structure data. These models can automate key parts of the data labeling process and save time while increasing accuracy.

AstraZeneca has been doing exactly this to use ML across all stages of research and development. Labeling data is time-consuming, especially given that it can take thousands of tissue sample images to train an accurate model.[30] To tackle this, the company is using a human-in-the-loop annotation service that's powered by ML and which will automate some of the most tedious parts of data labeling. This has resulted in less than half the amount of time being required to catalog samples.

Self-supervised learning in large language models could be a game changer here, because there's no need for data annotation to train these models. Also, these models are showing promise at ingesting different data modalities (such as text, images, and labs), and their output can also be multimodal.

This means that they can potentially ingest unlabeled radiological images and create models that can identify several abnormalities in those images. Most models to date have been task-specific, meaning that they're trained to identify one type of abnormality (e.g. pneumonia) on an X-ray using labeled data. The next generation of models may be able to carry out multiple tasks after being trained on a large amount of unlabeled data of different kinds.

2.7   Model Explainability

It's often difficult to explain the results from large, complicated algorithms in human terms. In other words, it's hard to say how the algorithm arrives at any given decision. This is related to the labeling issue in that the output of a model may be more easily explained by looking at the input data and how it was labeled. The idea is that human beings should be able to understand how any given algorithm makes its decisions or predictions. AI technologies will need transparency to justify a particular diagnosis, treatment recommendation, or outcome prediction.[5] Or, will they? If we observe that feeding more and better data into models results in their pattern recognition and predictability improving, do we have to fully understand how the model came to its conclusions? After all, we can test a model and investigate its output to see if it's making good predictions or accurately spotting issues. If it is—and if it's doing a better job than humans—should we refrain from using it, just because we can't explain how the model is arriving at its conclusions?

Large, complex models can make it more difficult for us to explain their results in human terms. Because of this, it can be hard for algorithms to receive certification in regulated industries like healthcare, finance, and aerospace. Regulators typically want rules and choice criteria to be clearly explainable (Figure 2.9).

This type of transparency is increasingly difficult with more powerful deep learning models. If they can absorb large amounts of multidimensional data, they can provide outputs that are beyond human processing capability and that aren't easy to explain. There will be a lot of debate about whether these outputs should be used to manage patients. We already give medications to patients with clear benefits and little side effects but we don't know exactly how those medications result in those benefits. Why should the algorithms be any different?

On the other hand, it will take time to prove that algorithmic recommendations are safe and superior. Once that happens, clinicians will become more comfortable using algorithms without being able to fully explain how they arrived at their results. There's some evidence that large language models trained on huge amounts of historical clinical literature can provide links to the studies that were used to create their output. This can allow clinicians to look up those references if there are questions about the validity of the output.

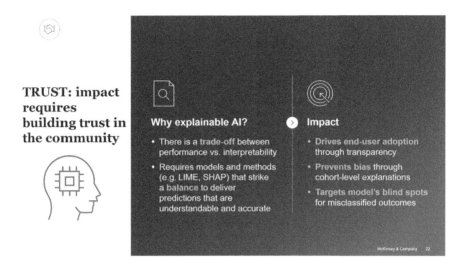

TRUST: impact requires building trust in the community

Why explainable AI?

- There is a trade-off between performance vs. interpretability
- Requires models and methods (e.g. LIME, SHAP) that strike a balance to deliver predictions that are understandable and accurate

Impact

- Drives end-user adoption through transparency
- Prevents bias through cohort-level explanations
- Targets model's blind spots for misclassified outcomes

McKinsey & Company   22

FIGURE 2.9   *(source: McKinsey & Company)*

Seymour Duncker told me, "At the moment, AI algorithms are mainly validated through retrospective studies, the gold standard being prospective trials. But we're missing health economics and outcomes studies akin to phase three clinical trials for drug development, demonstrating that the AI-enhanced clinical workflow is better than the current practiced standard." This will go a long way in making clinicians more comfortable with their use, even if they don't fully know how they arrived at their recommendations.

It's understandable for physicians to be wary of a black box providing recommendations for patient treatment, but if the algorithms can show *why* they're making their suggestions—along with their confidence in those recommendations—they'll be much more useful. That's why we should be aiming for explainability, allowing a complementary relationship between healthcare providers and technology companies. We need to remember that doctors go through years of specialized training and build upon that with real-world experience. It's unwise (and unrealistic) for us to expect them to accept treatment recommendations that come without any context. As part of transparency, we also need to provide clarity when it comes to the data that's used to train the algorithm in the first place. If the data used to train the AI isn't representative of how the technology will be used, that's a nonstarter and needs to be addressed head-on.[31]

There are already initiatives that aim to make healthcare models easier to understand and to uncover the key drivers for a model's output. One such example is Microsoft, which is developing a tool called Interpret ML that tries to better explain how models arrive at their outputs (Figure 2.10).

••• and an 'Explainable AI' output

ịᵥ̶ InterpretML

As the healthcare industry continues to move forward with AI implementations, the call for explainable AI has grown.

Doctors need more than a risk score; they need to consider the underlying factors that contributed to a model's prediction for their patient. model outputs produced by "black box" algorithms are notoriously difficult to explain.

Microsoft is working to fix this with interpretML, an open-source toolkit designed to bring clarity to model outputs.

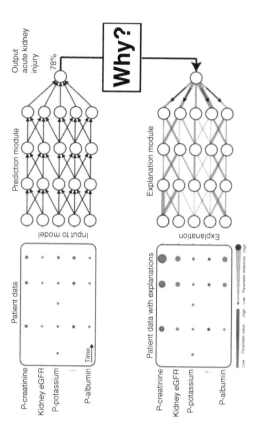

FIGURE 2.10 (*source: CB Insights*)

Mount Sinai Medical Center in New York used unsupervised learning on 700K EMR data to predict the onset and probability of diseases like schizophrenia.[32] If the model is doing a good job in these focused areas, why avoid using it just because we can't explain how it reached its conclusions? We know that deep learning models have superhuman capabilities when it comes to identifying patterns in data. Why wouldn't we use it to augment human capabilities?

As the accuracy of these models increases (due to the use of deep learning algorithms), the explainability goes in the opposite direction (Figure 2.11).

A recent project by Dr. Matthieu Komorowski and Prof. Aldo Faisal from Imperial College and NHS Trust London has taken AI to an exciting new level.[33] In critical care scenarios, AI algorithms have so far mostly been used to risk-stratify patients and to (often successfully) answer questions like: "Which patient will develop renal failure? Who will bleed after open heart surgery?" AI tools based on deep learning can predict critical medical events more reliably than traditional risk scores.

Komorowski and Faisal have done something completely different. Their algorithm, which they call "the AI Clinician," is making therapeutic suggestions to optimize the treatment of sepsis patients. These suggestions are about the administration of intravenous fluids and vasopressors, which is relevant because mortality amongst sepsis patients remains high and experts think that at least part of the difference in sepsis mortality between different hospitals can be attributed to suboptimal fluid and vasopressor therapy.

In the first step, the algorithm analyzed a dataset of more than 60,000 patients with early sepsis in relation to 48 parameters that are typically

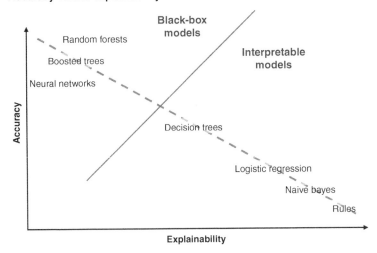

FIGURE 2.11   *(source: Gartner)*

measured and documented in intensive care units. This analysis led to 500 models that were then tested against another 16,000 patients to identify which model resulted in the highest level of patient safety and the lowest mortality. The winning model was then validated against another 17,000 patients. The researchers were able to show that sepsis mortality was lowest amongst patients where clinicians had prescribed vasopressors and fluids in line with recommendations from the winning model.

This research, which was published in *Nature Medicine*, is so outstanding because the researchers were able to identify the factors that determined the algorithm's decisions. The publication included a top-10 list of the parameters that were most relevant for recommendations on both fluid and vasopressor therapy. This meant that an intensive care doctor using the algorithm would be able to understand why any given approach was recommended. The "AI Clinician" at least partly explains itself. So far, the vast majority of deep learning algorithms are simply incapable of explaining their decisions.

The sepsis AI research project is an example of an AI tool that really does explain itself, but it doesn't use deep learning. Instead, it uses a different, highly computerized approach to ML called reinforcement learning which is based on Markov models.

Dr. Andreas Holzinger, Head of the Human-Centered AI Lab at the University of Natural Resources and Life Sciences in Vienna, says, "Explainable AI remains in the research stage, but the ability to explain is easier to reach with Markov models than with deep learning algorithms. Unfortunately, Markov models can't be used for all kinds of questions. They work well with very clear-cut, very focused questions, but less well with more general ones."

This is where the doctor comes back into the loop, where they can assess the algorithm's recommendation and form their own idea about whether a recommendation is relevant or makes sense. In clinical medicine, AI can be used in such a way that the doctor is in the driving seat while being assisted by various AI tools. It's similar to a driver who's assisted—but not replaced—by power steering.

It's widely accepted that it's important to create trustworthy AI through technologies or processes that make it easier for us to understand and interpret algorithms. There are already several major initiatives that aim to develop and promote trustworthy AI. Interpretable AI will almost certainly boost trust by tackling the black box problem and making sure that healthcare workers can understand how an AI has reached a particular recommendation. Then there are efforts to create clinical trial standards for AI algorithms. If they're done well, the innovations will help to boost the adoption of AI in the healthcare industry because people will be able to understand whether the algorithms reached their recommendations based on biased or incomplete data.

Another reason why transparency is important is that AI technologies have the potential for algorithmic bias, thereby reinforcing discriminatory practices based on race, sex, or other features.[4,5] If we have transparent training data and interpretable models, we'll be better placed to spot these biases. Ideally, ML could even help resolve healthcare disparities if it's designed to compensate for known biases.[5] Once again, all of this is aspirational and if we see models that are improving patient outcomes with low explainability, why wouldn't we use them?

This debate is especially salient because although some of these models have performed well in isolated validation studies, once they're put to work in clinical settings, their performance is less than stellar. The real test of whether a black box produces output that's superior to humans isn't in controlled settings (where many companies are currently validating their algorithms) but in the real world. We need to carefully study whether models' outputs are accurate, unbiased, and repeatable with different types of real-world data. This hasn't been done on a large scale with most of the models so far, and this will remain a barrier to the adoption of these models for the near future.[34]

2.8 Model Performance in the Real World

One of the key issues with AI is that algorithms developed in one institution or on one set of data might not perform as well when used at different institutions with different data. Researchers from the Icahn School of Medicine at Mount Sinai discovered that the same deep learning algorithms that could diagnose pneumonia in their own chest X-rays didn't work as well when they were used on imaging data from the Indiana University Network for Patient Care and the NIH.[32]

We're talking about how AI models still struggle to carry experience over from one set of circumstances to another. Companies typically need to dedicate further resources to train new models, even when they're being used in a similar set of circumstances to a previous model. This is especially true in healthcare, because each medical center has a unique population of patients that might be different than the one used to train an algorithm and thus the algorithm's output could be inaccurate. This has already been seen with some of the algorithms that were launched in institutions where they weren't developed. In many cases, the training sets for AI and ML algorithms are determined by geographical demographics. Hospitals and health systems only deal with patients from within the local area, and these unique populations naturally differ from one location to another. For example, there are health systems that are based in areas that don't have large communities of patients of color, and so they lack the representative data that's needed to train models to treat those populations. When this happens, training sets are skewed toward the demographics of whichever health system is providing the data.

It recently came to light that EHR vendor Epic's AI algorithms were underserving patients with serious illnesses. Epic is the nation's largest EHR vendor, and yet an investigation by STAT found that they were delivering both inaccurate and irrelevant information, contrasting sharply with the company's published claims.[35] Algorithms within the EHR aren't as scrutinized and the pathway for their review and approval isn't currently clear.

Many systems now have AI platforms to operationalize models inside the EHRs. This could theoretically include models developed by other vendors that can be imported into the EHR and then fed with the data within it. Given the poor performance of some of the models rolled out by Epic, many organizations will want the option to stay in their own EHR but use the best models that are out there. As we'll discuss later on in this chapter, the models developed on outside data should still be trained on local data (from your own EHR) before they're operationalized.

That's why ML developers should go out of their way to access training data from a diverse collection of organizations. The collection and identification processes need to be as thorough and purposeful as possible to avoid limited training data and ensure that it's as diverse and representative of the entire patient population as possible. Healthcare professionals have numerous and rigorous ways to evaluate the accuracy of these models, such as developing a test set that represents different populations.[36]

As AI models continue to experience difficulties while carrying experiences from one set of circumstances to another, the companies that develop them need to commit resources to training new models even when they're going to be deployed in use cases that are similar to previous ones. One promising response to this challenge is transfer learning, where AI models are taught to accomplish one task and then quickly applied to learning a similar but distinctly different task.

In the journal *PLOS*, researchers wrote, "Early results in using convolutional neural networks (CNNs) on X-rays to diagnose disease have been promising, but it hasn't yet been shown that models trained on X-rays from one hospital or one group of hospitals will work equally well at different hospitals. Before these tools are used for computer-aided diagnosis in real-world clinical settings, we must verify their ability to generalize across a variety of hospital systems. Estimates of CNN performance based on test data from hospital systems used for model training may overstate their likely real-world performance."[36]

The findings from Mount Sinai about the poor performance of their models on outside data also highlight that there's a lot of work remaining if we hope for AI technology to become ubiquitous in the healthcare industry. Moving forward, we'll need to validate algorithms across different companies and geographies to make sure that it's fit for purpose. This includes ensuring that it's appropriately labeled both for product uses and for academic literature.

Greg Wolff, executive director at UnaMesa Association, explains, "Google rolled out its diabetic retinopathy detection algorithm in Thailand to help with screening for the condition in a country without enough ophthalmologists. The algorithm performed well in controlled environments with high-quality images of the eye, but accuracy assessments from a lab only go so far. They don't teach us anything about how the AI will perform in the chaos of a real-world environment. Google's algorithm was designed to reject images that fell below a certain quality threshold. With nurses scanning dozens of patients an hour and often taking the photos in poor lighting conditions or with miscalibrated equipment, more than a fifth of the images were rejected in some locations. Also, because the system had to upload images to the cloud for processing, poor internet connections in several clinics caused delays. In subsequent studies in the US and elsewhere, the Google team demonstrated that a safe, reliable AI algorithm enabled a redesign of the clinical pathway. By providing immediate results to patients along with follow-up scheduling and counseling, the rate of adherence to recommended follow-on care increased dramatically while the time to follow-on care and treatment was significantly reduced, thereby leading to better outcomes."

This is further evidence that we'll require regular debugging, auditing, simulation, validation, and scrutiny if we plan to unleash AI algorithms in critical practice. It also underscores the need to require more evidence and robust validation to exceed the recent downgrading of FDA regulatory requirements for medical algorithm approval.[37] This is time-consuming and beyond the ability of most medical centers.

One of the key areas to examine AI models for good performance beyond their development environment is surveillance bias. Over-coding in clinical practice can lead to bias when you're looking for something and some of the people coded don't meet the clinical phenotype for that condition. For example, a dataset of people with sepsis might include people who didn't actually meet the clinical criteria for sepsis but were erroneously coded as having had it. In that case, your average sepsis patient could look less sick than they do in reality and your model would identify some people with sepsis who didn't have it. To identify the surveillance bias, you need to spend time carrying out clinical phenotyping of the coded patients to see if the coding data over-represented the sepsis population and/or underestimated severity. It's not an easy task, and few medical centers are prepared to take it on for every model they're rolling out. This represents an opportunity for the FDA and other public or private entities to take on this difficult process for AI models that will be used in clinical or operational settings.

2.9   Training on Local Data

The issue of the poor performance of models when they're used on new data in different institutions isn't a trivial one. An algorithm that only works in one institution won't go very far. Even a well-trained model might not be able to perform well when used on new data that represents a different patient population in a new geography. Local training of the models before putting them to use in real clinical settings will be important, and many medical centers lack such expertise.

This local training is important because some algorithms have local or culturally specific parameters that can't be generalized across other patient populations. Several studies have shown that local training of models is necessary. In a study of pneumonia patients, models trained on data from different sites performed better when trained on new data from those sites than when they used external data.[38]

The concept of irrational extrapolation has been a hot topic recently. Irrational extrapolation is the assumption that models trained on an easy-to-obtain set of patients or data can perform well on different types of patients or patients from different geographies.[39] It's highly recommended that algorithms deployed for clinical use be validated on local data.[40]

Seymour Duncker says, "At minimum, we need monitoring capabilities to detect how reliable an AI algorithm is in a given local context and based on that assessment, to determine whether local adaptation is required."

2.10 Bias in Algorithms

Algorithmic bias occurs in AI when the models' results can't be widely generalized. Most people think of algorithmic bias as happening due to preferences or exclusions in the training data, but bias can also be introduced due to the way that data is obtained, how algorithms are designed, and how the outputs are interpreted (Figure 2.12).

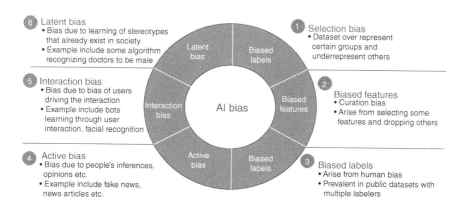

FIGURE 2.12   Different types of biases in AI algorithms *(source: Toward Data Science)[41]*

Bias can enter datasets in a variety of ways, including through patient-generated data, inadequate sample sizes, missing data, and misclassification and measurement errors. Today's AI technologies are largely built on human reasoning, and they therefore incorporate explicit and implicit bias in the delivery of care. AI is incapable of detecting that hidden bias and so it can inadvertently provide skewed, wrong, or unfair recommendations. Researchers say that a particularly difficult aspect of embedded bias is defining rules and ethical practices around fairness.[42]

The current state of healthcare data is a major source of bias introduction into AI models. Twenty-five percent of admission records are missing data, and that could have a huge impact on the robustness of their predictions, including mortality predictions. The challenge is that imbalances can be hard to assess. Common sources of bias include survey instrument bias (including sampling bias), confirmation bias, and technical bias, which includes faulty API or the ingestion of data and data governance problems.[43]

When you're combining data from different sources to build or validate a model, or in the real-world deployment of an already developed model, you can introduce several forms of bias. There's the implicit bias in each of the different forms of data, the portability issue where the algorithms don't account for different settings, and the difficulty that comes from defining the notion of fairness.[44]

As you can see, this issue deals with concerns that are more social in nature and which could therefore be harder to resolve. We'll need to learn how the processes used to collect the data can influence the behavior of the models they're used on. This will help us to avoid unintended biases due to training data not being representative of the larger population. Thus, facial recognition models trained on faces corresponding to the demographics of AI developers could struggle when applied to populations with more diverse characteristics.[44]

Seymour Duncker explains, "Interesting research by Dr. Marzeyh Ghassemi, who runs the Healthy ML group at MIT, shows that AIs which generate superhuman performance in the aggregate could underperform on subgroups and actually generate worse outcomes for them" (Figure 2.13).

Unfortunately, the bias we see in training data is only the tip of the iceberg. All of the data that we use are biased to some degree because they represent specific geographies and demographics, and certain diseases may be over- or underrepresented. The bias might not be deliberate, but that doesn't take away from the fact that it's there. In many situations, bias is unavoidable because of the way that measurements are taken, but we should still estimate the likelihood of error with each data point so that we can better interpret the results.

Modern AI developers often don't have access to huge, diverse datasets that they could use to train and validate new tools. Instead, they often use open-source datasets, but many of these datasets were trained using computer

Coverage bias
A selection bias example

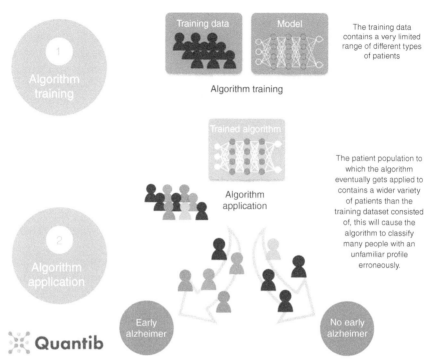

FIGURE 2.13   *(source: Quantib)*

programmers as volunteers, who are predominantly white. Algorithms are usually trained on single-origin data samples that have limited diversity, and that means that tech which seemed accurate during research will prove unreliable in the real world. It's rare for algorithms to have enough data on people from different races, genders, ages, and other demographics.

This will be an even bigger issue with the large language models that will probably be the future of medical algorithms. The unprecedented scale and complexity of the necessary training datasets will make it difficult to ensure that they're free of undesirable biases. Although biases already pose a challenge for conventional health AI, they're particularly relevant for large language models, which will need to be thoroughly validated to ensure that they don't underperform on particular populations such as minority groups. Furthermore, models will need to undergo continuous auditing and regulation even after deployment, as new issues will arise as models encounter new tasks and settings.

To visualize this, you can think of heights in the United States. If you collected data and put it on a graph, you'd find overlapping groups (or clusters) of taller and shorter people, which would broadly indicate adults and children. But we'd have to ask ourselves who was surveyed to get the data. If it was done during the week then it might miss people who were working. If it was done at medical offices, people without health insurance could be left out. If it was done in the suburbs, you'd get a different group of people than you would if you'd done it in the countryside or in the inner city. In other words, you need to ask: How large was the sample?[45]

AI algorithms are designed to spot patterns in data and to use them to create an output. There are many different kinds of AI, and each one has its own strengths and weaknesses. At the moment, deep learning is one of the most powerful kinds of algorithm that we have access to, and yet it's at its best when it's processing large, well-labeled datasets and with a precise output in mind. As we've already discussed, sometimes labeling is done by hand, while at other times, it's done using an algorithm that's trained for a different but similar task. This is called transfer learning and is generally a high-performing type of AI, but it can also introduce algorithmic bias.

Then there are algorithms that use auto-encoders, which process large amounts of data into smaller sets of features that are easier for models to learn from. The downside is that even though many techniques exist for the process of feature extraction, they can introduce bias by discarding information that could have increased the performance of the AI if it was available. This can lead to a biased algorithm even if the original dataset was unbiased.[45]

Medical AI bias can be a huge problem, because incorrect diagnoses or suggestions for the wrong therapies can be detrimental to patient health. Every bias that we've discussed has the potential to be a problem in the healthcare industry, but bias in data collection is perhaps the biggest of them all. That's because we usually only have access to the data that's generated from the patients that we see, or to the data from one or more medical institutions. These institutions, even taken together, may not represent the heterogeneity of the broader population.

But what about patients without insurance, or who for one reason or another don't seek medical attention when they're seriously ill? When that happens, how will models work when they're finally brought into the emergency room? There's a good chance that the AI will have been trained on people who weren't as sick as them, or who were younger or from some other demographic. There's also an increasing number of people who use wearable devices, which can provide data points such as the patient's pulse by measuring light reflections from the skin using photoplethysmography. Some of these algorithms witness a drop in accuracy when they're used by people of color.

Some of the pioneering work in this field has been done by Dr. Ziad Obermeyer at Berkeley. To address this, he and his collaborators have created an algorithm bias playbook.[46] As they state in the playbook, "Algorithmic bias is everywhere. Our work with dozens of organizations—healthcare providers, insurers, technology companies, and regulators—has taught us that biased algorithms are deployed throughout the healthcare system, influencing clinical care, operational workflows, and policy." They lay out a four-step process to inventory all of the algorithms in an organization, screen them for bias, retrain the biased algorithms, and set up structures to prevent future bias.

In an article for *Science*, Dr. Obermeyer and his colleagues lay out bias in risk models used to provide extra care to patients who need more care. The models use the amount of money currently spent on patients as a marker for risk. Because less money is spent on black patients who have the same amount of need, the algorithm falsely believes that black patients are healthier than equally sick white patients. Therefore, the model identifies a lower number of black patients to receive care, even when they need it.[47]

A company called AiCure is providing a solution that pharmaceutical companies are using to assess how patients are taking their medication during clinical trials. Through a combination of AI and computer vision that's powered by patients' smartphones, AiCure is able to make sure that patients receive the support that they need. It can also ensure that incorrect or missed doses are factored into the trial's data.

When the company first started in around 2011, its employees noticed that their facial recognition software wasn't working as intended on patients with darker skin. They realized that this was because they were using an open-source dataset that was built using people with fairer skin. To combat this, they rebuilt their algorithm from the ground up, recruiting black volunteers to submit video footage. Now, with more than one million dosing interactions recorded, AiCure's algorithms work with patients of all skin tones, which allows for unbiased visual and audio data capture.[48]

It's important for us to remember that no single dataset could represent the entire universe of available options. That's why it's so important for us to identify the target audience to begin with so that the training data can be tailored toward them. Another option is to train multiple versions of the same algorithm, with each version using specific datasets. If the output is the same across each of the models, they can then be combined. However, this approach requires a greater level of financial investment and so could be off-putting to some developers.

Speaking at HIMSS in 2021, Mayo Clinic Platform President Dr. John Halamka talked about some of the steps that could be followed to address some of the bias issues. He explained, "One key issue that must be solved first is ensuring equity and combating bias that can be baked into AI. The AI algorithms are only as good as the underlying data. And yet, we don't publish statistics describing how these algorithms are developed." According to Halamka, the solution is greater transparency—spelling out and sharing via technology the ethnicity, race, gender, education, income, and other details that go into an algorithm.[49]

As AI systems continue to gain prevalence in the healthcare industry, one option is to update the datasets they use for training so that they're increasingly tailored to their user base. This can introduce a number of unintended consequences, most notably that as the AI becomes more tailored to the user base, we increase the chances of introducing bias compared to the carefully curated data that we normally use to train them. The system could also become less accurate over time because the oversight needed to ensure the model's accuracy might no longer be in place out in the real world. A good example of this is the Microsoft ChatBot, which was designed to be a friendly companion but which, on release, rapidly learned undesirable language and behaviors and had to be shut down.[45]

There are many different approaches that are designed to eliminate bias in AI, and none of them are fool-proof (Figure 2.14). Options range from trying to create applications that are free of bias in the first place to collecting data in an unbiased way and designing mathematical algorithms to minimize its impact. One approach is to carry out external validation of AI models before they're deployed into the real world and used in a clinical setting. This could involve using large and diverse datasets to test the claims in new studies submitted for publication or regulatory approval and carefully testing the models' performance on external datasets.

We need to ensure that there's governance and peer reviews in place for all algorithms in the healthcare industry, because even the most tested algorithms still experience unexpected issues and outcomes. Like human beings, ML algorithms are never done learning. Unlike human beings, we need to ensure that we're constantly developing them and feeding them with more data if we want them to improve. Companies will need to be able to provide answers to important questions like, "How did the algorithm arrive at this conclusion? And how was it trained?" Ideally, algorithms should be tested using both common conditions and rarer scenarios. They should also be

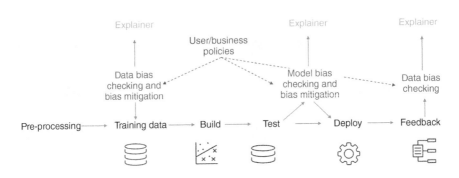

FIGURE 2.14 Proposed Workflow for Monitoring for Bias in AI Models
(source: Original Research)

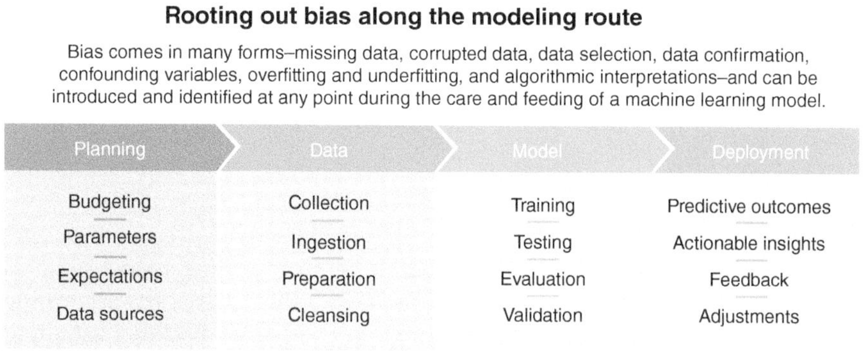

Rooting out bias along the modeling route

Bias comes in many forms–missing data, corrupted data, data selection, data confirmation, confounding variables, overfitting and underfitting, and algorithmic interpretations–and can be introduced and identified at any point during the care and feeding of a machine learning model.

Planning	Data	Model	Deployment
Budgeting	Collection	Training	Predictive outcomes
Parameters	Ingestion	Testing	Actionable insights
Expectations	Preparation	Evaluation	Feedback
Data sources	Cleansing	Validation	Adjustments

FIGURE 2.15   *(source: Original Research)*

exposed to a wide variety of populations and patient data before they're introduced into clinical settings (Figure 2.15).

In an interview with Healthcare IT News, Dr. Ziad Obermeyer made suggestions for minimizing the odds of algorithmic bias that could be harmful to patients. His suggestions included to ensure that there are people within each organization who are responsible for the strategic oversight of all algorithms. He also pointed out how important it is to have ways to quantify performance and bias, as well as that companies need to put these issues front and center for their mission and their strategic priorities. Algorithms are powerful tools to help to achieve our goals but also for staying on the right side of the law.[50]

In November 2022, the Mayo Clinic announced the launch of a new tool to identify potential biases in healthcare AI models. It's called Platform Validate and is designed to put an algorithm's credibility to the test, acting as a third party to confirm the AI's efficacy in meeting its intended clinical purpose. It does this by looking for disparities in the data used to train the AI model, such as age and ethnicity.

The idea here is that by providing information that's similar to nutrition and ingredient labels on food products, it can describe how an AI algorithm will perform in different scenarios, such as when faced with varying demographics across race, gender, and socioeconomic status.[51]

As you can see, this is deeply technical work that needs to be done to understand the data so that we can find bias and remove it. It will be important to develop standards and transparency. Model developers should explicitly lay out how they've thought about bias and its implications, as well as what they've done to address it. What technical choices were made? Did they set up systems that monitor the model's performance after launch? Is it doing what it's supposed to? Are the right people benefiting from it? And what are the ripple effects of using the model?

Seymour Duncker told me, "This relates to the idea of continuous learning, where you continuously measure the reliability of an algorithm and derive a signal when the algorithm needs to be retrained so that you can maintain the acceptable bounds of reliable operations. This is a concept that the FDA is considering with its total product lifecycle-based regulatory framework."

2.11   Responsible AI

Many of the issues that we've discussed here—such as bias, model explainability, transparency, and reliability—roll up into the concept of responsible AI (Figure 2.16). Responsible AI aims to ensure that key issues that can drive the appropriate use of AI are addressed as the technology becomes ubiquitous across different industries. Figure 2.17 is from a presentation of the World Economic Forum about the steps being taken to promote the responsible development and use of AI.

ML is particularly challenging because of the evolutionary nature of algorithms. In healthcare, new drugs and devices have a relatively well-established path of clinical trials for evaluation. ML algorithms don't, and they can also perform very differently from one day to another, as well as giving different results for different people in different contexts. This presents a challenge and a risk. If the model learns with time but some of the learnings lead to the introduction of bias (e.g. due to the real-world data it's operating on), ensuring responsible AI becomes very challenging.

As soon as we start to allow ML to play a role in clinical decisions, we're also introducing an element of real-time research that can't easily go through the rigor of traditional research evaluations. That means that right from the outset, during the initial conception and design, we need to think about the

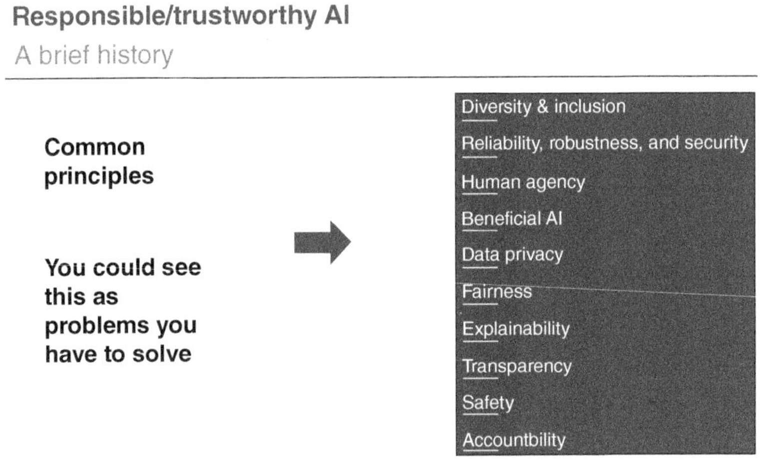

FIGURE 2.16   (source: World Economic Forum)

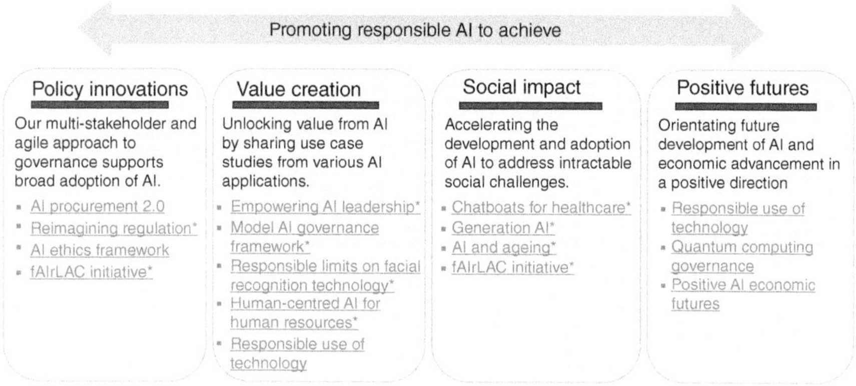

Promoting responsible AI to achieve

Policy innovations	Value creation	Social impact	Positive futures
Our multi-stakeholder and agile approach to governance supports broad adoption of AI.	Unlocking value from AI by sharing use case studies from various AI applications.	Accelerating the development and adoption of AI to address intractable social challenges.	Orientating future development of AI and economic advancement in a positive direction
• AI procurement 2.0 • Reimagining regulation* • AI ethics framework • fAIrLAC initiative*	• Empowering AI leadership* • Model AI governance framework* • Responsible limits on facial recognition technology* • Human-centred AI for human resources* • Responsible use of technology	• Chatboats for healthcare* • Generation AI* • AI and ageing* • fAIrLAC initiative*	• Responsible use of technology • Quantum computing governance • Positive AI economic futures

FIGURE 2.17   *(source: World Economic Forum)*

ethical implications of these technologies. In particular, we need to ask ourselves what will happen once a model is deployed, and we need to approach this from a range of different perspectives. It's alarmingly easy to get lost in the science of building models and to completely miss both the risks and the opportunities that those models create.

In healthcare, two of the most important processes for us to consider are risk assessments with the help of clinical resources and the traditional peer review approach, in which a data science specialist looks closely at the model and its assumptions to determine whether it's behaving appropriately.

In December 2022, The Coalition for Health AI released its *Blueprint for Trustworthy AI Implementation Guidance and Assurance for Healthcare*, which provides recommendations for ethical health AI guidelines to support high-quality care and increase AI credibility. The report outlines several elements that must be addressed to ensure that healthcare AI can be trusted: bias, equity, fairness, testability, usability, safety, transparency, reliability, and monitoring. Under this framework, bias, equity, and fairness are interrelated.[52]

Addressing issues in these areas requires leveraging health equity by design in all steps of AI policy, regulation, development, evaluation, and validation. Testability helps to provide a strong understanding of the model and its intended use, including where, why, and how it's used, as well as whether its performance can be verified as satisfactory within that context.

Safety aims to prevent adverse outcomes from a model's use, and transparency measures an algorithm's interoperability, traceability, and explainability. Reliability measures an AI's ability to perform its required function under certain conditions, while monitoring is concerned with ongoing surveillance of a model to look for and flag failures and vulnerabilities to minimize potential adverse effects.

One way to identify unexpected uses of a model is to ask clinicians how they intend to use it. For example, we'll need to consider whether a model designed to boost patient care could inadvertently penalize certain demographics. Alternatively, requiring additional personal data could exclude certain patient types or service beneficiaries.

If nothing else, we can demonstrate that we've carried out our due diligence by documenting what we hope to happen along with potential consequences and what actually happens out there in the real world. This will allow every model to continuously improve throughout its lifecycle and therefore ensure compliance with responsible AI.

References

1. Hang, et al. (2018). Big Data in Health Care: Applications and Challenges. Data and Information Management, 2(3), 175–197
2. Moor, M., Banerjee, O., Abad, Z. S. H., Krumholz, H. M., Leskovec, J., Topol, E. J., & Rajpurkar, P. (2023). Foundation models for generalist medical artificial intelligence. Nature, 616(7956), 259–265. https://doi.org/10.1038/s41586-023-05881-4
3. Timsina, P. and Kia, A. Machine learning platform at Mount Sinai health system (co-presentation). (2020, January 28). [Video]. YouTube. https://www.youtube.com/watch?v=aKAvj7njGw8
4. Char, D. S., Shah, N. H., & Magnus, D. (2018). Implementing machine learning in health care—addressing ethical challenges. New England Journal of Medicine, 378(11), 981–983. https://doi.org/10.1056/nejmp1714229
5. National Science and Technology Council Committee on Technology Council & Networking and Information Technology Research and Development Subcommittee. (2016). The National Artificial Intelligence Research and Development Strategic Plan. https://www.nitrd.gov/PUBS/national_ai_rd_strategic_plan.pdf
6. Topol, E. (2019). Deep Medicine: How Artificial Intelligence Can Make Healthcare Human Again (Illustrated ed.). Basic Books.
7. Ornstein, C., & Thomas, K. (2018, September 21). Sloan Kettering's cozy deal with startup ignites a new uproar. The New York Times. https://www.nytimes.com/2018/09/20/health/memorial-sloan-kettering-cancer-paige-ai.html
8. Revell, T. (2017, July 4). Google DeepMind's NHS data deal "failed to comply" with law. New Scientist. https://www.newscientist.com/article/2139395-google-deepminds-nhs-data-deal-failed-to-comply-with-law/
9. EUR-Lex – 32016R0679 – EN – EUR-Lex. (2016). EU Law.
10. Bill Text - AB-375 Privacy: personal information: businesses. (2018). California Legislative Information. https://leginfo.legislature.ca.gov/faces/billTextClient.xhtml?bill_id=201720180AB375
11. CMS advances interoperability & patient access to health data through new proposals | CMS. 2019, February 8). Centers for Medicare & Medicaid Services. https://www.cms.gov/newsroom/fact-sheets/cms-advances-interoperability-patient-access-health-data-through-new-proposals

12. Mandl, K. D. (2001). Public standards and patients' control: how to keep electronic medical records accessible but private Commentary: open approaches to electronic patient records commentary: a patient's viewpoint. BMJ, 322(7281), 283–287. https://doi.org/10.1136/bmj.322.7281.283

13. Jiang, F., Jiang, Y., Zhi, H., Dong, Y., Li, H., Ma, S., Wang, Y., Dong, Q., Shen, H., & Wang, Y. (2017). Artificial intelligence in healthcare: past, present and future. Stroke and Vascular Neurology, 2(4), 230–243. https://doi.org/10.1136/svn-2017-000101

14. Preparing for the future of artificial intelligence. (2016). Executive Office of the President & National Science and Technology Council Committee on Technology. https://obamawhitehouse.archives.gov/sites/default/files/whitehouse_files/microsites/ostp/NSTC/preparing_for_the_future_of_ai.pdf

15. He, J., Baxter, S. L., Xu, J., Xu, J., Zhou, X., & Zhang, K. (2019). The practical implementation of artificial intelligence technologies in medicine. Nature Medicine, 25(1), 30–36. https://doi.org/10.1038/s41591-018-0307-0

16. Soenksen, L. R., Ma, Y., Zeng, C., Boussioux, L. D. J., Carballo, K. V., Na, L., Wiberg, H. M., Li, M. L., Fuentes, I., & Bertsimas, D. (2022, December 9). Integrated multimodal artificial intelligence framework for healthcare applications. MIT. Retrieved December 9, 2022.

17. Tang, A., Tam, R., Cadrin-Chênevert, A., Guest, W., Chong, J., Barfett, J., Chepelev, L., Cairns, R., Mitchell, J. R., Cicero, M. D., Poudrette, M. G., Jaremko, J. L., Reinhold, C., Gallix, B., Gray, B., Geis, R., O'Connell, T., Babyn, P., Koff, D., Ferguson, D., Derkatch, S., Bilbily, A., Shabana, W. (2018). Canadian Association of Radiologists White Paper on artificial intelligence in radiology. Canadian Association of Radiologists Journal, 69(2), 120–135. https://doi.org/10.1016/j.carj.2018.02.002

18. Leroux, H., Metke-Jimenez, A., & Lawley, M. J. (2017). Towards achieving semantic interoperability of clinical study data with FHIR. Journal of Biomedical Semantics, 8(1). https://doi.org/10.1186/s13326-017-0148-7

19. Hong, N., Wen, A., Stone, D. J., Tsuji, S., Kingsbury, P. R., Rasmussen, L. V., Pacheco, J. A., Adekkanattu, P., Wang, F., Luo, Y., Pathak, J., Liu, H., & Jiang, G. (2019). Developing a FHIR-based EHR phenotyping framework: a case study for identification of patients with obesity and multiple comorbidities from discharge summaries. Journal of Biomedical Informatics, 99, 103310. https://doi.org/10.1016/j.jbi.2019.103310

20. Siwicki, B. (2021, June 9). What you need to know about data fluency and federated AI. Healthcare IT News. https://www.healthcareitnews.com/news/what-you-need-know-about-data-fluency-and-federated-ai

21. CB Insights. (2019, April 18). How AI is reshaping healthcare data. CB Insights Research. https://www.cbinsights.com/research/healthcare-ai-data-trends/

22. CB Insights. (2021, January 5). Healthcare AI trends to watch. CB Insights Research. https://www.cbinsights.com/research/report/ai-trends-healthcare/

23. Siwicki, B. (2021, June 3). Synthetic data boosts accuracy and speed of brain tumor surgery CDS. Healthcare IT News. https://www.healthcareitnews.com/news/synthetic-data-boosts-accuracy-and-speed-brain-tumor-surgery-cds

24. CB Insights. (2022, June 24). AI trends to watch in 2022. CB Insights Research. https://www.cbinsights.com/research/report/ai-trends-2022/

25. Hardesty, L. 2018, February 12). Study finds gender and skin-type bias in commercial artificial-intelligence systems. MIT News | Massachusetts Institute of Technology. https://news.mit.edu/2018/study-finds-gender-skin-type-bias-artificial-intelligence-systems-0212

26. Kuszko, J. 2021, December 13). What does synthetic data mean in healthcare's artificial intelligence revolution?The Medical Futurist. https://medicalfuturist.com/synthetic-data-in-healthcare-will-smarter-data-bring-the-a-i-revolution-in-healthcare/

27. Hashimoto, D. A., Rosman, G., Rus, D., & Meireles, O. R. (2018). Artificial intelligence in surgery: promises and perils. Annals of Surgery, 268(1), 70–76. https://doi.org/10.1097/sla.0000000000002693

28. C. (2020). The essential guide to quality training data for machine learning. Cloud Factory. https://www.cloudfactory.com/training-data-guide

29. CB Insights (2018). Top healthcare AI trends to watch

30. Siwicki, B. (2021, June 16). AWS leader talks about technologies needed to take precision medicine to the next level. Healthcare IT News. https://www.healthcareitnews.com/news/aws-leader-talks-about-technologies-needed-take-precision-medicine-next-level

31. Siwicki, B. (2021, April 28). How to help C-suite leaders and clinicians trust artificial. Healthcare IT News. https://www.healthcareitnews.com/news/how-help-c-suite-leaders-and-clinicians-trust-artificial-intelligence

32. Sullivan, T. (2018, November 8). Mount Sinai finds deep learning algorithms inconsistent when applied. Healthcare IT News. https://www.healthcareitnews.com/news/mount-sinai-finds-deep-learning-algorithms-inconsistent-when-applied-outside-imaging-data-sets

33. Komorowski, M., Celi, L. A., Badawi, O., Gordon, A. C., & Faisal, A. A. (2018 November). The artificial intelligence clinician learns optimal treatment strategies for sepsis in intensive care. Nature Medicine, 24(11), 716–1720. https://doi.org/10.1038/s41591-018-0213-5

34. Teodoridis, A. G. A. F. (2022, March 9). Why is AI adoption in health care lagging? Brookings. https://www.brookings.edu/research/why-is-ai-adoption-in-health-care-lagging/

35. Ross, C. (2022, February 28). Epic's AI algorithms, shielded from scrutiny by a corporate firewall, are delivering inaccurate information on seriously ill patients. STAT. https://www.statnews.com/2021/07/26/epic-hospital-algorithms-sepsis-investigation/

36. Zech, J. R. (2018, November 6). Variable generalization performance of a deep learning model to detect pneumonia in chest radiographs: a cross-sectional study. PLOS Medicine. https://journals.plos.org/plosmedicine/article?id=10.1371/journal.pmed.1002683

37. Miliard, M. (2018, July 10). As FDA signals wider AI approval, hospitals have a role to play. Healthcare IT News. https://www.healthcareitnews.com/news/fda-signals-wider-ai-approval-hospitals-have-role-play

38. Zech, J. R., Badgeley, M. A., Liu, M., Costa, A. B., Titano, J. J., & Oermann, E. K. (2018). Variable generalization performance of a deep learning model to detect pneumonia in chest radiographs: a cross-sectional study. PLoS Medicine, 15(11), e1002683. https://doi.org/10.1371/journal.pmed.1002683

39. Saria, S., Butte, A., & Sheikh, A. (2018). Better medicine through machine learning: what's real, and what's artificial? PLoS Medicine, 15(12), e1002721. https://doi.org/10.1371/journal.pmed.1002721

40. HIMSS. (2019). AI and imaging: your data as a strategic asset. https://365.himss.org/sites/himss365/files/365/handouts/552671993/handout-MLAI06.pdf

41. Shekhar, G. (2022, January 7). Bias detection in machine learning models using AmazonSageMakerclarify.Medium.https://towardsdatascience.com/bias-detection-in-machine-learning-models-using-amazon-sagemaker-clarify-d96482692611

42. Health Evolution. (2020, May 18). CEO Guide. https://www.healthevolution.com/ceo-guide/

43. HIMSS. (2019). Building a real-time community insights: engine for a healthcare system: challenges and opportunities. https://365.himss.org/sites/himss365/files/365/handouts/552672016/handout-MLAI13.pdf

44. Buolamwini, J., & Gebru, T. (2018). Gender shades: intersectional accuracy disparities in commercial gender classification. https://proceedings.mlr.press/v81/buolamwini18a/buolamwini18a.pdf

45. Siwicki, B. (2021, November 30). How AI bias happens – and how to eliminate it. Healthcare IT News. https://www.healthcareitnews.com/news/how-ai-bias-happens-and-how-eliminate-it

46. Obermeyer, Z., Nissan, R., Stern, M., Eaneff, S., Bembeneck, E. J., & Mullainathan, S. (2021). Algorithm bias playbook [Slides]. Ground. https://ground.news/article/ziad-obermeyer-and-colleagues-at-the-booth-school-of-business-release-health-care-algorithmic-bias-playbook-uc-berkeley-public-health

47. Ziad Obermeyer, Z., Power, B., Vogeliand, C., & Mullainathan, S. (2019, October 25). Dissecting racial bias in an algorithm used to manage the health of populations. Science, 366(6464), 447–453

48. Siwicki, B. (2021f, August 30). How one AI company works to reduce algorithmic bias. Healthcare IT News. https://www.healthcareitnews.com/news/how-one-ai-company-works-reduce-algorithmic-bias

49. Klimek, M. (2021, August 10). John Halamka on the 4 big challenges to AI adoption in healthcare. Healthcare IT News. https://www.healthcareitnews.com/news/john-halamka-4-big-challenges-ai-adoption-healthcare

50. Jercich, K. (2021, December 10). UC Berkeley's Ziad Obermeyer is optimistic about algorithms. Healthcare IT News. https://www.healthcareitnews.com/news/uc-berkeleys-ziad-obermeyer-optimistic-about-algorithms

51. Hale, C. (2022, November 15). Mayo Clinic launches digital referee for spotting potential bias in healthcare AI programs. Fierce Biotech. https://www.fiercebiotech.com/medtech/mayo-clinic-launches-digital-referee-spotting-potential-bias-healthcare-ai-programs

52. Kennedy, S. (2022, December 12). Coalition for Health AI unveils blueprint for ethical AI implementation. HealthITAnalytics. https://healthitanalytics.com/news/coalition-for-health-ai-unveils-blueprint-for-ethical-ai-implementation

CHAPTER 3

Barriers to AI Adoption in Healthcare

I**N THE LAST CHAPTER**, we discussed the many issues there are when it comes to building medical algorithm. Less than perfect data in the training, validation, or clinical deployment of models can result in the issues we touched on, such as model bias, gaps in performance, interpretability issues, lack of explainability, and more. We need to remember that these aren't the only issues that keep AI models from being developed or used in healthcare. A myriad of other technical, economic, regulatory, and business barriers exist (Figures 3.1 and 3.2). Many of these have yet to be addressed sufficiently so that the applications of AI in medicine can truly take off. In this chapter, we'll discuss many of those barriers and speculate on how they could be overcome.

According to a survey of over 12,000 participants by consultancy PriceWaterhouse Coopers (PwC), a lack of trust and the need for the human element were the biggest hurdles to using AI in healthcare.[2] Another survey by Klynveld Peat Marwick Goerdeler (KPMG) in 2020 revealed a number of areas of concern for healthcare executives in regards to AI.[3] One of these areas is that of talent. At the time of writing, only 47% of healthcare employees say that their employers offer AI training courses, a figure which is much lower than we see in other industries. This may be why only 67% of healthcare workers support AI adoption, which makes healthcare the lowest ranking industry. We can't build an AI-ready workforce from the top down. Instead, it will require huge changes to the way that we train and acquire talent.

AI Doctor: The Rise of Artificial Intelligence in Healthcare: A Guide for Users, Buyers, Builders, and Investors, First Edition. Ronald M. Razmi.
© 2024 Ronald M. Razmi. Published 2024 by John Wiley & Sons, Inc.

Barriers to AI in medicine

Short-term	Medium-term	Long-term
Training data and real-world data are often different leading algorithm to wrong conclusions	Trusting a program becomes even more dangerous over time as the training dataset gets older and clashes with the inevitable reality in medicine of changing practice, medications available, and changes in disease characteristics over time.	Machine learning algorithms are trained on fairly narrow datasets and unlike humans are unable to take into account the wider context of a patient's needs or treatment outcomes
Machine learning also doesn't have the same ability to weigh the costs and consequences of false positives or negatives the way a doctor would: they can't "err on the side of caution" like a human.	Machine learning can influence medical research: it can make "self-fulfilling" predictions that may not be the best course of action but over time will reinforce its decision making process.	They can "game the system," and learn to deliver results that appear successful in the short term but run against longer term goals.
Machine learning algorithms, especially those in the black box category, need some way to assess their own confidence in their predictions. Without attaching some degree of certainty, the machine learning application lacks a necessary "fail-safe."		A continuously learning autonomous system will eventually experiment with pushing the boundaries of treatments in an effort to discover new strategies, potentially harming patients.

FIGURE 3.1   *(source: Original Research)*

High initial capital requirement
Potential for increased unemployment
Difficulty in deployment
Reluctance among medical practitioners to adopt AI
Ambiguous regulatory guidelines for medical software
Lack of curated healthcare data
Concerns regarding privacy and security
Lack of interoperability between AI solutions
State and Federal Regulations

FIGURE 3.2   **Challenges to AI Adoption in Healthcare** *(source: Global Market Insights[1])*

It's particularly critical for our industry to attract people who understand how AI can be used to solve complex problems.

Cost is another major barrier. It's not been long since healthcare providers needed to make huge investments to meet electronic health record (EHR) requirements, and so we shouldn't be surprised if they're resistant to adopting AI. It will require even more investment for them to get AI off the ground, and the companies that are already struggling due to COVID-19 are likely to be slow to allocate funding to AI programs.

This might explain why over half (54%) of executives think that so far, AI has increased the overall cost of healthcare. That's also why most healthcare decision-makers are still struggling to figure out where and how to invest in AI so that they can get the greatest gains for their businesses. They know how difficult it is to determine what return-on-investment will look like. The same survey found that 75% of respondents were concerned that AI could threaten the privacy and security of their patient data, while 86% said that their organizations were taking care to protect patient privacy as they implemented AI algorithms.

Another major group of stakeholders is also skeptical of the use of AI in healthcare, with only 20% of physicians saying that AI has changed the way they practice medicine, according to a recent survey.[4] According to Medscape's survey of 1500 doctors from across Europe, Latin America, and the United States, the majority of physicians were anxious or uncomfortable with AI. US physicians were the most skeptical (49%), with 35% of European physicians and 30% of Latin American physicians saying the same.

The survey also found that physicians are more comfortable with using AI tools in their personal lives than they are at work. Half of US physicians use Google Home, Amazon Echo, or other, similar devices, but only 7% of them use it in healthcare settings. The adoption rate is even worse in Europe and Latin America, where more than three quarters of physicians don't use voice-controlled technologies for any reason.

Only 19% of physicians would be willing to use voice technology during a consultation with a patient, while nearly a third of them thought that their role could be threatened by AI algorithms. The good news is that despite all of that, doctors are still interested in its potential. 70% of respondents said that they thought AI-powered software would help to make their decisions more accurate.

The rest of the survey's findings are interesting, too. For example, two thirds of responding physicians said they'd use AI in the future if it was better than humans for diagnostics, although only 44% think that it will be as good as or better than human physicians at diagnostics. 68% believed that AI-powered software would mean they could spend more time on other tasks.

So how do physicians envisage themselves using AI software? Well, 54% are interested in using it to look up drug information, 53% would check for drug interactions, and 52% would look up treatment guidelines. The survey also revealed that physicians are worried about how AI tools will handle sensitive patient information, as well as whether it might be biased. In particular, doctors are distrustful toward AI-powered software that's created by pharmaceutical companies.

Barriers for Companies Developing AI in Healthcare Applications

1. **The fragmented US healthcare system:** AI companies in healthcare will need to work hard if they want to obtain data to train their models. This might mean interfacing with health systems and universities, bringing data together from multiple disparate datasets. This process can take many years.

2. **Bad data ruining companies:** Even if an AI company is able to obtain the healthcare data that it needs, there's a good chance that the data will

be of a low quality and need cleaning. Bad data leads to bad models, and that can be the beginning of the end for healthcare startups.

3. **Determining where to invest funding:** Because the applications often provide ancillary services, the total potential market for many healthcare AI applications is relatively small.

4. **Receiving adoption:** It's extremely difficult for AI companies in the healthcare industry to get their services adopted by providers unless they're also delivering vertical care. However, receiving adoption while delivering care vertically can also be tough, because companies need to build their own provider group and delivery infrastructure.

5. **Showcasing better clinical outcomes:** It all comes back to the outcomes that these tools are able to deliver. If an AI company is struggling to communicate how its services can provide better patient outcomes, it will struggle to win providers and investors over.

6. **Payers don't normally reimburse:** As soon as a provider is interested in an AI company's clinical benefit, it will ask who's paying. Most health AI companies aren't reimbursed by insurance, and providers are operating on thin margins, so it can be difficult for companies that have a value proposition of cost savings rather than adding revenue to get their services adopted by providers.

7. **User onboarding:** Unless an AI healthcare company can seamlessly integrate its service with a provider's existing workflows, its adoption will be relatively slow.

8. **Finding a working business model:** it is easier to sell AI solutions to providers if they only pay based on their usage of the solution. However, this represents significant risk to the company as adoption of new technologies usually takes a long time and the company may not survive this business model. Flat fee contracts are less risky for startups, but they're harder to sell to providers.

In his seminal paper in Nature, Dr. Eric Topol wrote about the mountain of challenges facing AI in healthcare, including regulatory barriers, interoperability with legacy hospital IT systems, and serious limitations on access to the crucial medical data needed to build powerful, health-focused algorithms in the first place.[5] We discussed some of these issues in the last chapter and it's fair to say that when it comes to AI, data issues reign supreme. Until you solve those, you don't have to worry about much else. Assuming that you've addressed the data issues, you can move on to dealing with some of the other key barriers.

Speaking at the 2021 The Healthcare Information and Management Systems Society (HIMSS) conference, Mayo Clinic Platform President, Dr. John Halamka, pointed to four main challenges that could slow AI's adoption in healthcare:[6]

1. **Gathering valuable data**—such as GPS information from the phones and other devices that people carry as well as wearables—and incorporating it into healthcare algorithms.

2. **Creating institutionalized discovery** so that even people without AI experience are empowered to engage with algorithm development.

3. **Validating algorithms to ensure that they're fit for purpose** across different organizations and geographies. The algorithms also need to be labeled in such a way that they make sense from both a product and an academic point of view.

4. **Getting information and advice to physicians in real time** while they're in front of their patients through improvements to workflow and delivery.

As you can see, some of these are related to the issues we touched on in the last chapter and are data-related. However, other issues mentioned, such as organizational mobilization and workflow issues, will also need to be addressed before AI is successfully adopted in healthcare.

3.1   Evidence Generation

The first critical issue is the evidence needed to support the use of these algorithms.[1,7] It's absolutely critical that any new approach to the practice of medicine be fully studied to ensure that it's safe and effective. This isn't just an academic issue that's insisted on by the elites who want to create a high bar for new innovation or for them to lead studies that will be done at their institutions, thus generating income for their research and departments. Many extremely promising diagnostic or treatment approaches in the past haven't resulted in any benefits or have even harmed patients, and only well-designed trials uncovered these issues (Figure 3.3).

Evidence-based medicine revolves around conscientiously and judiciously using the evidence that's currently available to make decisions about healthcare practices. We need a similar paradigm if we're to deploy evidence-based AI on the healthcare front line.

Watson for Oncology, IBM's AI algorithm for cancer, provides a great example of this. Watson for Oncology is used around the world to recommend treatments for cancer patients, but the algorithm itself is based on a small number of synthetic records with very limited access to real data from oncologists. Many of its treatment recommendations were erroneous, such as using bevacizumab in a patient with severe bleeding. This is an explicit contraindication and a "black box" warning for the drug.[8] It highlights how algorithms could potentially cause harm to patients, which would constitute a case of medical malpractice. At the moment, we typically deal with a single doctor making a mistake that hurt a patient. In the future, we'll have to come

Although algorithms are being created, research to establish their clinical impact is to come

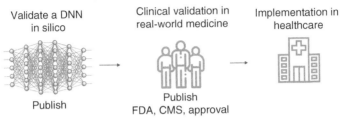

From AI algorithm to changing medical practice

Validate a DNN
in silico

Clinical validation in
real-world medicine

Implementation in
healthcare

Publish

Publish
FDA, CMS, approval

The need to publish results in peer-reviewed journals after validation in real-world environment
must be addressed before AI solutions can gain widespread adoption in healthcare

FIGURE 3.3   *(source: Original Research)*

to terms with the vast risks posed by a machine learning (ML) algorithm that's used in thousands of healthcare settings throughout the world.

My discussions with many of the experts in the field have highlighted the fact that well-designed, large-scale, multicenter trials are yet to be carried out. These types of trials would establish the efficacy and safety of these algorithms in real-world settings where there are different types of patients. Also, the algorithm would be tested to see whether it could generate its output during normal clinical workflows while staying timely and being based on realistically available inputs (data). Another challenge is that algorithms are constantly being improved and modified, so the algorithm that was tested might not be the same as the one that finally makes it into production.

A key reason for why these studies haven't been carried out is that it costs a lot of time and money, so they're beyond the means of research centers and small companies. For larger companies to invest capital, they'll need a clear path to a return-on-investment, and that's not as clear for algorithms as it is for drugs and medical devices. Intellectual property protections aren't very strong for algorithms and the barriers to entry are low.

Experts emphasize the importance of doing well-designed trials to establish the benefits of AI models. Many medical AI pioneers have told me that the current state of research is chaotic with a wide range of quality and publications scattered throughout clinical and computer science journals. Dr. Ted Shortliffe of Columbia University's College of Physicians and Surgeons and Editor in Chief Emeritus at the Journal of Biomedical Informatics indicated that high-quality studies will need to be designed to examine these algorithms based on their impact on one or more of these areas:

- Improvement of outcomes
- Improvement of efficiency

- Great workflow integration
- Cost reduction
- Better referral pathways

Dr. Aaron Kesselheim of Harvard University, who has expertise in the healthcare industry's regulatory process, indicated that prospective trials involving several centers with diverse patient populations and datasets would provide far more convincing data about the quality of these models. Professor Peter Szolovits of MIT indicated that the current quality of papers published in this area reflects the underlying research, which is often early-stage or which revolves around studies that are retrospective and not outcome-based.

Of course, doing real-world studies isn't easy and the questionable return-on-investment might not be the only reason why they're not being done. Dr. Armin Zadeh, Associate Professor of Medicine at John Hopkins University, says that the current state of healthcare data may serve as a barrier to the short- and medium-term adoption of AI technologies. In real-world settings, the data to run the algorithm will need to be available at the right moment to generate an output and if it's not, it won't help the clinician or the user when its help is needed. So, if you design a trial, you need to be sure that the data flow is air-tight. If it's not, the study might not show the benefits of your algorithm. In that situation, you'll have invested time and money but failed to show any benefits!

These types of trials aren't just needed for the adoption of these models by clinicians. Insurance companies (both public and private) demand solid evidence before they agree to pay for these technologies. In healthcare, it's difficult to drive the adoption of innovation if it's not paid for. Dr. Zadeh says that as long as the promised impact on patient outcomes isn't shown in well-designed trials, reimbursement will be difficult to secure and thus medical centers will be slower to make purchases.

There's some evidence to show that large technology companies like Google are realizing that trials could be their ticket into the large healthcare sector and so they're moving toward doing trials in partnership with academic medical centers. This is good news and a strong step toward driving clinical adoption and securing reimbursement.

Evidence-based AI isn't exclusive to showing that AI algorithms will improve patient outcomes, improve clinical workflows, or lower the cost of care. There's currently a large amount of variability that comes into play when risk-mitigating AI development and deployment. That's why we need a paradigm for the development and implementation of AI, similar to what we have for evidence-based medicine, to launch an evidence-based AI movement for health and healthcare.[9]

An article in the *Journal of the American Medical Informatics Association* mapped known AI risks to evidence-based best-practice mitigation strategies that could alleviate them.[10] Some of these risks include issues around data security, data privacy, transparency, workflow integration, and user feedback. Fortunately, evidence-based AI risk mitigation practices already exist for three key areas: data selection and management, algorithm development and performance, and trust-enhancing business practices and policies.

Some of these practices include data encryption, secure mobile hardware, detailed provenance records, performance surveillance, models that account for casual pathways, human-in-the-loop practices, and adherence to data governance policies. Professional organizations or associations are critical in leading the field in reviewing available evidence, translating the evidence into practice guidelines, and educating AI developers and implementers about the need to adhere to such guidelines.[9]

For us to move forward, it would help if governments would create purchasing rules that explain how evidence-based AI solutions would be favored by public sector healthcare companies. This would send a strong signal to the market and make a huge difference to companies that sell software to the public sector. However, the government would need to find or create a system that could verify that solutions adhere to evidence-based standards for deployment and development.

The government may even decide to regulate AI solutions, such as how the United States' Food and Drug Administration operates its Software as a Medical Device (SaMD) certification program. This voluntary program allows developers who use AI to have their software assessed and certified by demonstrating a culture of excellence and a commitment to the ongoing monitoring of software performance after it's shipped and used in the real world.[9]

3.2   Regulatory Issues

Before any new technology can be used in healthcare, it has to be deemed safe and effective by certain regulatory bodies. The United States, the EU, Japan, and other advanced countries have robust requirements for such approvals. This has historically been the case for drugs and medical devices. However, now the question is, what level of evidence should be required for the approval of medical algorithms? After all, unlike drugs and medical devices, these algorithms change over time as they're exposed to more data along with feedback based on their output. Since there's ongoing change to the algorithms, how often should they be resubmitted for review and approval? Should you require large-scale, real-world trials to approve these algorithms, similar to what we do with biopharma and medical devices?

So far, regulatory bodies, such as the Food and Drug Administration (FDA), have required only smaller, retrospective studies that show that the algorithm works as promised in the narrow area that it's trained in and that the results are close to the accuracy of humans. This allows developers to start marketing their algorithms to clinicians. It doesn't mean that insurance companies would pay for it (most won't if there's no evidence that it improves patient outcomes in a real-world setting or that it lowers the cost of care) or that clinicians would consider the evidence to be sufficient for them to buy and use it.

This is both a driver and a barrier. By allowing clearance without requiring large-scale trials to show real-world efficacy, we'd allow models to be launched, observed, and improved in the real-world setting. But that would also act as a barrier, because the medical community doesn't necessarily see FDA approval as a signal to start using a model, since the evidence required for that is far below what's normally required to start using a new innovation in practice.

In my discussions with experts, there's a wide range of opinions on this approach. Predictive Health's Chief Medical Officer, Dr. Joel Brill, indicated that the FDA is looking at safety and effectiveness and that it won't require proof of improved patient outcomes. This would allow the medical community to start using these technologies and to generate evidence for their use. This approach makes sense for technology that will change over time with use, so creating high barriers for initial approval doesn't make sense when the technology isn't going to have the same level of efficacy or safety over time. Dr. Kesselheim indicated that the FDA's approach will have negative long-term consequences for these technologies and that it doesn't lead to the establishment of high standards for AI-based products. This could lead to issues that will slow the adoption of these technologies.

For example, given the low evidence standard required to approve these technologies, organizations will each make their own decision about whether the specific product has enough evidence for them to use it. Given this approach, each health system and its experts will make their own decisions about each technology and its level of evidence. This can lead to more fragmented uptake and slower long-term adoption. According to Dr. Kesselheim, post-marketing surveillance of these technologies will be vital, since the approved models might not be trained on enough data or appropriately diverse data to ensure optimal performance in the real world. Also, payers will need to use a case-by-case basis to review it because FDA clearance doesn't necessarily give universal confidence to all stakeholders.

Baku Patel, former head of the FDA's digital health unit, laid out the rationale for the lighter-touch approach by the FDA. He indicated that the review of AI-based technologies includes evaluation of the data used to train and validate models and that the FDA is looking to improve through novel ways of independently assessing the data before the models are trained. He also suggested that given the ongoing technological improvement of these models, the FDA will require post-marketing surveillance of approved technologies. I'll discuss this further in the next chapter.

The FDA is also creating a way for the users of these technologies to provide feedback. Patel suggested that the thresholds for clearance should be matched to the claims and risks for those products and that the tools will evolve over time. That's why real-world exposure is needed to improve the models. Substantial equivalence clearance is used for the clearance of follow-on submissions with the same intended use but something different in terms of performance or application. Another avenue being explored is the preregistration of AI technologies that are aiming for FDA submission. One barrier is that AI researchers use classifiers that often don't know what hypothesis they're aiming for, which makes it harder to predict the endpoints discovered for the purposes of preregistration. Patel indicated that one idea is for the submitters to place their data (for training and validating the model) in escrow so that experts could review the data and opine on its integrity, size, and diversity.

Another major issue is the concept of learning AI. Learning AI means that the model's performance and output change over time as it ingests more data, creates more output, and receives feedback. This happens in many of the AI models currently in use in consumer industries like shopping, entertainment, and real estate. However, in healthcare, the concept of learning AI could have unintended consequences that could pose a risk to patients. As such, novel regulatory pathways need to be created.

Back in February 2020, the FDA announced that it had used the De Novo pathway to authorize marketing for the first AI-based cardiac ultrasound software. This breakthrough device is notable not only for its pioneering intended use but also for the manufacturer's utilization of a predetermined change control plan to incorporate future modifications.[11] This is a framework that's designed to support modifications to an AI/ML-based SaMD. The SaMD pre-specifications aim to describe *what* the manufacturer plans to change through learning. Then there's the algorithm change protocol, which explains *how* the algorithm will learn and change without compromising on safety or efficacy.

Within the industry, we use the term "good machine learning practice" to describe a set of best practices for AI that are equivalent to the best practices for engineering or system development. These cover data management, feature extraction, training, interpretability, evaluation, and documentation. The creation and development of these practices will be vital to guide the healthcare industry through product development and to provide oversight for complex products through the manufacturer following a well-established set of standards.

3.3   Reimbursement

Reimbursement is critical for any new healthcare technology. If a new diagnostic or therapeutic technology isn't paid for by insurance, there's little chance that it will gain widespread adoption. Medical innovation is expensive and beyond the reach of most patients or even medical centers if it's not reimbursed. For decades, companies that have developed new solutions have done so with clear plans to show their benefits and thus secure reimbursements. Most public and private payers have established criteria and processes to make decisions about reimbursing new medical innovations. Usually, there has to be a fully demonstrated benefit to the patients or providers for a clinical innovation to receive a positive reimbursement decision, and this has to be shown in well-designed trials. We've already addressed the lack of such studies for AI in healthcare, and this promises to slow the adoption of such technologies.

Although the FDA only requires safety and efficacy metrics to approve AI technologies, health plan require outcome data to issue new codes. Dr. Zadeh says that physicians will be aware of the impact of AI technologies on their incomes and if they see an adverse impact, they'll be slow to adopt or will continue with current approaches. This is important in the context of reimbursement since it's possible that part of the reimbursement for these technologies will go to the physicians, driving their willingness to use them. What about the threat to physicians' jobs and income? I don't see any threat in the near future. For example, radiologists can review the whole scan and have a global perspective while an algorithm only reads one area and looks for a specific type of issue. We're a long way away from a future where multiple algorithms run a scan to look for abnormalities without the need for a radiologist.

The same concepts apply to health system economics. Reimbursement is relevant for buyers, as well as for physicians. My discussions with health system executives indicated that these technologies will be used in niches for the near future but that the economics of health systems will continue to push the money-making procedures. They spoke about how health systems will be careful to assess the impact of such technologies, but that if they make physicians more productive and satisfied, they'd invest without reimbursement. Health systems are heavily dependent on procedures and thus will incentivize physicians to continue using them. This can include investments in technologies, such as AI, to assist in performing colonoscopies. Increased physician satisfaction and productivity will be a major driver of adoption, even without reimbursement.

For AI systems to work at their best, they'll need ongoing maintenance in terms of incorporating increasing amounts of patient data, as well as updating algorithms and ensuring that they work with the existing hardware and software. This may require ongoing upgrades to the equipment and investment in personnel training and means that health systems will need to find some sort of funding mechanism or have a clear return on investment (ROI) before investing in AI technologies. This could present a huge challenge because it's not currently clear how AI technologies will be reimbursed.

Business incentives aren't the only way to advance healthcare, but there's no denying the fact that they've historically been a key driver of change.

The problem is that it's still not clear whether AI-based technologies are actually adding value to the healthcare industry. Large-scale clinical trials with emerging algorithms are yet to take place. As such, their benefits are speculative at best.

The idea of advanced technologies with huge amounts of unrealized potential is hardly new. Key examples in the healthcare industry include gene therapy, genomic-led personalized medicine, and use of EHRs, which have all been touted as having the ability to revolutionize the delivery of healthcare. So far, it's easy to argue that their potential has exceeded their performance, but each of these fields is continuing to witness ongoing advancements as well as continuing promise when it comes to the future.

It's still early days for AI-based tech in healthcare. Initial investments from government, academia, and the tech industry are continuing to grow, but we're yet to see whether this growth will be sustained in the future and it will likely depend upon the success of early applications. As such, the near-term implementation of AI in healthcare is by no means certain and we may encounter another AI winter, even if only in healthcare.

3.4   Workflow Issues with Providers and Payers

One of the key issues with the use of digital technologies in healthcare has been that they need a reliable feed of data to perform as expected and their output needs to be timely so that clinicians can benefit at the right time. If not, their long-term adoption is in serious doubt since they won't provide the intended benefits at the right moment. If you're familiar with the state of data in healthcare, you'll know that this isn't an easy task. Healthcare data is fragmented, often chaotic, and mostly unstructured. One of the major hurdles we need to overcome is to ensure that the new algorithms fit into existing workflows. Dr. Zadeh indicated that the disorganized nature of the data in provider institutions is a barrier, not only for developing these models but also for operationalizing them in different centers. He says that these technologies need to have frictionless workflows or facilitate better workflows for physicians to adopt their use. Fitting into existing workflows means that they won't cause delays or result in extra steps for clinicians.

In radiology, which many see as the initial frontier for healthcare AI to improve patient care, key barriers include IT implementation and integrating into legacy systems. One example of this is AiDoc's AI solution for the diagnosis of intracranial hemorrhage on head computed tomography (CT) scans. My discussions with some of the pilot sites indicated that although the algorithm identified subtle hemorrhages that could potentially be missed by radiologists, the initial setup and implementation took a long time and was taxing on the IT staff. The multiple interfaces that had to be created between the scanner, the cloud, and the picture archiving and communication system (PACS) system weren't simple. Also, the algorithm had a high false-positive rate, which created extra work and scrutiny for the clinicians and resulted in serious discussions about whether long-term use was worth the effort.

At present, many of the algorithms that have FDA approval aren't suitable for the front lines of clinical practice. This is for two reasons: first, these AI innovations by themselves don't change existing clinical workflows and the incentives that enable those workflows.[12] In other words, we need to remember that adding AI to existing workflows doesn't necessarily mean that it will change people's behaviors. Second, most healthcare companies don't have the infrastructure to feed the necessary data into these algorithms at the point of care. It's imperative to train the algorithms to (i) "fit" the local practice patterns, a requirement prior to deployment that's rarely highlighted by current AI publications and (ii) interrogate them for bias to guarantee that the algorithms perform consistently across patient cohorts, especially those who weren't adequately represented in the training data.[13, 14] In addition, ongoing evaluation and retraining must continue after implementation to reflect practice patterns which inevitably change over time.[15]

One of the other issues is the fact that these algorithms are often in the cloud and so medical center data would need to leave the institution to be examined by the algorithm. This puts the security and privacy of patient data at risk. Many institutions are uncomfortable with the routine traffic of patient data out of their firewalls due to security and privacy issues. As such, this could serve as a barrier for them adopting AI technologies in the short term.

For decision support systems, the AI should deliver advice and information to physicians in real time when they're in front of their patients. If the data that the algorithm needs is fragmented, not yet entered into the system, or initially unstructured, the algorithm won't be able to provide its output in a timely manner. These types of issues could make the algorithm obsolete.

Everyone should acknowledge that there will be a certain degree of resistance among clinicians when considering AI. Much of this could stem from the challenges clinicians faced during the implementation of EHRs. Clinicians will be hesitant to adopt tools that they perceive as trying to replace them (though most experts believe clinicians have little cause for concern) or that will end up increasing their workload. Moreover, clinicians will also have deep concerns about the validation of AI recommendations and will need to evaluate the clinical use of AI in much the same way they'd evaluate a new drug therapy or diagnostic tool. Approaching AI adoption as if it were a therapy will help to create a model for clinician acceptance.

Another workflow and implementation issue is taking an algorithm that was trained on external data and deploying it on local data, because we'll need to ensure that it performs as expected on the local patient population. Selecting that data and further training the model will take work and create extra friction, which will mean a lower amount of short and medium-term adoption by health systems and clinicians.

Figure 3.4 highlights some of the challenges that providers and payers will encounter in their journey to leverage AI-based solutions.

One of the most heated debates is about whether AI will replace large portions of the healthcare workforce. Estimates vary on the overall impact. The Royal College of Physicians projects that actual job loss could be less than 5%, while Gartner predicted that AI would lead to the creation of 2.3 million jobs in 2020, more than the 1.8 million it's estimated to have replaced.[16]

Payers and providers need to overcome a few challenges to best leverage ML techniques

Challenges	Potential organizational solutions
Lack of artificial intelligence (AI) strategy	• Investor-like approach to funding AI use cases • Dedicated AI leader with strong Analytics Interpreter bench
Fragmented data storage and tech limitations	• Shared, inexpensive computing resources • Investment in data infrastructure and storage system • Strong data governance for quality and traceability
Tight talent market	• Home-grown data science and translator talent • Shared service model across the organization for AI/ML
Disbelief in AI's potential	• "Quick-win" use cases leveraging existing datasets

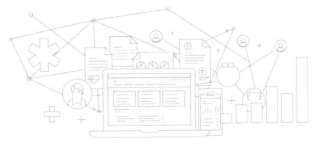

FIGURE 3.4   *(source: CMS 2016 US Healthcare Expenditure Estimate)*

3.5   Medical-Legal Barriers

Another possible barrier is the medical-legal implications of using AI algorithms that make predictions and provide recommendations. Clinicians could rely on these to make key decisions about patient management. What if there are issues with the recommendations? What if the patient is harmed by physicians following those recommendations? Who's responsible for the AI errors? Consider an algorithm that flags patients for sepsis risk before physicians or nurses would notice based on patterns in their vital signs. The algorithm might miss some cases and falsely flag others. If clinicians depend too heavily on the algorithm to generate alarms, they're still responsible if a patient becomes septic.

As AI capabilities are incorporated into medical care, the responsibility for clinical decisions can become unclear, and in that gray area lies potential liability if adverse events occur. Organizations must be vigilant to understand how those decisions play into a patient's care. Take, for example, a radiologist who depends on AI to make the first pass of images to find those that require further review. If the AI misses an image that shows an abnormality, a plaintiff might successfully challenge the trust that the physician placed in the algorithm. The downside is that after the standard of care expands to include AI for reading images, radiologists who miss a malignancy could be held liable for not using AI in the evaluation.

If a medical device uses a biased algorithm and leads to less than ideal outcomes for patients, they could then make a claim against the manufacturer or the health organization that used it. Meanwhile, clinicians who use new devices in a healthcare setting but who don't account for how outcomes can vary across different groups of people could find themselves on the wrong end of a malpractice lawsuit. We'll need to do what we can to address these kinds of legal risks, but that's no easy feat because the risks involved will vary depending upon the situation.

When an organization is going to subscribe to or implement a tool, it should screen the vendor. This will include asking questions about how algorithms were developed and how the system was trained, including whether it was tested on representative populations.[17] If the tool is going to directly interact with patient care, the device should be built into the process of obtaining informed consent.

The mutability and opaque nature of AI makes it difficult to determine liability for malpractice claims and professional regulatory standards. Health systems that choose to implement AI before the case law on these issues is established might increase the risk of litigation. This is a concern when products are developed without a complete understanding of how they'll be used in a healthcare environment.[16]

It's important to remember that almost all of the medical algorithms approved to date are considered to be assistive devices. This means that their job is to help the physician make better patient management decisions, while the clinician is ultimately responsible for those decisions. This creates a dilemma. If the physician doesn't know how the AI algorithm came to its conclusions, how can they feel legally protected when using it to make important decisions that affect patients' lives?

A salient example of this is the IBM Watson recommendations for oncology that proved to be not just erroneous but to go against explicit black box warnings. This could have caused harm to the patients as a result of the algorithm's recommendations, but the decisions were ultimately made by the physicians and they bore the ultimate legal responsibility for what happened to the patients.

Then there are the potential legal issues around data. This can include sharing data by providers with vendors that are developing AI solutions or moving data out of medical centers to run AI models. The potential for privacy and security breaches and data-sharing arrangements that profiteer from patient data is real. Google and Chicago Medical Center were named in a class action lawsuit when a former patient said the organizations failed to properly de-identify sensitive medical data.[16] Memorial Sloan Kettering also faced backlash with IBM Watson in 2012 with documents alleging that Watson made unsafe recommendations about how to treat patients with cancer. In a separate incident, ProPublica and The New York Times exposed that three members of the cancer center's board held investments in Paige.AI, founded in early 2018 with $25 million in venture capital.

The investment included an exclusive deal for Paige.AI to use Memorial Sloan Kettering's archive of 25 million patient tissue slides—an arrangement that received backlash from pathologists at Memorial Sloan Kettering, who weren't too pleased that the founders had been given shares in a company that relied on their work, data, and expertise. These and other early partnerships between healthcare organizations and AI companies have gained highly unfavorable attention, largely because of fears of data misuse. This is likely to continue as patient privacy advocates critique the contract structure of vendor–provider data analytics partnerships. The crucial issue is whether enough has been done to protect against the patient's identity being recovered through assimilation of the anonymized medical record with other data that the AI company has access to.

The more that AI becomes a black box, the riskier it is from a legal perspective. When AI is implicated in a medical error, liability becomes a concern. Healthcare organizations need to validate data that underlies an AI algorithm, particularly if it's their own data, as well as the conclusions that the AI draws from the data. Even if the exact reasoning process isn't known, healthcare organizations should be prepared to evaluate the results, just as they would for human clinicians or for therapeutics or diagnostics.

There must be a mechanism in place to monitor AI performance and review and correct failures in specific cases and across populations.

Health systems will also be forging partnerships with companies developing medical AI algorithms. Often, providing those companies with health data is the main contribution that the health system makes to the partnership. All that data could represent a target for bad actors.[18] When health systems transfer protected data to an outside company, it opens them up to privacy and security issues, so they'll need to make sure that their systems are designed to protect them against attacks. Some hospitals that have been attacked by ransomware have had to deal with both the attackers and with lawsuits from patients, who argue that health systems should be taking greater care to protect their information.[19-21]

Providers should also be aware of whether an AI product is "locked." In other words, will it always work the same way or is it designed to learn and change as it acquires more data and collects feedback on its performance? A process that changes—even if it's theoretically improving—requires more vigilance than one that doesn't. An AI algorithm that works one way on specific cases, and months later works differently, poses major quality control challenges, particularly if clinicians become dependent on the AI's recommendations.[16]

One possible answer is that if the algorithms have been through large-scale, well-designed clinical trials in the real world and performed to expectations, that could provide comfort and legal protection for the clinicians who use them. Also, since there's significant work underway to come up with technologies that will make the models more explainable, it's possible that in the near future, clinicians will have a greater understanding of the logic behind the model, which could serve as their legal protection.

3.6   Governance

Health systems and care providers must be vigilant in ensuring that the models they implement foster better care and promote health equity without bias. Efforts must include a legal, regulatory, and compliance review to decide who's in charge of various elements, as well as how to avoid patient harm. The governance teams will need to work with clinical and scientific experts to verify and ensure that any algorithms have been vetted and tested, as well as to set guidelines for obtaining patients' permission to use AI and informing them about the role AI plays in diagnosis or treatment. Whether appointing a Chief AI Officer or another executive to lead AI efforts, organizations need to bring in people who understand data and analytics, as well as the nature of the healthcare industry, at the highest levels of the organizations.

In January 2020, Google Health—which is an arm of the search engine giant that focuses on healthcare research, clinician tools, and healthcare partnerships—released an AI model which was trained on more than 90,000 mammogram X-rays. The company claimed that the algorithm achieved better results than human radiologists and said that it could recognize more false negatives than other tools. This is important because these false negatives are mammograms that look healthy but which contain breast cancer.

However, Google's work was rebutted by a score of experts who were affiliated with organizations like Harvard University, Stanford University, McGill University, and the City University of New York. In their contribution to the journal *Nature*, they said that Google failed to share detailed methods and code and that this "undermines its scientific value."[22] As if that wasn't enough, they also noted that Google's research model lacked details like a description of its development, along with the data and training that was used. Google omitted the definition of several hyper-parameters for the model's architecture (the variables used by the model to make diagnostic predictions), and it also didn't disclose the variables used to augment the dataset on which the model was trained.[23]

Much of the data that we're using to train AI algorithms for disease diagnosis could perpetuate inequalities, in part because of how reticent developers are to release code, data, and techniques. A team of UK scientists found that almost all eye disease datasets come from patients in North America, Europe, and China, meaning eye disease-diagnosing algorithms are less certain to work well for racial groups from underrepresented countries.[24] A study of a UnitedHealth Group algorithm determined that it could underestimate the number of black patients in need of greater care by half.[25] A growing body of work suggests that skin cancer-detecting algorithms tend to be less precise when used on black patients, in part because AI models are trained mostly on images of light-skinned patients.[26]

A lot of the concerns about AI in healthcare are around how models could reinforce bias and inequities. This is one of the many reasons why we need to create diversity amongst development teams and strong governance by the users of AI in healthcare. Then there's the data that's used to train the system. In healthcare, many of the common data inputs—such as claims data and clinical trial data—reflect biases in how care has been delivered in the past.[27] If health systems do not have strong governance, algorithms with bias can result in worsening of inequities in their institutions.

In a recent paper in the *Journal of the American Medical Informatics Association*, its authors asserted that bias in AI models could worsen the disproportionate impact that the COVID-19 pandemic has had on people of color.[28–30] They explained, "If not properly addressed, propagating these biases under the mantle of AI has the potential to exaggerate the health disparities faced by minority populations already bearing the highest disease burden. These tools are built from biased data reflecting biased healthcare systems and are thus themselves also at high risk of bias—even if explicitly excluding sensitive attributes such as race or gender."

On top of the basic challenges that we face is that models that haven't been sufficiently peer-reviewed could run into other, unforeseen road blocks after being deployed in the real world. Scientists at Harvard found that algorithms trained to recognize and classify CT scans could become biased to scan formats from certain CT machine manufacturers.[31] Meanwhile, a Google-published whitepaper revealed challenges in implementing an eye disease-predicting system in Thailand hospitals, including issues with scan accuracy.[32]

All of this point to the fact that implementing AI models isn't as easy as finding or developing a good model, connecting it with your information systems and letting it do its magic. Health systems need to have a robust governance process in place to vet the models before they're used and to monitor their effectiveness and output.

3.7 Cost and Scale of Implementation

The large language models that will most likely be the future of medical AI represent special challenges for their users. General Medical Artificial Intelligence (GMAI) models can be challenging to deploy, requiring specialized, high-end hardware that could be difficult for hospitals to access. Many large language models will need to be deployed locally in hospitals or other medical settings, removing the need for a stable network connection and keeping sensitive patient data on-site. Also, their size will require increased computational costs for the organizations using them. Given the state of legacy hardware and software in healthcare, these challenges will require new solutions for healthcare organizations to be able to implement them.

Some of these solutions could include reducing the model size through techniques, such as knowledge distillation, in which large-scale models teach smaller models that can be more easily deployed under practical constraints. Even then, the deployment of AI in healthcare will require all organizations (such as providers, payers, and life science companies) to upgrade their data collection and storage, their hardware strategy and their software portfolio. Given that these models will become the price of admission for most processes in healthcare, these investments have to be undertaken at some point so that organizations can prepare themselves for the future.

3.8 Shortage of Talent

One of the most challenging aspects of AI deployment has been the recruitment and retention of data science talent. Creating an AI-ready enterprise will require organizations to build a team of data custodians: experts at blending information sources, providing feedback on new data sources, and doing the requisite analytics to address issues that arise. To begin with, an analytics team will consist of data scientists, AI engineers, data engineers, data governance experts, and specialists in data entry. Teams can grow and evolve as the needs for AI expand.

The construction and optimization of AI models is still something of an art form, and experts need to define use cases and think about how the algorithms can be incorporated into clinicians' daily workflows. The supply of AI talent is far outstripped by the demand, with some estimates finding that there are less than 10,000 people with the skills that are needed to tackle the most serious AI problems. Competition for them is fierce among the tech giants.[33]

Managing AI initiatives calls for a new kind of expertise as well as rigorous standards. We'll need significant amounts of a very specific type of expertise for us to design, implement, and sustain AI models in healthcare. We're talking about something much more complicated than logical decision support rules, and health systems will need centralized expertise and tools.

One example of this is OhioHealth, where a health system used a hub-and-spoke design for their model using a centralized team of data scientists along with clinical informatics, program management, and monitoring. Each different business unit and clinical project team was responsible for a different element of identifying use cases, designing workflows, and managing change.

References

1. Global Market Insights. (2017). "Healthcare AI Market Size, Competitive Market Share & Forecast, 2024."
2. PricewaterhouseCoopers. (2016). Survey Results. PwC. https://www.pwc.com/gx/en/industries/healthcare/publications/ai-robotics-new-health/survey-results.html
3. KPMG. (2020). Living in an AI world 2020 report: taking the temperature of artificial intelligence in healthcare. https://assets.kpmg/content/dam/kpmg/tw/pdf/2020/05/healthcare-living-in-and-ai-world.pdf

4. Healther Landi (2019). Nearly half of U.S. doctors say they are anxious about using AI-powered software: survey. Fierce Healthcare. https://www.fiercehealthcare.com/practices/nearly-half-u-s-doctors-say-they-are-anxious-about-using-ai-powered-software-survey

5. Topol, E. J. (2019). High-performance medicine: the convergence of human and artificial intelligence. Nature Medicine, 25(1), 44–56. https://doi.org/https://doi.org/10.1038/s41591-018-0300-7

6. Klimek, M. (2021, August 10). John Halamka on the 4 big challenges to AI adoption in healthcare. Healthcare IT News. https://www.healthcareitnews.com/news/john-halamka-4-big-challenges-ai-adoption-healthcare

7. Artificial Intelligence in Healthcare Market. (2020). Markets and Markets. https://www.marketsandmarkets.com/Market-Reports/artificial-intelligence-healthcare-market-54679303.html

8. Ross, C., & Swetlitz, I. (2018, July 30). IBM's Watson supercomputer recommended 'unsafe and incorrect' cancer treatments, internal documents show. STAT. https://www.statnews.com/2018/07/25/ibm-watson-recommended-unsafe-incorrect-treatments/

9. Siwicki, B. (2022, February 23). Why healthcare needs an evidence-based AI development and deployment. Healthcare IT News. https://www.healthcareitnews.com/news/why-healthcare-needs-evidence-based-ai-development-and-deployment-movement

10. Roski, J., Maier, E. J., Vigilante, K., Kane, E. A., & Matheny, M. E. (2021). Enhancing trust in AI through industry self-governance. Journal of the American Medical Informatics Association, 28(7), 1582–1590. https://doi.org/10.1093/jamia/ocab065

11. U.S. Food & Drug Administration (FDA). (2021). Artificial Intelligence/Machine Learning-Based Software as a Medical Device Action Plan. FDA. https://govwhitepapers.com/whitepapers/artificial-intelligence-machine-learning-based-software-as-a-medical-device-action-plan

12. Rajkomar, A., Dean, J., & Kohane, I. (2019). Machine learning in medicine. New England Journal of Medicine, 380(14), 1347–1358. https://doi.org/10.1056/nejmra1814259

13. Panch, T. (2019, August 16). The "inconvenient truth" about AI in healthcare. Nature. https://www.nature.com/articles/s41746-019-0155-4

14. Gijsberts, C. M., Groenewegen, K. A., Hoefer, I. E., Eijkemans, M. J. C., Asselbergs, F. W., Anderson, T. J., Britton, A. R., Dekker, J. M., Engström, G., Evans, G. W., de Graaf, J., Grobbee, D. E., Hedblad, B., Holewijn, S., Ikeda, A., Kitagawa, K., Kitamura, A., de Kleijn, D. P. V., Lonn, E. M., ... den Ruijter, H. M. (2015). Race/ethnic differences in the associations of the Framingham risk factors with carotid IMT and cardiovascular events. PLoS One, 10(7), e0132321. https://doi.org/10.1371/journal.pone.0132321

15. Fry, E., & Schulte, F. (2021, June 7). Death by a Thousand Clicks: Where Electronic Health Records Went Wrong. Fortune. https://www.fortune.com/longform/medical-records/

16. Health Evolution. (2020, May 18). CEO Guide. Health Evolution. https://www.healthevolution.com/ceo-guide/

17. Jercich, K. (2021, October 28). FDA releases "guiding principles" for AI/ML device development. Healthcare IT News. https://www.healthcareitnews.com/news/fda-releases-guiding-principles-aiml-device-development

18. Jercich, K. (2021, August 27). CISA releases guidance on protecting data from ransomware attacks. Healthcare IT News. https://www.healthcareitnews.com/news/cisa-releases-guidance-protecting-data-ransomware-attacks

19. Jercich, K. (2021, June 23). Scripps Health hit with class action suits after ransomware attack. Healthcare IT News. https://www.healthcareitnews.com/news/scripps-health-hit-class-action-suits-after-ransomware-attack

20. Jercich, K. (2021, October 18). Florida health system hit with proposed class-action lawsuit over. Healthcare IT News. https://www.healthcareitnews.com/news/florida-health-system-hit-proposed-class-action-lawsuit-over-data-breach

21. Jercich, K. (2021, October 29). Machine learning can revolutionize healthcare, but it also carries. Healthcare IT News. https://www.healthcareitnews.com/news/machine-learning-can-revolutionize-healthcare-it-also-carries-legal-risks

22. Haibe-Kains, B., Adam, G. A., Hosny, A., Khodakarami, F., Shraddha, T., Kusko, R., Sansone, S. A., Tong, W., Wolfinger, R. D., Mason, C. E., Jones, W., Dopazo, J., Furlanello, C., Waldron, L., Wang, B., McIntosh, C., Goldenberg, A., Kundaje, A., Greene, C. S., ... Aerts, H. J. W. L. (2020). Transparency and reproducibility in artificial intelligence. Nature, 586(7829), E14–E16. https://doi.org/10.1038/s41586-020-2766-y

23. Wiggers, K. (2020, October 14). Google's breast cancer-predicting AI research is useless without transparency, critics say. VentureBeat. https://venturebeat.com/ai/googles-breast-cancer-predicting-ai-research-is-useless-without-transparency-critics-say/

24. Knight, W. (2020, October 11). AI Can Help Diagnose Some Illnesses—If Your Country Is Rich. WIRED. https://www.wired.com/story/ai-diagnose-illnesses-country-rich/

25. Obermeyer, Z., Powers, B., Vogeliand, C., & Mullainathan, S. (2019). Dissecting racial bias in an algorithm used to manage the health of populations. Science, 366(6464), 447–453

26. Lashbrook, A. (2018, August 16). AI-Driven Dermatology Could Leave Dark-Skinned Patients Behind. The Atlantic. https://www.theatlantic.com/health/archive/2018/08/machine-learning-dermatology-skin-color/567619/

27. Siwicki, B. (2021, April 28). How to help C-suite leaders and clinicians trust artificial. Healthcare IT News. https://www.healthcareitnews.com/news/how-help-c-suite-leaders-and-clinicians-trust-artificial-intelligence

28. Jercich, K. (2020, August 18). AI bias may worsen COVID-19 health disparities for people of color. Healthcare IT News. https://www.healthcareitnews.com/news/ai-bias-may-worsen-covid-19-health-disparities-people-color

29. Cases, Data, and Surveillance. (2020, February 11). Centers for Disease Control and Prevention. CDC.

30. Röösli, E., Rice, B., & Hernandez-Boussard, T. (2020). Bias at warp speed: how AI may contribute to the disparities gap in the time of COVID-19. Journal of the American Medical Informatics Association, 28(1), 190–192. https://doi.org/10.1093/jamia/ocaa210

31. Biondetti, G. P., Gauriau, R., Bridge, C. P., Lu, C., & Andriole, K. P. (2022). "Name that manufacturer". Relating image acquisition bias with task complexity when training deep learning models: experiments on head CT. Journal of Digital Imaging (Springer Journal).

32. Beede, E. (2020, April 25). Healthcare AI systems that put people at the center. Google.

33. Chui, M., Manyika, J., Miremadi, M., Henke, N., Chung, R., Nel, P., & Malhotra, S. (2019, November 20). Notes from the AI Frontier: Applications and Value of Deep Learning. McKinsey & Company. https://www.mckinsey.com/featured-insights/artificial-intelligence/notes-from-the-ai-frontier-applications-and-value-of-deep-learning

CHAPTER 4

Drivers of AI Adoption in Healthcare

WE'RE FORTUNATE IN THAT there are many factors driving the development and adoption of artificial intelligence (AI) healthcare solutions (Figure 4.1). Before we talk about anything else, we should start by noting that the main driver of AI adoption in the healthcare industry is the fact that more data than ever before is available in digital formats. Without that, we wouldn't have much to talk about. Then we can move on to topics like improved machine learning (ML) methodologies, increased computing power, cloud computing, healthcare resource shortages, the opportunity to reduce costs, precision medicine, and more.

We'll start with technical issues, such as the availability of data and increasing computing power, because without these, we wouldn't be able to use AI to improve outcomes and cut costs. The issues of outcomes and costs aren't new and will continue into the distant future if we don't use AI or other technologies to address them. However, given the huge amounts of money we invest in healthcare and the fact that our outcomes aren't commensurate with our investments, there's an increasing appetite for any technologies that could address this imbalance.

The main macroeconomic drivers for growth in healthcare AI include ever-increasing individual healthcare expenses, aging populations, and the imbalance between patients and the healthcare workforce. In 2014, the global expenditure on healthcare increased to 9.9% of the total gross domestic product (GDP), up from 9% in 2000. The United States had the world's single highest rate of healthcare expenditure at 17.8% of its GDP in 2015.

Meanwhile, the world's population is aging, with the number of people aged 60 or above due to grow by 56% from 2015 to 2030, compared to a 16.4% increase for the number of people as a whole.[2] It should go without

AI Doctor: The Rise of Artificial Intelligence in Healthcare: A Guide for Users, Buyers, Builders, and Investors, First Edition. Ronald M. Razmi.
© 2024 Ronald M. Razmi. Published 2024 by John Wiley & Sons, Inc.

The Key Drivers of AI Adoption in Healthcare

Adoption of AI in research areas
Increasing range of future applications
Reduced workload and increased quality of care
Growing demand for precision medicine
Growing number of cross-industry partnerships
Shortage of health workforce to meet patient demand
Need to reduce increasing healthcare costs

FIGURE 4.1   *(source: [1]/Global Market Insights)*

saying that an aging population will place our healthcare system under a huge amount of strain. At the same time, the United States is dealing with an ongoing shortage of nurses and technicians, with a number of vacancies for nurses due to exceed 1.5 million by 2025. The trend toward consolidation in US healthcare has meant that larger health systems which combine hospitals, clinics, and ancillary services are now a dominant form of care delivery. This is resulting in increased investments in technologies that can improve operations and care delivery at these health systems.

Many healthcare pundits hope that AI will help medical practitioners to more efficiently achieve their tasks with less human intervention. Reducing the amount of human-performed activities that patients need is likely to be a critical factor when it comes to meeting this ever-increasing patient demand. It could also improve the quality of care by digesting data and identifying patterns, helping with diagnosis and treatment selection, and reducing costs and mistakes due to more intelligent automation. All of this means that there are increasing public and private investments to realize the future potential for AI, and regulatory and reimbursement bodies are taking positive steps to facilitate its adoption.

4.1   Availability of Data

AI needs access to large amounts of digital data, and for the first time in human history, the healthcare industry is producing just that (Figure 4.2). A lot of this data is unstructured and fragmented, which is a major issue. With that said, we're heading in the right direction, and there's enough structured data in radiology, pathology, and ophthalmology for us to start developing and deploying the initial set of AI applications. Also, the emergence of AI solutions is highlighting how data should be captured and organized to facilitate the use of AI. As more and more providers see the benefits of AI, the value

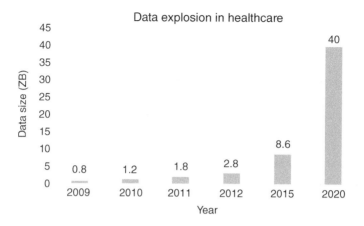

FIGURE 4.2   *(source: Hang et al.[3])*

of the extra effort to capture and organize data will become more obvious. It's estimated that only 5% of healthcare data has been analyzed so far.[4]

4.2   Powerful Computers, Cloud Computing, and Open Source Infrastructure

Another major driver for the emergence of AI in healthcare is the fact that we now have more powerful computers with stronger Graphic Processing Units and cloud computing. You need a lot of computing power to do the type of analytical heavy lifting that AI algorithms do. Cloud computing allows algorithms to be deployed in a central place in cyberspace and to receive the data they need to do their jobs. This makes it more feasible to implement algorithms in medical centers because developers don't need to physically go to each center to install their algorithms. However, even with cloud computing, local Information Technology (IT) work needs to be done to deploy a new algorithm, but if they're just making connections to the cloud, they have considerably less work to do at each center. This is important as the economics of developing and deploying models will need to make sense to attract companies.

One of the major challenges of developing and deploying models is the huge amount of biomedical data that's needed and which often resides in different systems and in multiple different formats. For example, data used for computational chemistry and molecular simulations can consist of millions of data points and require billions of different calculations if it's to provide a useful output. This means that if all of this data is stored in different systems, the work of collecting the data from each system and combining it all is a challenge.

To maximize the opportunities we have in healthcare when it comes to analytics and ML, we'll need to securely and compliantly boost access to data while simultaneously enhancing usability. When it comes to big datasets being used for research and development, we can turn to large-scale cloud services which could transfer hundreds of terabytes of data and millions of files at speeds that are as much as ten times faster than open source tools allow. We'll need to tap into storage gateways to make sure that all of this data is stored securely while making it available to collaborators who are supposed to have access to it. Cloud-based hyperscale computing and ML enable organizations to collaborate across datasets, create and leverage global infrastructures to maintain data integrity, and more easily perform ML-based analyses to accelerate discoveries and de-risk candidates faster.[5]

The availability of open source algorithmic development modules like TensorFlow also lowers the cost and technical barriers for companies. If each company had to create their own development modules, there would be far fewer companies and institutions involved in healthcare AI.

4.3   Increase in Investments

Figure 4.3 shows the rapid rise in investments in healthcare AI over the last decade. This only represents private investments, but we can safely say that public investments in AI have also increased dramatically.

It's important for us to see commercially successful applications of healthcare AI in the near future as there's always concern that large investments without commensurate return could mean that investors will stop pouring money into the sector.

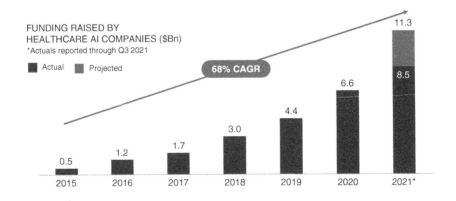

FIGURE 4.3   *(source: [6]/CB Information Services)*

4.4   Improvements in Methodology

In the first chapter, we talked about how key methodological issues in AI have been addressed in the last decade, and that's been a key driver in the performance of these algorithms.[7–10] The recent launch of ChatGPT has captivated people, and its ability to generate text that's sophisticated and to the point is an indication that the pace of progress is accelerating. This is coupled with other advances, such as AI''s superhuman abilities to recognize objects in images, to pick up trends and patterns in large datasets, and to generate art and music. If AI can effectively solve everyday problems in a manner that's accessible to everyone, its growth will be all but assured.

Large language models could be the breakthrough that makes this happen. Their ability to ingest large amounts of data and to learn from it using self-supervision—without the need to annotate all of the data—means that models will be able to train on much larger datasets and at a faster speed than we've seen to date. It is possible that these language models could further be trained on industry-specific data and become very effective at performing tasks that are currently being done by humans. This is critical at a time of an aging working population and shortages across industries, especially healthcare. The initial use cases in healthcare in administration and decision support are showing significant promise.

4.5   Policy and Regulatory

4.5.1   FDA

In late 2023, President Biden issued an Executive Order on Artificial Intelligence. While it's not focused on healthcare, it does contain healthcare-specific language and aims to address the accountability of how AI technology is developed and deployed. The order provides a pathway for the industry and the federal government to begin to address issues around privacy, security, safety and equity in the use of AI while continuing to advance innovation. Many of the elements of the executive order involve issues such as privacy, security, safety, and data sharing. Issues that are very relevant in healthcare AI. As part of the Executive Order, the Department of Health and Human Services is directed to develop a system of premarket assessment and postmarket oversight of AI-enabled healthcare technology.[11]

As far back as 2017, it became obvious that an increasing number of AI-enabled devices were getting FDA clearance. That trend has only accelerated over the last six years. Figures 4.4 and 4.5 show the significant increases in the number of AI-enabled solutions with Food and Drug Administration (FDA) approvals or clearance in recent years.[12]

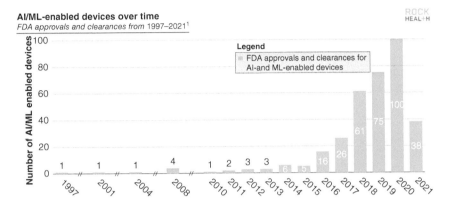

FIGURE 4.4   *(source: Rock Health)[12]*

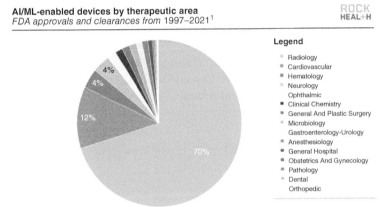

Note: 1. 2021 includes FDA approvals and clearances for AI-and ML-enabled devices through June 17. 2021
Source: FDA list of Artificial Intelligence and Machine Learning (AI/ML)-Enabled Medical Devices as of 09/22/2021

FIGURE 4.5   *(source: [12]/American Association for Physician Leadership)*

This is simultaneously a driver and a sign of growth in the healthcare AI sector. The FDA has formulated new policies that allow for the easier clearance of these technologies, but it's looking at safety and effectiveness as opposed to patient outcomes. We discussed in the last chapter how there are people on both sides of the argument when it comes to whether the FDA is helping the growth of these technologies by adopting more relaxed policies than the ones used for pharmaceuticals or medical devices, or whether it's actually hurting the long-term prospects of the sector. We discussed this in the previous chapter, but it's worth revisiting a few of those points here.

There are those who believe that since algorithms change over time and learn from the feedback they receive and the increasing amounts of data flowing toward them, the FDA should determine their safety and effectiveness and allow them to be used in real world settings so that their collective experience builds up over time. Others believe that although the FDA's lighter touch is allowing for a faster rollout of these technologies, it could lead to significant issues down the road. For example, technologies that are developed on narrow datasets could underperform when deployed in new medical centers with more diverse patient populations. This could lead to a model that isn't trained on enough data and which provides false results.

If this happens, health systems could apply the brakes on adopting these technologies until the FDA adopts higher standards, which could set the field back several years while these issues are adequately addressed. This point of view also has some validity, and the current FDA approach might actually end up slowing the long-term adoption of these technologies.

The FDA's vision is that they'll be able to use appropriately tailored regulatory oversight to allow AI and ML-based software as a medical device (SaMD) products to deliver safe and effective ways to improve the quality of care that patients receive. In February 2020, the FDA announced it was using the De Novo pathway to provide marketing authorization for the first AI-powered cardiac ultrasound tool. This device is notable for the manufacturer's utilization of a predetermined change control plan to incorporate future modifications.[13]

Baku Patel, who was once the FDA's Chief Digital Health Officer of Global Strategy and Innovation, says that the lighter touch is informed by the fact that these aren't static technologies. The idea is that by ensuring safety and acceptable efficacy, we can get these technologies in the hands of users to assess how they perform in the real world and receive the type of feedback that will help shape regulatory policy moving forward. He explained that the thresholds used for clearance are matched to the claims and risks for those products.

The De Novo process is a risk-based classification process which provides a pathway to classify novel medical devices for which general and/or special controls provide a reasonable assurance of safety and effectiveness for the intended use, but for which there's no legally marketed predicate device.[14] If a medical device receives a class I or class II classification through a De Novo request, they can be marketed and used as predicates for future 510(k) pre-market notification submissions.

Healthcare software is considered to be a medical device by the FDA, which means that it's subject to the same regulations as physical products like pacemakers or contact lenses. That was fine back in the day, when most medical software was the firmware for these devices, but it's no longer suitable for the modern world. Software can be created, iterated, and updated much more quickly, and indeed the pace of innovation for new products like AI diagnostic tools depends almost entirely on how quickly they can be iterated upon. At the moment, approval timelines for medical devices range from three to six months, and delays are common and can push that back to a year. This timeline is simply unacceptable for modern software.

That's where pre-certification comes in, providing another way for healthcare software to receive clearance. The idea is that instead of the FDA reviewing the company and its products for every iteration, it will essentially certify a company and its processes as conforming to its principles of excellence. Once a company has achieved this certification, any of their products which fall below a certain risk threshold will be able to either go through a streamlined review or to skip the pre-market review entirely (Figure 4.6).

In 2023, the FDA released draft guidance to provide recommendations for lifecycle controls in submissions to market ML-enabled device software functions. In this document, *Marketing Submission Recommendations for a Predetermined Change Control Plan for Artificial Intelligence/Machine Learning-Enabled Device Software Functions*, the FDA proposes ensuring that AI/ML-enabled devices "can be safely, effectively and rapidly modified, updated and improved in response to new data." The document aims to lay out the requirements for companies to continue improving their AI-enabled solutions without having to keep submitting new applications to the FDA. These include detailed descriptions of planned device modifications, explanations of the methodologies

FDA pre-certification

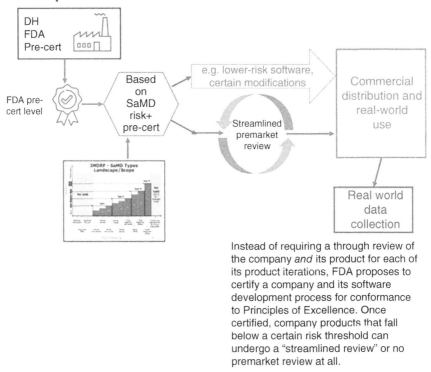

Instead of requiring a through review of the company *and* its product for each of its product iterations, FDA proposes to certify a company and its software development process for conformance to Principles of Excellence. Once certified, company products that fall below a certain risk threshold can undergo a "streamlined review" or no premarket review at all.

FIGURE 4.6   *(source: Adapted from[15])*

that will be used to develop, validate, and implement those modifications, and assessments of the benefits and risks of the planned modifications.[16]

The FDA says that its streamlined review and no review options through the pre-cert program will enable them to be more agile and to help patients to access new and updated SaMD products much more quickly. This has always been the vision at the heart of the pre-certification program, with the goal of software manufacturers being able to release FDA-regulated software as quickly as they can develop it, especially if modifications are low risk.[15] Developers can use the SaMD pre-specifications to describe which aspects the manufacturer plans to change through ML. They can also use the algorithm change protocol to explain how it will learn while still being safe and effective.

It's perfectly reasonable to be concerned about how these devices will be regulated. However, it's not going to be easy to regulate them. There are all sorts of challenges, ranging from labeling the devices to describing the data that was used, the relevance of its inputs, the logic that it uses, the role it's supposed to play, and the evidence there is to show that it's performing as intended.

We also need to remember that the issue of algorithmic bias isn't exclusive to AI and ML. It's just that many of these algorithms are difficult to "see" into and given that these solutions will have an important role to play in the healthcare industry, it becomes especially important for us to understand them. On top of that, bias is potentially more likely because AI and ML tools are developed and trained using historical datasets, which means they can hold a mirror up to the biases that are already present there.

The FDA knows that it's crucially important for new healthcare solutions to work across a racially and ethnically diverse patient population, which means that they'll need new and improved methodologies for identification and improvement. This will include being able to identify and eliminate bias, as well as showing evidence of the robustness and resilience of the algorithms when it comes to dealing with changing inputs and conditions.[13]

Fortunately, manufacturers will be able to gather real-world performance data on how SaMDs are being used, and this will help them to understand use cases, opportunities for improvements, and the proactive changes they need to make to address safety or usability concerns. Real-world data collection and monitoring is an important mechanism that manufacturers can use to miti- gate the risk involved with AI/ML-based SaMD modifications in support of the benefit–risk profile in the assessment of a particular marketing submission.[13]

It's clear that the agency is growing more comfortable with reviewing these solutions and that the time from filing to clearance is getting shorter. This was apparent in the time difference between the two algorithms approved for Aidoc over the span of three years. After the approval of their second algorithm for the diagnosis of pulmonary embolism, Aidoc CEO, Elad Walach, said that the company's previous work with the FDA had helped to create a more reliable and efficient regulatory pathway leading to the new approval, which took a year less than their first clearance.[17]

4.5.2   Other Bodies

In 2021, the World Health Organization issued a report about AI in Healthcare called *Ethics & Governance of Artificial Intelligence for Health*, which came about as the result of eighteen months of discussions between experts from the Ministries of Health and thought leaders in the fields of law, human rights, ethics, and digital technology. The report found that even though new AI technologies have a great amount of potential for the healthcare industry, their developers need to put ethics and human rights at the heart of everything they do.

The report also does a great job of spotlighting the ethical challenges and the risks that come along with using healthcare AI, as well as providing six principles that can be followed to make sure that AI works for the public benefit of every country. Alongside this, they provided recommendations for the governance of healthcare AI which is designed to maximize the technology's potential while holding both public and private sector stakeholders accountable for their software. They also need to be responsive to the healthcare workers who'll rely on the tech, as well as the people and the communities that will be most affected by its usage.

The six principles are[18]:

1. Protecting human autonomy
2. Promoting human well-being and safety and the public interest
3. Ensuring transparency, explainability, and intelligibility
4. Fostering responsibility and accountability
5. Ensuring inclusiveness and equity
6. Promoting AI that's responsive and sustainable

The International Medical Device Regulators Forum (IMDRF) is one of the organizations that's leading the charge to provide guidance. Formed by a group of medical device regulators who aim to unify international regulation, it has members from countries like Australia, Canada, Brazil, China, South Korea, Japan, Singapore, Russia, and the United States. As part of its remit, the IMDRF has provided a range of key definitions for SaMD, as well as a framework for regulators in the industry. It suggests using an iterative process based on real-world performance data, which is similar to what the FDA is doing. It also says that low-risk SaMD applications might not need independent review.

In April 2023, the Coalition for Health AI released its first blueprint for the effective and responsible use of AI in healthcare. Its objective is to generate standards and robust technical and implementation guidance for AI-guided clinical systems. The *Blueprint for Trustworthy AI Implementation Guidance and Assurance for Healthcare* aims to ensure ethical, unbiased, and appropriate use of the technology, to combat algorithmic bias and to define fairness and efficiency goals up front.[19]

The American Medical Informatics Association (AMIA) has also proposed a framework for the regulation of AI decision support software.[20] The AMIA has said that adaptive clinical decision support (CDS) (that is, clinical decision support tools that train themselves and adapt based on new data) will present unique challenges when it comes to their development and implementation. We can expect adaptive CDS to become the new norm, but it will still need to be managed and supported by new, globally agreed-upon approaches, and independent oversight that don't exist at the time of writing.

According to the AMIA, we'll need new, more flexible oversight structures that can evolve alongside the healthcare ecosystem. These structures will need to be distributed throughout the world and supported by a range of key organizations. We'll also need new organizational competencies so that we can evaluate and monitor adaptive CDS in patient settings. The FDA is currently working on new policies for marketed adaptive CDS tools, but a number of algorithm-driven tools have already been developed without any guidance or oversight.

The AMIA is calling for two key pillars in the oversight of AI solutions:

1. **Transparency in how adaptive CDS is trained:** This would require standards for how decision support algorithms are trained, "including the semantics and provenance of training datasets ... necessary for validation prior to deployment."

2. **Communications standards:** To convey specific attributes of how the model was trained, how it was designed, and how it should operate in situ.[18]

The AMIA has also suggested that new groups should be created to govern AI at specific healthcare organizations, as well as leading calls for a new system that could provide oversight across organizations. It appears from their statements that they feel that the current FDA-cleared products can't promise data integrity and algorithmic clarity. This goes back to the issue we alluded to earlier with the two schools of thought on the FDA's role in clearing healthcare AI applications. The AMIA is of the opinion that the FDA isn't asking for enough before clearing these solutions.

In 2020, *Guidelines for Clinical Trial Protocols for Interventions Involving Artificial Intelligence: The Standard Protocol Items: Recommendations for Interventional Trials (SPIRIT)-AI Extension* was released to provide more structure and standards for the increasing number of clinical trials for AI-based clinical interventions.[21] The standards have also been updated for reporting the results of trials involving AI interventions through the release of *Consolidated Standards of Reporting Trials–Artificial Intelligence (CONSORT–AI extension).*[22]

The SPIRIT-AI extension includes over a dozen new items that are vital additions to the clinical trial protocols for AI tools. Each of these fifteen new items will need to be routinely reported as well as and on top of the core items from SPIRIT 2013. SPIRIT-AI encourages investigators to document clear descriptions of the AI, including the skills that are required for it, the instructions which need to be followed, the setting in which it will be used, how the input and output data should be handled, and how people should react to errors. The idea is for SPIRIT-AI to ensure transparency and completeness for clinical trials for AI models. Editors, peer reviewers, and the general readership will be able to use it to understand, interpret, and appraise the designs and bias risks of clinical trials.

The CONSORT–AI extension has 14 new items that should be reported alongside the core items that were outlined by CONSORT 2010. As part of its recommendations, CONSORT–AI asks investigators to provide the same set of descriptions and instructions for use.

Health technology companies like Philips and Ginger have been collaborating with major health providers to develop a new standard to be used to promote trust in healthcare AI solutions. Convened by the Consumer Technology Association (CTA), a working group made up of 64 organizations set out to create a new standard that identifies the core requirements and baselines to determine whether AI solutions in healthcare are trustworthy.[21] The standard has been accredited by the American National Standards Institute.[22]

CTA president and CEO, Gary Shapiro, says, "AI is providing solutions, from diagnosing diseases to advanced remote care options, for some of healthcare's most pressing challenges. As the US healthcare system faces clinician shortages, chronic conditions and a deadly pandemic, it's critical that patients and healthcare professionals trust how these tools are developed and their intended uses."

Driven by consensus, the standard essentially aggregates human trust, technical trust, and regulatory trust. Human trust looks at factors related to human interaction and the way they perceive the AI tool, such as how easy it is to use and explain and how autonomous it is. Technical trust deals with data access, privacy, and security, as well as the quality of the data and whether it's biased. It also looks at the way that the system has been designed and trained to deliver its results. Regulatory trust is gained through compliance by industry and based upon clear laws and regulations and information from regulatory agencies, federal and state laws, and accreditation boards and international standardization frameworks.[23]

4.6   Reimbursement

If you want adoption of any technology in a meaningful way in the long term, you need the public and private entities to pay for it. Most modern technologies are out of the reach of the majority of the population in terms of cost. Paying for healthcare is a major headache for most governments in advanced economies and those brave enough to become private insurance companies have to make trade-off decisions on which solutions to cover and which ones not to cover. AI technologies are in their nascence in healthcare and so far there is not much track record to indicate how they will be reimbursed in the long term. However, there has been recent progress in this area. This bodes well for the timeline of the adoption of these technologies.

There is some history in this area, such as mammography computer-aided diagnosis (CAD), an older form of AI which aimed to help with the detection of breast cancer. Mammography CAD first gained popularity in the 2000s, when the Centers for Medicare and Medicaid Services (CMS) started reimbursing CAD-aided mammography scans. Thanks to the CMS, providers were reimbursed for an additional $10 or so if they used CAD instead of doing a standard reading. With this reimbursement, within a decade almost every screening mammogram in America is read with CAD assistance (Figure 4.7).[25]

When CMS released its 2022 physician fee schedule, it established the first national pricing for autonomous AI diagnostics.[26] This was intended for the IDx-DR service to be used in physicians' offices (CPT code 92229) and to create equitable access throughout the country. You can find this ruling on page 114 of the Federal Register Document in a section called "e. Establishment of Value for Remote Retinal Imaging (CPT Code 92229)." This is particularly significant because it's the first time that the agency has ever announced a national price for autonomous AI services.

Digital Diagnostics is the IOWA company that created IDx-DR, the first autonomous AI in healthcare technology approved by the FDA. IDx-DR is an AI-based diagnostic tool that's designed to be used at the point of care to

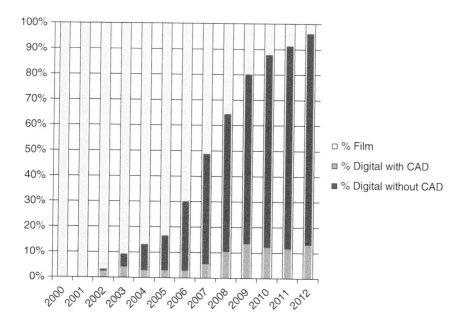

FIGURE 4.7   Breast Mammograms in the United States
(source: [25]/The Healthcare Blog)

detect diabetic retinopathy and diabetic macular edema. The statistics show that only 15% of diabetics receive their annual diabetic eye exam, despite it being strongly recommended, and this is linked to widespread blindness, especially amongst certain patient populations such as black and Hispanic communities.[27] This happens because if the disease is undiagnosed, it's also left untreated.

In early 2018, Viz.ai received FDA clearance for a deep learning system that could detect blockages in the large blood vessels that supply the brain on computed tomography (CT) scans.[28] What's interesting about this system is that it differed from the purely diagnostic systems that other start-ups were producing. Instead of only providing diagnosis, it was also equipped for triage and fast response. If it saw a blockage, it directly contacted the radiologist and the specialist who could fix the problem.[29]

In the United States, the CMS approved reimbursement for the Viz.ai system in September 2020, marking the first reimbursement for AI-augmented medical care. Viz's system was granted a new technology add-on payment of up to $1040 per use in patients with suspected strokes.[25]

To secure this reimbursement, Viz.ai produced clinical evidence for the benefits of their system. These benefits included faster notification times for the clot-busting specialist, faster transfer times from peripheral hospitals to central hospitals, and a faster overall time for the clot-busting procedure. They were also able to provide evidence of a range of improved metrics including a better modified Rankin score (mRS) during discharge, an improved National Institute of Health (NIH) Stroke Score on day five, and an improved mRS score on day 90. These scores are widely used in stroke trials and summarize the degree of damage/disability following a stroke.[25] Viz.ai's metrics proved that patients with ContaCT had better outcomes than those that went without.

It's clear that physician organizations such as the American College of Radiology are taking serious notice of these technologies and are leading the charge in creating the economic case for how they'll impact their members. Reimbursement experts indicated to me that the creation of the new CPT codes will be engineered by physician organization in such a fashion that the reimbursement of their members will be protected.

Thought leaders in health system economics have told me that these technologies will be used in niche indications for the near future but that the economics of health systems will continue to push the money-making procedures. Health systems will need to assess the impact of these technologies, but if they make their physicians more productive and more satisfied, they'll invest without reimbursement. Health systems are heavily dependent on procedures and thus will incentivize physicians to continue using them as first line.

As for physicians and their offices, experts suggest that if AI technologies can help physicians to increase their income by enabling them to take care of more patients, adoption rates will be brisk. However, if the technologies don't boost their income and there's no approved reimbursement, physicians won't buy them for their offices but will push hospitals to buy them instead.

All of this is encouraging and a positive sign of things to come. Although we're only talking about a couple of algorithms, these cases show that with clear benefits and strong evidence, reimbursement will be made available. This will be critical for the long-term adoption of these technologies.

4.7 Shortage of Healthcare Resources

As Figure 4.8 shows, there's an increasing imbalance between the health workforce and the demand for clinical services. This imbalance is due to a number of factors such as the aging workforce within healthcare, competition from other sectors of the economy, the aging population with higher healthcare needs, high burnout rates amongst clinical workers, and more. This imbalance can present a significant challenge to the healthcare system's ability to meet the increasing needs of an aging population. AI is uniquely positioned to help with this imbalance in the coming years and decades.

As you can see from Figure 4.9, AI can assist in a diverse array of areas in healthcare and help to provide intelligent automation. This cannot only reduce the need for human hours in providing care but also reduce the number of mistakes, which are a cause of lower quality care and worse patient outcomes.

The pandemic has accelerated the number of valuable resources leaving the healthcare system. Burnout is one of the key drivers of the clinician shortage. By assisting doctors and nurses with tasks that can be automated such as

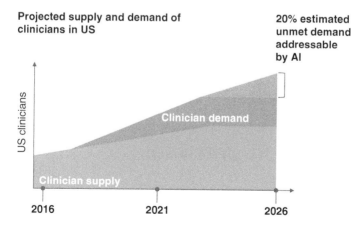

FIGURE 4.8   AI can help with the projected shortage of US clinicians
(source: Accenture)

Application	Value
Robot-assisted surgery	$40B
Virtual nursing assistants	$20B
Administrative workflow assistance	$18B
Fraud detection	$17B
Dosage error reduction	$16B
Connected machines	$14B
Clinical trial participant identifier	$13B
Preliminary diagnosis	$5B
Automated image diagnosis	$3B
Cybersecurity	$2B
TOTAL = $150B	

FIGURE 4.9   **Projected Top 10 Applications by Value Delivered** *(source: Accenture)*

administration, documentation, and data collection, burned-out doctors and nurses can free up time and do fewer routine tasks such as typing, ordering, and checking numbers. It's well documented that the high rate of physician burnout leads to medical errors. It also reduces the amount of time they're able to spend with patients and on research, rather than on routine tasks.

More time means more happiness for people and doctors. AI can free up time for doctors, as long as the automation doesn't put them under additional pressure to see more patients and be more productive. It's estimated that AI could free up to 25% of clinician time across different specialties. This increased amount of time could mean less hurried encounters and more humane interactions, including more empathy from happier doctors. This is important because empathy has been shown to improve outcomes by boosting patient adherence to the prescribed treatments, increasing motivation, and reducing anxiety and stress.

4.8   Issues with Mistakes, Inefficient Care Pathways, and Non-personalized Care

We can't afford to underestimate the many issues that are slowing the adoption of AI in healthcare, which includes fragmented data, misaligned economic incentives, and legacy IT systems. These issues are leading to less than ideal medical practice and producing patient outcomes that are far from optimal, wasting resources with duplicative tests and variable decision-making. We end up dealing with inefficiencies in delivering and receiving care as well as care that's not longitudinal and which doesn't help patients to follow their treatment plans.

This massive waste of resources is due to the lack of standardization and the imbalance of resources that we discussed in the last section, as well as the fact that the healthcare system was never designed to care for patients outside of the clinical setting. We've increasingly realized that to achieve the best outcomes, we need to help patients to follow the prescribed treatment plans on an ongoing basis in their daily lives. But it's a challenge for a healthcare system that was designed to care for patients when they're ill to take on the extra task of caring for them outside of the clinical setting.

There's already a shortage of human resources, and so for us to rise to this new challenge, we'll need technology and automation. Emerging technologies such as sensors, software, analytics, and AI can perform many of the tasks that would be unrealistic for the current healthcare system to do at scale to improve the quality of patient outcomes. These technologies can collect data from patients, analyze it, identify opportunities to intervene, and involve healthcare providers only when their input is needed. This would help us to get more done while simultaneously introducing intelligence and consistency when it comes to *how* those things are done.

Currently, any analysis of the healthcare system would show a high cost of care with poor outcomes as a result of a number of factors, including mistakes in diagnosis, wrong or too many treatments, poor decision-making by physicians due to lack of time, variable quality of training, difficulty taking statistical factors in mind (Bayesian theorem), inadequate or fragmented data, treatments that aren't individualized based on clinical trials, and more.[3] There are more than 12 million significant missed diagnoses per year on medical imaging. An alarmingly high percentage of imaging is unnecessary, and healthcare resources are badly stretched, especially now with COVID.

This is why there's a significant opportunity to improve care using AI. The ability of AI to improve patient outcomes, reduce healthcare costs, and facilitate precision medicine and ongoing patient management outside of the clinical setting sets it apart from other promising technologies in healthcare.

In a survey by Klynveld Peat Marwick Goerdeler (KPMG), many healthcare executives expressed interest and optimism about the potential impact of AI in their businesses.[30] 89% of people said that AI was already boosting the efficiency of their systems, while 91% said that it was increasing the access that patients had to care. Those in the healthcare industry were particularly optimistic about how AI could help with disease diagnosis. 68% of respondents said they were confident that AI would become effective at diagnosing illness and conditions, while 90% thought that AI would improve patient experience. They expected to see the biggest impact on the fields of diagnostics (47%), electronic record management (41%), and robotics (40%).

AI software can be used to assist the healthcare system by extracting relevant insights and helping with medical imaging and diagnostics, in-patient care and hospital management, virtual assistance, precision medicine, lifestyle management and monitoring, patient data and risk analysis, and research.[31] Although many of these will take years to fully achieve their potential, they'll be drivers of a future with healthcare that's far more effective and cost-efficient.

For health systems and life science companies to start realizing the full potential of AI, we'll require partnerships within the healthcare system and cross-industry partnerships with entities that have significant technology expertise. These partnerships are being announced with increasing frequency.

In December 2021, AI researchers from UC Berkeley, Mayo Clinic, and Duke University unveiled their new health AI partnership. The partnership's mission statement explains, "There's an urgent need to cultivate capabilities across healthcare delivery settings to conduct AI software procurement, integration and lifecycle management."[32] To tackle this need, they're developing an online curriculum which aims to educate IT leaders by working with a range of stakeholders like policymakers, regulators, users, and payers. The entire curriculum is designed to be open source and freely available online, with the goal of "decentralizing the high concentration of technology [and] regulatory expertise" from some of the United States's leading health systems. They'll use it to develop guidelines to help organizations to make smarter decisions and will focus on two main subsets of healthcare AI—diagnosis and treatment decisions, and prioritization of resources for care management programs.

More than a dozen major health systems, with millions of patients in 40 states, are banding together to launch Truveta, a new data-driven initiative that focuses on collaborative approaches to precision medicine and population health.[33] The aim is to innovate care delivery and to develop new therapies by searching through the billions of clinical data points that are available. Truveta can use automation to provide continuous learning to physicians, pharmaceutical developers, and researchers. There are fourteen health systems participating in Truveta, and they can provide a rich source of data from a wide geographic footprint to enable advancements in the development and integrity of AI algorithms. This is vital, because studies have shown that "under-developed and potentially biased models" can worsen care.[34]

Given the expertise of technology companies when it comes to data, software, and AI, we can expect them to see healthcare as one of their most promising growth sectors. Their participation has already led to various initiatives and partnerships with healthcare entities. In December 2020, Google launched a new Android app—Google Health Studies—that streamlines study participation for consumers and provides transparency around how their data is being used for health research.[35] Apple also has clinical research and data-sharing capabilities on its iPhone devices.

Meanwhile, Google has launched its Healthcare Interoperability Readiness Program, which aims to make it easier for healthcare companies to understand their data and to standardize it so that it can be integrated across different systems. Back in April 2020, the company opened up its Cloud Healthcare API and quickly took on a number of health systems and medical centers, including the Mayo Clinic. Further underscoring its commitment to the healthcare industry, Google has also started working with electronic health records (EHR) companies like Meditech to migrate their systems and data to the cloud. It's said that this work could eventually result in a two-way data flow, with EHR companies incentivized to integrate their patient-generated data with Google's software.

Meanwhile, the continued adoption of mobile devices means that Google and Apple are now at the heart of the healthcare data ecosystem. Our mobile devices mean that we can start to gather previously unavailable data in real time.

Google's Verily has partnered with healthcare entities such as Stanford Medical Center and Duke University School of Medicine on Project Baseline. This project aims to map human health using data to accelerate finding treatments for more medical conditions. Part of Project Baseline's aim is to better match patients with clinical research that's relevant to their issues. Patient-generated data, like the data created by Project Baseline, could potentially create "digital twins" and remove the need for a control group. If this happens, it could help to reduce the recruitment bottlenecks we often see in clinical trials (Figure 4.10).

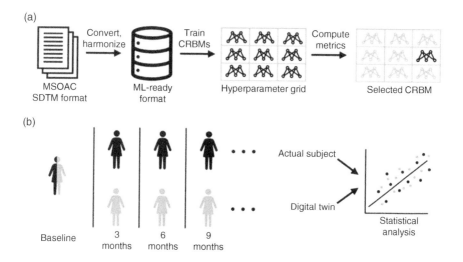

FIGURE 4.10   Digital Twins *(source: CB Information Services³⁵)*

References

1. Global Market Insights (2017). Healthcare AI Market Size, Competitive Market Share & Forecast, 2024
2. The World Population Prospects: 2015 Revision. (2015). Latest Major Publications - United Nations Department of Economic and Social Affairs. https://www.un.org/en/development/desa/publications/world-population-prospects-2015-revision.html
3. Hang, et al. (2018). Big Data in Health Care: Applications and Challenges. Data and Information Management, 2(3), 175–197
4. Topol, E. (2019). Deep Medicine: How Artificial Intelligence Can Make Healthcare Human Again (Illustrated ed.). Basic Books.
5. Siwicki, B. (2021, June 16). AWS leader talks about technologies needed to take precision medicine. Healthcare IT News. https://www.healthcareitnews.com/news/aws-leader-talks-about-technologies-needed-take-precision-medicine-next-level
6. CB Insights. (2022, March 9). State Of AI Q3'21 Report. CB Insights Research. https://www.cbinsights.com/research/report/ai-trends-q3-2021/
7. Krizhevsky, A., Sutskever, I., & Hinton, G. E. (2017). ImageNet classification with deep convolutional neural networks. Communications of the ACM, 60(6), 84–90. https://doi.org/10.1145/3065386
8. Dean, J., Corrado, G., Monga, R., Chen, K., Devin, M., Mao, M., Ranzato, M., Senior, A., Tucker, P., Yang, K., Le, Q., & Ng, A. (2012). Large Scale Distributed Deep Networks. NeurIPS Proceedings. https://papers.nips.cc/paper/2012/hash/6aca97005c68f1206823815f66102863-Abstract.html
9. Sutton, R. S., & Barto, A. G. (1998). Reinforcement Learning: An Introduction (Adaptive Computation and Machine Learning) Adaptive Computation and Machine Learning series (second edition). A Bradford Book.
10. Goodfellow, I., Pouget-Abadie, J., Mirza, M., Xu, B., Warde-Farley, D., Ozair, S., Courville, A., & Bengio, Y. (2020). Generative adversarial networks. Communications of the ACM, 63(11), 139–144. https://doi.org/10.1145/3422622
11. Landi, H. (2023, November 9). 'Devil is in the details' for Biden's AI strategy, but some experts are skeptical about efforts to regulate the technology. Fierce Healthcare. https://www.fiercehealthcare.com/ai-and-machine-learning/devil-details-bidens-ai-strategy-some-experts-are-skeptical-about-efforts?utm_medium=email&utm_source=nl&utm_campaign=HC-NL-FierceHealthTech&oly_enc_id=1016C4538789G4F
12. Dives, D., Croxen, J., Kaganoff, S., With help from:, & Golden, I. (2021, October 12). Pulse check: An analysis of the FDA's list of AI- and ML-enabled devices | Rock Health.
13. U.S. Food & Drug Administration (FDA). (2021). Artificial Intelligence/Machine Learning-Based Software as a Medical Device Action Plan. US Food and Drug Administration. https://govwhitepapers.com/whitepapers/artificial-intelligence-machine-learning-based-software-as-a-medical-device-action-plan
14. Center for Devices and Radiological Health. (2022, August 25). Evaluation of Automatic Class III Designation (De Novo) Summaries. U.S. Food and Drug Administration. https://www.fda.gov/about-fda/cdrh-transparency/evaluation-automatic-class-iii-designation-de-novo-summaries

15. Shukla, M. (2019, January 9). FDA Pre-Cert v1.0 Explained: 2019 and the Promises of Years to Come. Medium.

16. Fox, A. (2023, April 4). FDA drafts AI-enabled medical device life cycle plan guidance. Healthcare IT News. https://www.healthcareitnews.com/news/fda-drafts-ai-enabled-medical-device-lifecycle-plan-guidance

17. Ventech Solutions and MedCity News. (2019, May 16). Aidoc gets FDA nod for AI pulmonary embolism screening tool. MedCity News. https://medcitynews.com/2019/05/aidoc-gets-fda-nod-for-ai-pulmonary-embolism-screening-tool/

18. Ethics and Governance of Artificial Intelligence for Health. (2021). World Health Organization. https://www.who.int/publications-detail-redirect/9789240029200

19. Fox, A. (2023, April 6). CHAI publishes its blueprint for AI in healthcare. Healthcare IT News. https://www.healthcareitnews.com/news/chai-publishes-its-blueprint-ai-healthcare

20. Petersen, C., Smith, J., Freimuth, R. R., Goodman, K. W., Jackson, G. P., Kannry, J., Liu, H., Madhavan, S., Sittig, D. F., & Wright, A. (2021). Recommendations for the safe, effective use of adaptive CDS in the US healthcare system: an AMIA position paper. Journal of the American Medical Informatics Association, 28(4), 677–684. https://doi.org/10.1093/jamia/ocaa319

21. Rivera, S. C., Liu, X., Chan, A. W., Denniston, A. K., & Calvert, M. J. (2020). Guidelines for clinical trial protocols for interventions involving artificial intelligence: the SPIRIT-AI Extension. BMJ, m3210. https://doi.org/10.1136/bmj.m3210

22. Liu, X., Rivera, S. C., Moher, D., Calvert, M. J., & Denniston, A. K. (2020). Reporting guidelines for clinical trial reports for interventions involving artificial intelligence: the CONSORT-AI Extension. BMJ, m3164. https://doi.org/10.1136/bmj.m3164

23. Landi, H. (2021). AHIP, tech companies create new healthcare AI standard as industry aims to provide more guardrails. Fierce Healthcare. https://www.fiercehealthcare.com/tech/consumer-technology-association-launches-new-healthcare-ai-standard-as-industry-aims-to

24. Consumer Technology Association®. (2021). The Use of Artificial Intelligence in Health Care: Trustworthiness (ANSI/CTA-2090). Consumer Technology Association/American National Standards Institute.

25. Liu, C. (2020, September 10). The Medical AI Floodgates Open, at a Cost of $1000 per Patient. The Health Care Blog. https://thehealthcareblog.com/blog/2020/09/10/the-medical-ai-floodgates-open-at-a-cost-of-1000-per-patient/

26. Department of Health and Human Services Centers for Medicare & Medicaid Services 42 CFR Parts 403, 405, 410, 411, 414, 415, 423, 424, and 425. (2022). Code of Federal Regulations. Department of Health and Human Services. https://www.ecfr.gov/current/title-42/chapter-IV

27. Benoit, S. C., Swenor, B. K., Geiss, L. S., Gregg, E. W., & Saaddine, J. B. (2019). Eye care utilization among insured people with diabetes in the U.S., 2010–2014. Diabetes Care, 42(3), 427–433. https://doi.org/10.2337/dc18-0828

28. Office of the Commissioner. (2018, February 13). FDA Permits Marketing of Clinical Decision Support Software for Alerting Providers of a Potential Stroke in Patients. U.S. Food and Drug Administration. https://www.fda.gov/news-events/

press-announcements/fda-permits-marketing-clinical-decision-support-software-alerting-providers-potential-stroke

29. Siwicki, B. (2021, May 10). Mass General Brigham and the future of AI in radiology. Healthcare IT News. https://www.healthcareitnews.com/news/mass-general-brigham-and-future-ai-radiology

30. Kent, J. (2020). 53% of Execs Say Healthcare Leads Artificial Intelligence Adoption. Healthcare IT Analytics

31. Ltd, R. A. M. (2021). Artificial Intelligence in Healthcare Market by Offering (Hardware, Software, Services), Technology (Machine Learning, NLP, Context-aware Computing, Computer Vision), Application, End User and Geography - Global Forecast to 2027. Research and Markets Ltd 2022. https://www.researchandmarkets.com/reports/5116503/artificial-intelligence-in-healthcare-market-by?utm_source=dynamic&utm_medium=GNOM&utm_code=gstppz&utm_campaign=1404802+-+Artificial+Intelligence+in+Healthcare+Market+with+COVID-19+Impact+Analysis+by+Offering%2c+Technology%2c+End-Use+Application%2c+End-user+and+Region+-+Global+Forecast+to+2026&utm_exec=jamu273gnomd

32. Miliard, M. (2021, December 15). Duke, Mayo Clinic, others launch innovative AI collaboration. Healthcare IT News. https://www.healthcareitnews.com/news/duke-mayo-clinic-others-launch-innovative-ai-collaboration

33. Miliard, M. (2021, February 12). Truveta, formed with big-name health systems, aims for AI-powered. Healthcare IT News. https://www.healthcareitnews.com/news/truveta-formed-big-name-health-systems-aims-ai-powered-data-advances

34. Jercich, K. (2020, August 18). AI bias may worsen COVID-19 health disparities for people of color. Healthcare IT News. https://www.healthcareitnews.com/news/ai-bias-may-worsen-covid-19-health-disparities-people-color

35. CB Insights. (2022, August 16). The Future of Clinical Trials: Trends to Watch in 2022 and Beyond. CB Insights Research. https://www.cbinsights.com/research/briefing/clinical-trials-trends/

PART II

Applications of AI in Healthcare

CHAPTER 5

Diagnostics

DIAGNOSTICS IS the first frontier for artificial intelligence (AI) in healthcare. Much of what happens in healthcare is about collecting data (symptoms, exam data, labs, genetics, etc.) and interpreting it to make determinations about a patient's health or medical issues. We've developed great capabilities in diagnostic testing over the last century. Often, a piece of data can clinch a diagnosis, such as a CT scan that shows a stroke or bleed in the context of a patient with neurological issues or a urinalysis that shows a urinary tract infection in someone with lower abdominal pain.

Lab results often have a normal range and if something is out of that range, the abnormal result is used to diagnose the cause of an issue. Sometimes, the interpretation is much more subjective and requires careful examination of an X-ray or an MRI scan, looking for abnormalities in different areas such as the bones, kidneys, or abdomen. This is a prime area for AI algorithms to assist clinicians. AI could also help when there's a large amount of information to interpret (e.g. genetics) or a combination of information from different sources. It's my opinion that with the explosion of medical information about each individual, AI will soon be a necessity and not a luxury, allowing us to interpret what all of this information means for each individual.

Let's see what AI is capable of, as well as what the short-term applications are and what will be possible in the long term but is currently inaccessible due to the variety of issues we've discussed.

5.1 Radiology

This is the first area for us to look at because images are digital files with structured data that can be used to develop and validate models to perform a narrow task such as finding a tumor on a CT scan or a fracture on an X-ray.

AI Doctor: The Rise of Artificial Intelligence in Healthcare: A Guide for Users, Buyers, Builders, and Investors, First Edition. Ronald M. Razmi.
© 2024 Ronald M. Razmi. Published 2024 by John Wiley & Sons, Inc.

The infrastructure that's been created for digital imaging yields itself well to incorporating algorithms into that workflow. That means it's possible, but it doesn't mean it's easy. Health systems have many priorities with limited resources, so incorporating an AI algorithm into radiology systems is still difficult. However, out of the many possible applications of AI in healthcare, this is one that's currently possible. In addition to radiology, some of the other early applications of AI in healthcare include the use of images to screen for or diagnose conditions. Here, we're not necessarily talking about radiology images because we'll be able to use images from a cell phone, such as facial images for stress levels or skin images for dermatologic conditions.

The largest and fastest-growing source of data in the healthcare industry is medical imaging, which accounts for 90% of all healthcare data. Despite the fact that we have all of this data, over 97% of it is unanalyzed and unused. Estimates suggest that there were 4.7 billion diagnostic imaging scans in 2019, a number that's forecast to grow at approximately 3% per annum over the next five years. X-ray exams accounted for most of these scans in 2020, but others such as MRI and CT are forecast to grow at a faster rate over the coming years, as they have over the last decade.[1]

Reading these scans involves radiologists carefully studying each image and finding abnormalities based on their training. There are 800 million medical scans in a year that result in 60 billion images. The estimated error rates are that 2% are false positives and 25% are false negatives. Interpreting all of this medical imaging data could lengthen turnaround times and cause delays between image acquisition, diagnosis, and care. These delays could then cause patients' health to further decline, especially when it comes to critical conditions where rapid analysis and escalation are of paramount importance.

One of the initial benefits of AI is that it could allow us to detect life-threatening events much earlier and ensure higher accuracy in reading these studies. If a patient presents with a stroke or a collapsed lung, an algorithm that can immediately look for abnormalities and alert the radiologist if it finds something could lead to faster life-saving interventions. If an algorithm augments a radiologist in finding hard-to-spot tumor or spinal stenosis, it can lead to a diagnosis that would have otherwise been missed.

The algorithms can give radiologists a boost in reading scans. Radiomics is the study of scans for hidden findings and signatures. Algorithms can help us to better access these findings and lead to deeper quantification of what's on the scans in the near future. Deep learning could be used to identify incidental findings, and it could also help radiologists manage their workloads, enhance the quality of scans, and reduce the number of retakes, which can lead to unnecessary exposure to radiation. Deep learning is also showing promising results in image reconstruction from the imaging modalities.[1]

AI is rapidly gaining traction in the field of radiology. Clinical adoption of AI by radiologists has gone from 0% to 30% from 2015 to 2020, according to a study by the American College of Radiology (Figure 5.1).[2, 3]

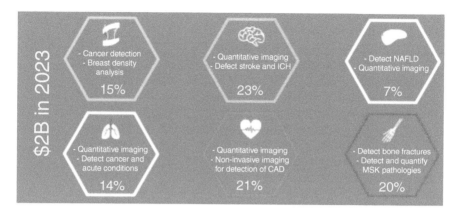

FIGURE 5.1   AI in Radiology *(source: Signify Research)²*

There are, of course, certain issues that would stop AI algorithms from being the only entity that reads a scan. First, the current algorithms are trained to perform a narrow task such as finding tumors, hemorrhages, or fractures. That means that they won't be able to identify other things that might be present on a scan. This not only presents a major clinical issue but also offers up legal considerations. It's the radiologist's responsibility to report on all visible abnormalities on a radiologic study. That means that while an algorithm could help a radiologist perform a narrow task like finding a fracture, it would miss everything else. That's why a radiologist needs to read the study and be ultimately responsible for the final report.

The emergence of large language models and a new generation of algorithms that can be trained on large, unlabeled datasets that can perform more than one task could usher in a new era. The promise of these algorithms is that they can perform multiple tasks when trained on a large number of unlabeled radiological images. That means that these models could identify multiple abnormalities on a radiological study, which would certainly be of more help to radiologists. However, even with these new, flexible models, radiologist supervision will most likely be necessary. On top of that, these models will require large, diverse datasets to train on, something that isn't easy to get in healthcare. Also, given their flexibility in performing multiple tasks, it's more challenging to anticipate potential failures. Validating these models will be more difficult and more time-consuming.

Verifying these models' outputs will be difficult, too. For example, conventional models may consider only a radiological study or a whole-slide pathology image when classifying a patient's cancer. In each case, a radiologist or pathologist could verify whether the model's outputs are correct. However, these larger and more flexible models could consider both radiology images and pathology slides and create an initial diagnosis and classification, as well as a treatment recommendation. In this case, a multidisciplinary panel (consisting of radiologists, pathologists, oncologists, and additional specialists) may be needed to judge the model's output. Fact-checking large language models (LLMs') outputs therefore represent a serious challenge, both during validation and after models are deployed.

Another issue with the current task-specific models is that reading a scan and knowing what an abnormality means often requires context. Did the patient have surgery in that area before? If so, that may explain unusual findings on a scan. Was there a nodule there before? Well, if there was and it looks identical now, the likelihood of a tumor is significantly reduced. This lack of full context could keep the algorithms from fully translating what they find on a scan into what it actually means, although emerging large language models that can accept multimodal inputs could potentially address this issue. One report highlighted the potential for a digital radiology assistant that could do an initial read of a scan and look for multiple abnormalities while taking patient history into account. These assistants could generate an initial report and provide examples of detected abnormalities.[4]

Machine learning (ML)-based pattern recognition tools are perfectly suited to medical imaging, but adoption amongst healthcare providers runs at a notoriously slow pace. This is due to a lack of trust in AI amongst clinical staff, unclear value propositions, complex data integration as a result of siloed and proprietary platforms, and the difficult process of obtaining regulatory approval. In the near future, the algorithm will most likely do initial reading, segmentation, and annotation, as well as any quantification before a radiologist reads the study. For the next generation of models to read an entire scan and annotate it before a radiologist review, the issues of validation and verification will need to be addressed and we'll require clinical evidence of positive impact on patient outcomes.

The reported accuracy of current single-task algorithms in radiology has varied from 0.56 to 0.99.[2] However, this has been steadily improving and the current questions around the use of algorithms in radiology are less about their accuracy and more about their clinical value. Proving the accuracy of an algorithm is very different to demonstrating clinical efficacy. Only prospective studies in real-world settings can establish that. Not many of these studies have been performed to date, and the only ones so far are in diabetic retinopathy, wrist fracture, breast cancer histology, colonic polyps, and congenital cataracts.[2]

It's well-established that algorithms can read a scan immediately upon completion and therefore can provide an initial interpretation much faster than a radiologist. In studies to date, this is 150 times faster (1.2 versus 177 s).[2] This can be extremely important in the context of time-sensitive clinical issues, such as strokes, fractures, and collapsed lungs.

The benefits of AI in rapidly and accurately reading radiological studies to improve patient care have been shown in the context of COVID. A recent study detailed the use of an AI tool to rapidly detect COVID-19 by analyzing chest CTs.[5] The system had been developed using a dataset with more than 10,000 CT scans from patients with COVID-19, influenza, and community-acquired pneumonia. The system, which used a deep convolutional neural network, was able to achieve an area under the receiver operating characteristic curve (AUC) of 97.81% for multi-way classification on a test cohort of 3199 scans, as well as an AUC of 92.99% and 93.25% on two publicly available datasets, CC-CCII and MosMedData. In a reader study involving five radiologists, the AI system outperformed the radiologists in more challenging tasks at a speed order of magnitude above them. In the reader study, the average reading time of radiologists was 6.5 minutes, while that of the AI system was 2.73 s. This could significantly improve the productivity of radiologists.[5]

A series of studies have investigated how deep learning algorithms could detect abnormalities in radiology, yielding promising results. qXR, Qure.ai's chest X-ray interpretation tool, can automatically detect and localize up to 29 abnormalities, including those that could indicate lung cancer.[6] There are several features of chest radiographs (e.g. sharply circumscribed nodules or masses, those with irregular margins and those with ill-defined lesions) that could indicate the presence of lung cancer. The CE-marked qXR algorithm can detect lung cancer nodules with a high level of accuracy in under a minute, and it can also mark the size and position of the nodules. It can help clinicians to spot minuscule nodules which could be missed even by experts. A Qure.ai study demonstrated a 17% improvement in sensitivity compared to radiologist readings when using AI to interpret chest X-rays. These kinds of early detection aids could have considerable long-term benefits and lead to a lower cost per life-year saved.

Seymour Duncker, who's worked with Qure.ai's algorithms, indicates that, "The qXR algorithm also nicely demonstrates that not all algorithms are of equal quality. During the early days of COVID-19, before rapid tests became widely available, dozens of special purpose algorithms were hastily trained to use x-rays to identify and triage COVID-19 patients. While demonstrating seemingly good results under highly constrained conditions, few of these studies held up to further scrutiny, let alone providing a path to deployment. Using the qXR algorithm, one could make use of a specific signature of symptomatic COVID-19 cases, which is a high degree of opacity on both lungs. In a field study conducted at Grupo Angeles Hospitales in Mexico, we were able to validate that a generic high quality algorithm such as qXR that wasn't specifically trained on COVID-19 could potentially be used to triage patients. While the use case was short-lived (rapid tests became available not long after), it shows the power and versatility of well-trained, robust algorithms."[7, 8]

AI can also be helpful in teleradiology, which uses the electronic transmission of radiological images to move them from a scanning organization to a reading organization so that the latter can provide diagnostic interpretation and reporting. In 2019, less than 2% of the world's 4.7 billion diagnostic imaging scans fell into this category.

However, several drivers will contribute to this penetration rate increasing significantly over the next five years. These drivers include[9]:

- Radiologist shortages in certain regions.
- Increased demand for more specialized modality reads, such as CT and MRI, that require radiologists with specific skills.
- Demand for out-of-hours reporting, especially in time-critical applications like neurology.
- Longer read times for more specialized modalities (e.g. CT versus X-ray).
- Increased use of cloud-based technology, allowing simpler IT implementation for teleradiology.
- Changes in legislation that support reading services being provided out of country and by third parties.
- Increasing numbers of imaging IT vendors offering workflow tools that are designed specifically for teleradiology applications.

One final driver, not mentioned above, is that of technological advances, and those relating to AI in particular.

Three of the most important factors that heavily influence the success of teleradiology reading service providers are[9]:

- The speed that radiologists working for teleradiology service providers perform and report on their reads.
- The accuracy of the reports produced by radiologists.
- The workflow and decision support processes that service providers put in place to ensure urgent reads are prioritized and reported on quickly.

Over time, AI can be used to support and improve all three. The first two bullets (i.e. speed and accuracy) will become increasingly important as diagnostic imaging scans become increasingly focused on more complex and time-consuming procedures. For example, 11.5% of global diagnostic imaging procedures in 2019 were CT scans. This ratio has been increasing steadily over the last decade and is projected to reach 14% of all diagnostic imaging scans in 2024. Conversely, X-rays accounted for 61% of all scans in 2019, a figure that's projected to fall to approximately 55% in 2024. The emerging larger models that can identify multiple abnormalities while taking patient context into account and generating an initial report can have a tremendous impact on improving radiologists' workflows.

Even though X-rays accounted for most of the scans that were carried out, it's estimated that they accounted for less than 20% of radiologist reading time because of faster reading times per scan. The net effect of the changing scan types over the next five years is that with diagnostic procedures increasing, the procedures that take the longest amount of time to report are growing the fastest, thus increasing the amount of demand there is for radiologists. AI can provide a huge competitive advantage for teleradiology service providers that can reduce read times while simultaneously maintaining (or even improving) accuracy.

Teleradiology reading service providers have been exploring how AI can be used to improve workflows and decision support. For example, US teleradiology service provider vRad has been working with Qure.ai on worklist prioritization, specifically in relation to intercranial hemorrhage on head CT scans. Other examples include Real Time Medical of Canada collaborating with Google Cloud to develop AI-assisted workload balancing tools, I-Med Radiology Network of Australia implementing AI tools for worklist triage for brain hemorrhages, pulmonary embolisms, and C-spine fractures, and Global Diagnostics Group, again of Australia, partnering with Aidoc to implement AI-based workflow solutions supporting care management pathway development.[9]

The potential benefits of AI in radiology aren't limited to better and faster reading of the scans. AI can also help us to acquire better images and at a faster rate. Facebook has an MRI initiative that's been creating models that can create equally detailed and accurate MRIs while using a quarter of the raw data that's traditionally required. Because they only need a quarter of the data, they can be carried out nearly four times faster. A team of independent radiologists compared the AI-generated images with traditionally captured images and couldn't tell which were created using the new method.[10] Subtle Medical has developed AI technology that uses image processing techniques to speed up MRIs and PET scanning processes and enhance the quality of the images that are obtained (Figure 5.2).

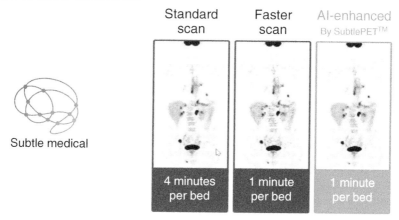

FIGURE 5.2   AI allows for imaging using less radiation *(source: Subtle Medical, Inc.)*

Also, a number of companies are embedding AI in ultrasound machines that help primary care offices perform the study without having received full training. The AI can guide the user to acquire better quality images. Examples of these companies include Butterfly, Caption, and Exo.

5.2 Pathology

If a radiology scan suggests a mass that could indicate whether something's serious or not, the next step is to take tissue from that mass and examine it. When a radiologist suspects cancer, a biopsy is taken and that sample is taken to a pathology lab. At the lab, a team processes the sample into glass slides so that a pathologist can examine it. The pathologists often spend hours at the microscope, tapping into their years of pattern recognition expertise to see if the images before them contain cancerous cells.

The field of pathology is critical to both the diagnosis and treatment of many cancers, yet the tools of the trade haven't been upgraded much in 100 years. We still turn biopsies into physical slides, have pathologists view them on microscopes for hours on end and rely on memory to find problems. By comparison, radiology went through a digital revolution 20 years ago and now digital X-rays enable remote readings and teleradiology (including overnight readings from across the globe).

If discrete digital imaging files are the initial frontier for AI in healthcare, pathology could be one of the first specialties to benefit. That's because it involves looking at tissue samples to find subtle abnormalities that could indicate disease, and the shape of those abnormalities could tell us what's causing the disease along with how aggressive it is. It seems tailor-made for AI.

Much like radiology, pathology is about the interpretation of pictures. However, there are also some differences. While radiology images are pure pictures created by X-ray or MRI, pathology images are actual tissue samples taken from patients. This tissue needs to be prepared with certain materials and then viewed under a microscope. Because of that, the slides aren't necessarily photographed or digitized to create a structured data file for AI to examine.

One of the main reasons why pathology lagged behind in the move to digital was how expensive it is to digitize slides. Each image has to be incredibly high resolution so that it can be zoomed in on and searched, like a detailed satellite image. That's why the technology required for pathology image storage has needed to catch up with the market's demands.

Four factors came together to make digital pathology a must-have instead of a nice-to-have. First, COVID-19 sent pathologists home and challenged them to figure out new remote workflows. Second, cloud storage got cheaper and more robust, allowing for the sharing of massive images. Third, the development of advanced AI has enabled pathologists to better appreciate the potential benefits of a digital pathology system. Finally, cancer cases are on the rise and pathologists are on the decline, creating a critical gap that's only going to grow in coming years.

This is creating momentum for what needs to be done to make pathology ready for the AI revolution. The first step would be to digitize as many of the slides as possible (called whole slide imaging) and then to use those to train AI algorithms that can assist in the interpretation of pathology images. Well, I'm happy to report that there's a significant push to make pathology digital. As a matter of fact, being able to train and use AI models to improve and accelerate the reading of pathology images might have been an accelerant. Another factor that's made pathology a slower turf so far for AI is that there's less agreement between pathologists when it comes to the reading of pathology slides and thus it's not as easy to create training datasets as it is with radiology.

AI's use in pathology so far has led to a number of interesting observations.[11] Reading a pathology image requires a combination of speed and accuracy. Pathologists who take their time and carefully examine the image seem to have better accuracy and have been shown to be equivalent to algorithms, but algorithms can produce their results much faster. However, pathologists who work alongside algorithms have improved accuracy and significantly more speed, giving us the best of both worlds. Much like with radiology, where AI might be able to help us to acquire the images, algorithms could be useful in pathology to improve the quality of out-of-focus images. Also, as molecular diagnostics becomes part of the diagnosis and classification of path results, machines can integrate information about omics (DNA sequence, RNA sequence, proteomics, methylation patterns, etc.) into the final diagnosis. This is especially true of the emerging large language models that promise to accept multimodal inputs, look for multiple abnormalities on pathology slides, create initial reports, and provide context for reported findings. AI can ingest and analyze all of this information to yield better diagnosis and has been shown to be effective in relating specific mutations to treatments.

In 2021, the Food and Drug Administration (FDA) issued its first clearance for an AI-based cancer diagnosis tool. This clearance was given to Paige, a company from New York that was founded in 2018 using data and technology from Memorial Sloan Kettering Cancer Center. The product, Paige Prostate, analyzes slides of biopsied prostate tissue to spot the hallmarks of malignant cells and highlights the sections of prostate biopsies that are the most likely to contain cancer cells.[12] It can then assign them to a trained professional for further review. One of the benefits of the software is the increased efficiency of the diagnostic workload for pathologists. It's imperative for us to do this because those workloads are growing at a rapid rate.

It's projected that we'll see a 60% rise in the number of global cancer cases in the next 20 years, and the number of pathologists that are available is unlikely to keep pace. Fortunately, AI software could help to increase the productivity of the pathologists that we do have, ultimately saving lives.

The FDA approval was due to a clinical study by 16 pathologists who evaluated the software. Each pathologist examined cancerous and benign tissue slides, both with and without Paige Prostate. The samples that the pathologists used were gathered from over 150 different institutions so that they could test how the AI performed across a range of hospitals, geographies, and demographics.

Final patient diagnoses are based on a range of information, including multiple biopsies and examinations, but even with that in mind, the AI software was able to improve cancer detection by an average of 7.3%. The software also helped to cut the number of false-negative diagnoses by 70% and false-positive diagnoses by 24%.[12]

5.3 Dermatology

Consistent with radiology and pathology, dermatology is another specialty where a lot of the diagnosis comes down to a visual inspection of the skin and doing pattern recognition. This is good fit for AI, although the diagnosis will need to take other factors into consideration such as patient symptoms, other exam findings, and lab results. However, given that the skin's appearance is a big part of the diagnosis, AI can provide a huge amount of assistance to the dermatologist. There's significant activity in this area involving Google and start-up companies that are focusing on developing solutions.

In some initial studies, algorithms outperformed dermatologists on both skin lesion images and dermascopic digital images.[13] Esteva et al. used a convolutional neural network (CNN) on 129,000 dermatological lesions to classify whether the lesion was a benign seborrheic keratosis versus a keratinocyte carcinoma or a benign nevus versus a malignant melanoma.[14] This study found that the model performed at about the same level as a panel of 21 professional dermatologists. Most skin lesions are diagnosed by Primary Care Physicians (PCPs) with significantly less expertise, so the use of the algorithm could represent significant improvements in accuracy and detection.[15]

One of the most interesting developments in this area has been the release of Google's tool to help people get an initial idea of what their skin issue might be.[16] Google's new tool helps users to identify skin conditions by analyzing images that are uploaded into Google's portal.[17] To use this web-based application, which provides AI-powered dermatology assistance, its users are tasked with uploading three high-quality photographs of the area of concern from different angles. After that, the tool asks its users a number of questions about skin type, the duration of the issue, and any other symptoms that the patient is experiencing so that it can narrow down possibilities. The AI model analyzes this information and draws from its knowledge of 288 conditions to provide a list of possible diagnoses.[16]

Every time it finds a matching condition, the AI tool shows dermatologist-reviewed information, as well as matching images from the internet and the answers to some of the most commonly asked questions. Its users are then able to save or delete their results, as well as to donate them to Google's research team. There are two billion people on this planet who suffer from dermatological issues, and there aren't enough specialists to go around. That's one of the reasons why many people start by going straight to Google, but it can be difficult to describe what your skin looks like with words alone. That's why researchers spent three years to build this AI-powered virtual assistant.

Along the way, Google published a number of peer-reviewed research papers that validate the model. In a study published in Nature in 2021, the AI system was shown to be as good as a dermatologist at identifying 26 skin conditions, and more accurate than nurses and primary care physicians.[13] A recent paper published in JAMA Network Open demonstrated that Google Health's AI tool might help clinicians to diagnose skin conditions more accurately in primary care practices, where most skin diseases are initially evaluated.[15]

One of the main challenges of using ML tools to detect skin conditions is that they need high-quality images of the skin. There's also the fact that training these models requires a diverse set of images that reflect the range of pigmentations in human skin. It can be a challenge to recognize the signs of disease in different skin types. For example, increased blood flow appears red in lighter skin and brown in darker skin. Images need to be taken with care and properly illuminated so that we can see the subtle redness or differences in complex conditions across all skin types.[18]

5.4 Ophthalmology

Ophthalmology is another specialty where the examination of the eye (including the fundus) is a huge part of screening and diagnosis. As such, if there was a way to create high-quality digital pictures of the fundus (which there is!), AI algorithms could be used to identify and monitor conditions.

The FDA has already approved the first autonomous AI system to screen for diabetic retinopathy.[19] This system, IDX-DR by Digital Diagnostics, has shown to be very accurate at detecting diabetic retinopathy on fundus photographs. When combined with a device to take photo of the fundus, the algorithm can detect more than mild diabetic retinopathy. The AI system takes images that have been captured by a retinal camera and uploads them to a cloud server for analysis. Within a couple of minutes, the software can provide a result that indicates either that more than mild retinopathy is present and that the patient needs to be referred to a specialist or that the screen was negative and should be repeated in a year. The software is notable in that it was the first AI-based diagnostic system to be authorized by the FDA for commercialization in the United States that can provide a screening decision without the need for clinician interpretation.[20]

Google also has developed a system that can auto-detect diabetic retinopathy from a fundus photograph. In two validation sets of 9963 images

Google's algorithms are matching doctors

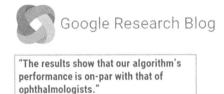

Google Research Blog

"The results show that our algorithm's performance is on-par with that of ophthalmologists."

Performance of the algorithm (black curve) and eight ophthalmologists (colored dots) for the presence of referable diabetic retinopathy based on 9,000+ images.

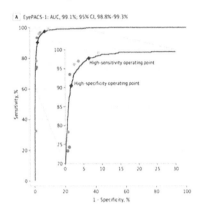

CBINSIGHTS

FIGURE 5.3   *(source: CB Information Services)*[22]

and 1748 images, at the operating point selected for high specificity, the algorithm had 90.3% and 87.0% sensitivity and 98.1% and 98.5% specificity for detecting referable diabetic retinopathy.[21] The study's conclusion was that deep learning algorithms had a high level of sensitivity and specificity for detecting diabetic retinopathy and macular edema in retinal fundus photographs (Figure 5.3).

Moore's Field Eye Hospital partnered with Google's DeepMind to develop optical coherence tomography (OCT) algorithms for the eye. They can diagnose most retinal diseases—diabetic retinopathy, age-related macular degeneration (AMD), glaucoma, and 50 more—with a combination of high-quality photos of the eye and deep learning algorithms. Smartphone attachments can enable remote OCT or fundoscopic photos, coupled with an algorithm to diagnose emerging eye conditions.

Also, AI algorithms can assess the risk of cardiovascular disease by looking at the same fundoscopic photos and examining the vessels for evidence of vascular disease. This can provide a window into the body and in the future, the use of smartphone eye exams may become part of the ongoing screening and management of chronic conditions.

AI models have shown promise when it comes to predicting the potential progression of early AMD to clinically significant disease.[23, 24] Millions of people show signs of early AMD and yet have excellent vision, and so the path of progression to advanced AMD with legal blindness is variable and difficult to quantify. The good news is that AI can automatically analyze imaging biomarkers to provide personalized predictions of how someone's early AMD is likely to progress.[23, 24] A color fundus image allows for the categorization of AMD to none/early AMD or intermediate/advanced AMD with accuracy that's comparable to expert ophthalmologists.

A deep learning model called DeepSeeNet has been developed to classify patients with AMD depending on how severe their symptoms are.[25] Trained on 58,402 images and tested on 900 more, DeepSeeNet did a better job of patient classification than retinal specialists with a high AUC when detecting large drusen (0.94) and pigmentary abnormalities (0.93). However, it had a slightly lower performance when detecting late AMD (accuracy 0.967 versus 0.973; kappa 0.663 versus 0.754). DeepSeeNet simulated the human grading process and showed high accuracy with increased transparency when it came to automatically assigning patients to AMD risk categories. This shows how much potential there is for deep learning tools to enhance clinical decision-making for patients with AMD, especially when it comes to detecting it early and predicting the risks of them developing late AMD.

Although all of this is very promising, it is worth remembering the issues Google encountered when launching their eye algorithm in Thailand with regard to low image quality and poor internet connection. As such, in spite of the great promise in this specialty, some of these other issues may slow down the pace of adoption.

5.5   Cardiology

As a cardiologist with expertise in AI, I can see a whole range of areas where AI could improve the field. But my excitement is less about AI adding more accuracy to the imaging studies performed when assessing cardiac patients and more about adding intelligent automation to the practice of cardiology. Cardiovascular disease is the number one killer in America and number two in the world. Much of this is due to lifestyle factors, the lack of adequate early screening and intervention, cumbersome diagnoses, and the scarcity of specialists.

We have good interventions available to prevent, slow, or treat heart disease. We just need to identify those at risk and intervene sooner. If AI algorithms can allow us to use modern technologies such as cell phones, telehealth, and intelligent bots to collect data, diagnose, and intervene in a more streamlined fashion, we can significantly lower the burden of cardiovascular disease. That means less suffering and lower costs. As such, careful thinking about how AI algorithms can be applied to data from unconventional channels to diagnose disease will be required to ensure these solutions gain traction and can scale up. The most promising aspect of emerging large language models is their ability to accept multimodal inputs such as patients' risk factors for heart disease, available images and output from their wearables and apps, and how they can use that data to identify risk and recommend actions. The current single-task models are more limited in the type of input they can accept per model, but these new models will change the paradigm.

Some of the early efforts at using AI in cardiology involve augmenting the cardiologists by interpreting some of the commonly performed tests such as electrocardiograms (ECGs) and echocardiograms.

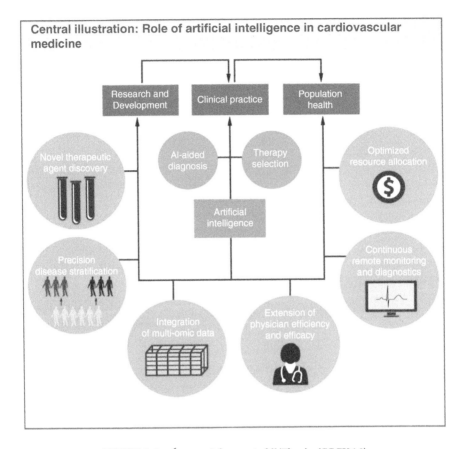

FIGURE 5.4   *(source: Johnson et al.[26]/Elsevier/CC BY 4.0)*

At the moment, when an ECG is performed, a rules-based algorithm provides an initial interpretation that's often ignored by the cardiologist (due to its rudimentary findings and lack of robustness). The early evidence suggests that deep neural network algorithms can vastly improve on this reading. There's also emerging evidence that AI algorithms can be effective at using data from cell phone-based rhythm detection systems to diagnose arrhythmias (Figure 5.4).

AliveCor has a watch-based system for diagnosing atrial fibrillation. The band is a sensor and uses an accelerometer to match activity level with heart rate and rhythm. If they're not concordant, it alerts the patient to place their thumb on the band to record its rhythm. Back in 2014, AliveCor received 501(k) clearance for its afib algorithm. Users who receive a positive result are encouraged to print it out and to confirm their results with a board-certified cardiologist.[20]

Within twelve months, AliveCor had also been given clearance for two other algorithms: its Normal Detector, which reassures users that their ECG is abnormality-free, and its Interference Detector, which alerts people if interference is compromising their ECG tests.[20, 27]

AliveCor and Mayo Clinic researchers have been working together to use AI to create a mobile device that could identify if patients are at risk of a sudden cardiac death. This collaboration has been a major breakthrough when it comes to monitoring the health of the electrical recharging system in patients' hearts. The researchers determined that a smartphone-enabled mobile electrocardiogram (EKG) device can rapidly and accurately determine a patient's QTc, an EKG finding that can provide clues to the heart's electrical system. This can help with identifying patients at risk of sudden cardiac death from congenital long QT syndrome or drug-induced QT prolongation.[28]

Clinicians evaluate QTc (the heart's rate-corrected QT interval) and use it to determine how healthy the heart's electrical recharging system is. If the QTc is equal to or longer than 50 ms, it could lead to dangerously fast heartbeats or even cause sudden death. For the last century, QTc monitoring and assessment has relied on EKGs, but this research shows that it might be time for a change.

The ability of the algorithm to recognize clinically meaningful QTc prolongation via a mobile EKG device is roughly as powerful as EKG assessments made by a trained expert in conjunction with a commercial laboratory. The new device was able to detect QTc values of greater than or equal to 500 ms at an 80% sensitivity rate, meaning that fewer cases of QTc prolongation were missed. It also achieved 94.4% specificity, meaning that if a case was detected, it was almost certainly real.

Using simplified ECG data taken from an Apple Watch, researchers at the Mayo Clinic were also able to use an AI algorithm to spot people whose hearts were having trouble pumping blood out to the rest of their body.[29] Low ejection fraction is often a prelude to or a part of heart failure and needs to be addressed to avoid continued deterioration. Researchers at the clinic previously demonstrated that they could use AI to detect cases of low ejection fraction using a hospital-based ECG machine, which requires 12 leads and multiple electrodes to be wired to the patient's chest. Now, they've shown they can tune the system to get the number of leads down to one. Participants from 11 countries signed up for the study over email. More than 125,000 ECGs were logged over a period of six months. According to the researchers, the test demonstrated an area under the curve of 0.88, a measure of prediction accuracy about equivalent to a treadmill-based cardiac stress test.

As cardiac imaging is a big part of managing cardiac patients, we can expect AI to play a key role in reading these images to augment the cardiologist and allow them to be more accurate, faster, and to make better decisions. Our dreams of automated processing and high-level machine-based interpretation for cardiac imaging are rapidly becoming a reality. If we apply ML to the huge stockpile of quantitative data that's generated per scan and integrate it with clinical data, we'll be able to facilitate a move to more patient-specific interpretation. These developments are unlikely to replace interpreting physicians but will provide them with highly accurate tools to detect disease, risk-stratify, and optimize patient-specific treatment.[30]

According to another study, when Mayo Clinic partnered with Israeli start-up Beyond Verbal, which analyzes the acoustic features in a patient's voice, they were able to identify unique features in the voices of patients with coronary artery disease (CAD). The study found two voice features that were strongly associated with CAD when subjects were describing an emotional experience.[31]

Meanwhile, Google is working to help providers to use retinal images to detect cardiovascular issues. They've published a paper that details how their ML algorithms could identify the risk of cardiovascular issues through an analysis of the blood vessels in patients' eyes. The images below are fundus images of the eye, with the green lines being the areas that the neural network used to make its predictions (Figure 5.5).[32]

In a study assessing a new treatment of cholesterol, medical AI company Owkin and biotech company Amgen worked together to show that ML models are more accurate than traditional clinical methods at predicting the risk of severe cardiovascular diseases. The study included 13,700 participants in the placebo group of an Amgen clinical trial evaluating the cholesterol drug Repatha. Owkin's AI algorithms accurately identified which patients were at the highest risk of death, heart attack, or stroke over the next three or more years.[33] Throughout the study, Owkin tested several approaches to AI and used hundreds of different clinical variables. The best-performing model tapped into metrics like age, smoking status, medical history, kidney function, cholesterol count and diabetes, but it also picked up on less-common

Images of the fundus of the eye
Green areas represent blood vessels the neural network is analyzing

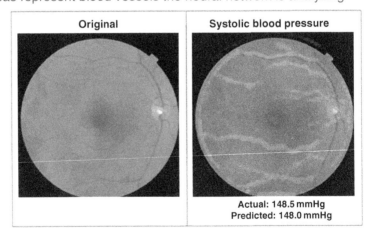

FIGURE 5.5   *(source: Poplin et al.[31]/Springer Nature)*

variables that could help physicians to predict which patients are most at risk of cardiac events.

Subtyping (also called precision phenotyping) of cardiovascular disease is one of the most promising uses for unsupervised learning. Precision medicine in cardiology is different to precision medicine in other fields. With cancer, for example, a series of somatic genetic mutations could clearly define a before and after state. In cardiology, most diseases are slow, multi-morbid, heterogeneous, and chronic, with pathogenesis beginning decades before the disease actually manifests. This is compounded by the fact that many cardiologic diseases, such as heart failure and CAD, are relatively broadly defined and can be arrived at through different pathophysiological mechanisms. Unsupervised learning allows to us enable precision cardiology by learning subtypes of monolithic disease concepts, and ultimately it will help us to treat these subtypes differently and thus lead to improved outcomes.[26]

Researchers from the Smidt Heart Institute at Cedars-Sinai have created an AI tool to help identify hypertrophic cardiomyopathy and cardiac amyloidosis.[34] These two conditions are difficult for even the most seasoned cardiologist to accurately identify, which is why patients often have to wait for years or even decades before they're correctly diagnosed. Fortunately, AI tools can identify disease patterns that can't be seen by human beings and then use them to predict the right diagnosis. After being applied to over 34,000 clinical images, the algorithm focused on features like the size of heart chambers and the thickness of heart walls and used them to identify particular patients that were likely to have cardiac diseases. It was able to spot high-risk patients with a greater amount of accuracy than a trained clinician.

The AI algorithm is also able to process ultrasound videos and to distinguish between heart conditions that resemble either each other or more benign conditions. For example, cardiac amyloidosis (caused by deposits of an abnormal protein in the heart tissue) and hypertrophic cardiomyopathy (which causes the heart muscle to thicken and stiffen) can resemble each other on ECG scans, but their treatments differ significantly.

Another interesting cardiac application of AI was shown in Denmark. Using voice data from calls to Denmark's health emergency hotline, an algorithm was developed to identify cardiac arrest and provide resuscitation instructions.[35] The algorithm analyzed the words, tone of voice, and background noise and correctly predicted cardiac arrest in 93% of cases vs. 73% for humans. It also did this in an average of 48 s, making it 30 s faster than humans. Both the algorithm and humans have the same rate of false positives: 2%. This was made possible because Copenhagen Emergency Medical Service (EMS) has a great audio archive since they record EMS calls and track outcomes.

This is the perfect recipe for an AI solution: a large dataset and a human benchmark that's already available. Now, they're working on other conditions such as strokes and CAD.

5.6   Neurology

We previously touched on algorithms that can predict strokes from atrial fibrillation and characterize plaques in carotid arteries. These fall under the bucket of cardiovascular or neurological diseases. Other neurological applications include the assessment of acute ischemic strokes or intracranial hemorrhage. Viz.ai, a company that uses AI algorithms to do an initial read of head CT scans to identify strokes and alert radiologists and neurologists, became one of the first AI companies to receive an insurance code and reimbursement for their technology.

MaxQ AI's Accipio Ix is an AI workflow tool designed to help clinicians to prioritize adult patients that are likely presenting with acute intracranial hemorrhage.[20] The algorithm has been cleared by the FDA and automatically retrieves and processes non-contrast CT images to provide a case-level indicator. This is what's used to determine which cases are most in need of expert review and medical diagnosis.

AI can also be applied to multiple sclerosis, a disease that currently has no known cure. We're also not entirely sure what causes it, although we know that it occurs because the immune system attacks the myelin sheath in the brain, leading to memory loss, deterioration of muscle control, and other unpleasant symptoms. Google's Verily has teamed up with Brigham and Women's Hospital and Biogen, a biotech company, to carry out a longitudinal study which aims to understand how the disease progresses over time. This combines data from participants wearing a study watch with clinical data fed into Verily's ML algorithms to improve detection and understand what causes the disease to progress and flare up.[36]

Meanwhile, researchers from the Duke University have created an app called Autism & Beyond, which uses the front camera on an iPhone and runs it through facial recognition software to screen children for autism. Similarly, nearly 10,000 people use the mPower app, which provides exercises like finger tapping and gait analysis to study patients with Parkinson's disease who have consented to share their data with the broader research community.[37]

A team from the Stevens Institute of Technology has created an AI tool that has greater than 95% accuracy at diagnosing Alzheimer's disease, removing the need for in-person testing and expensive scans. The algorithm can also explain how it arrived at its conclusions, which makes it easier for human physicians to check its accuracy. Alzheimer's can affect the way that people use language, such as with patients replacing nouns with pronouns or struggling to express themselves. The team designed an explainable AI tool that uses attention mechanisms and a convolutional neural network to accurately identify well-known signs of Alzheimer's, as well as subtle linguistic patterns that were previously overlooked.[38]

The algorithm was trained using text describing children stealing cookies from a jar, which had been written by both healthy subjects and known

Alzheimer's sufferers. Each sentence was converted into a unique numerical sequence that represented a specific point in a 512-dimensional space. This meant that even the most complex of sentences could be given a numerical value, which made it easier for the algorithm to analyze the structural and thematic relationships between different sentences. Using those vectors along with handcrafted features, the AI gradually learned to spot differences between sentences composed by healthy or unhealthy individuals and was able to determine with significant accuracy how likely any given text was to have been produced by a person with Alzheimer's.[38, 39]

In the future, AI tools may be able to diagnose Alzheimer's using any text, from emails to social media posts.[40] However, to develop such an algorithm, researchers would need to train it on many different kinds of texts produced by known Alzheimer's sufferers instead of just picture descriptions.[41]

Combinostics, a neurology technology company, creates a Dementia Differential Analysis report based on the findings of head MRIs. Existing technologies only compare against cognitively normal reference data. The AI-enabled tool goes one step further, quantifying and evaluating patients' MRI data against the distributions of key dementia-specific biomarkers and reference data from 2000 patients who have been diagnosed with a neurodegenerative disease, which includes Alzheimer's disease, frontotemporal dementia, and vascular dementia. This means that in the near future, based on digital biomarkers, a most likely diagnosis will be generated from radiology or other forms of diagnostic study.[42]

5.7   Musculoskeletal

In musculoskeletal medicine, AI promises to play a key role in the coming years and decades. In addition to interpreting radiological studies such as X-rays and MRIs, AI will also help with remote monitoring and assisting patients with their therapies. There are already highly valued companies that use AI to monitor and provide feedback to patients with musculoskeletal issues doing home physical therapy (e.g. Sword and Hinge).

Because of the large number of X-rays that radiologists have to read, patients often have to wait for hours in the emergency room before they can be seen, evaluated, and treated. Fracture interpretation errors represent 24% of all of the harmful diagnostic errors in the ER. These errors and inconsistencies with the diagnosis of fractures are most common between 5 p.m. and 3 a.m., due in part to physician fatigue.

One of the first musculoskeletal AI systems to be approved by the FDA is Imagen's Osteodetect. Osteodetect is a piece of computer-aided detection and diagnosis software that's designed to detect wrist fractures in adult patients by analyzing two-dimensional X-rays for signs of distal radius fractures, which is a common type of wrist fracture.[43] The software helps providers to detect and diagnose by marking the location of the fracture on the image, but it's an adjunct tool that doesn't aim to replace clinician review or their clinical judgment.

Studies demonstrated that the readers' performance in detecting wrist fractures was improved using the software, including increased sensitivity, specificity, and positive and negative predictive values when aided by OsteoDetect, as compared with their unaided performance according to standard clinical practice.[43]

Gleamer AI demonstrated that their algorithm could quickly detect and flag X-rays with positive fractures, helping hospitals to reduce missed fractures by 29%.[44] In this retrospective diagnostic study, 480 X-rays were analyzed by 24 readers who assessed them with and without AI. To simulate a real-life scenario, the study included readers from a range of disciplines, from radiologists and orthopedic surgeons to emergency physicians, rheumatologists, family physicians, and physician assistants, all of whom were used to reading X-rays in clinical practice. Each reader's diagnostic accuracy, with and without the use of AI, was compared against the gold standard. They also assessed the diagnostic performance of AI on its own.

The AI model was trained using a large dataset of X-rays from multiple hospitals to identify pelvis, torso, limb, lumbar spine, and rib cage fractures. It was able to increase sensitivity by 16% for exams with one fracture and by 30% for those with multiple fractures. It could quickly detect and flag X-rays with fractures so that radiologists could prioritize them.

5.8   Oncology

Oncology promises to be one of the many medical specialties where AI can have a huge long-term impact. That's because there are many different types and subtypes of cancer and the successful diagnosis and subtyping of each could lead to better and more personalized management. As a matter of fact, the successful long-term management of cancer will come down to identifying the genetic abnormalities that predispose or lead to that type of cancer and directing therapies to those specific abnormalities. That means analyzing the huge amounts of genetic and other data to identify patterns and link them to individual cancer types. This is perfect for AI, because handling large amounts of multidimensional data and finding patterns is what it's made for.

Given all of the inputs that large language models can accept (e.g. images, text, genomics), they may have their biggest impact in oncology. Also, there are already ChatGPT-style models which are being developed on medical data and which are showing great promise in successfully extracting insights from medical literature. This could mean finding relationships that we weren't aware of before and insights that could accelerate the diagnosis and treatment of cancer

When I speak with oncologists, many indicate that finding new targets will be one of the key contributions of AI. To do that, we'll need large datasets such as proteomics, genomics, transcriptomics, and histologic data. This data is increasingly available, but it's not necessarily in a form that makes it ready to be fed to AI algorithms. Another area would be to find subtle patterns in histopathology data that aren't noticed or looked for by pathologists. Also, a good source of data in oncology is in vitro data, generated in lab by observing the responses to different interventions. In those situations, AI algorithms might be able to see things that normal observation methods can't.

Some of the applications we can expect to see in oncology include (Figure 5.6):

- The increasing number of biological matters and better ways to measure this matter mean that AI can better help to understand disease. AI needs multidimensional data and this data is increasingly becoming available. AI can help to construct new medicines, find new targets and patient populations and identify combination therapies.

- Digital twin technology will be important in oncology, and it can be enabled by the combination of multimodal data and AI. The immune function will be better understood and new therapies developed.

- AI can lead to better diagnostics by picking up on subtle patterns that aren't visible to human eyes.

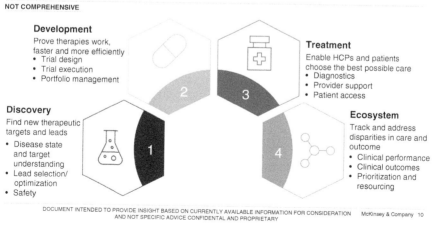

AI can touch everything in oncology – however each application requires specific data and tools

NOT COMPREHENSIVE

Development
Prove therapies work, faster and more efficiently
- Trial design
- Trial execution
- Portfolio management

Treatment
Enable HCPs and patients choose the best possible care
- Diagnostics
- Provider support
- Patient access

Discovery
Find new therapeutic targets and leads
- Disease state and target understanding
- Lead selection/ optimization
- Safety

Ecosystem
Track and address disparities in care and outcome
- Clinical performance
- Clinical outcomes
- Prioritization and resourcing

DOCUMENT INTENDED TO PROVIDE INSIGHT BASED ON CURRENTLY AVAILABLE INFORMATION FOR CONSIDERATION   McKinsey & Company 10
AND NOT SPECIFIC ADVICE CONFIDENTAL AND PROPRIETARY

FIGURE 5.6   *(source: McKinsey & Company)*

5.8.1   Diagnosis and Treatment of Cancer

The detection of cancer has become easier because of the use of AI and deep data mining. Researchers from the Oregon State University successfully used deep learning to extract information from gene expression data that, in turn, helped them to classify different types of breast cancer cells.[45] The authors were able to extract genes from the data that were useful for cancer prediction and also as cancer biomarkers and for breast cancer detection. In an attempt to use AI for the classification of skin cancer, Esteva et al. used CNNs to automatically classify tumors. The performance of the CNN was comparable to that of the dermatologists, which highlights the promise of this approach as a way to classify types of skin cancer.[14]

5.8.2   Histopathological Cancer Diagnosis

Histomorphology has been revolutionized by precision histology. With advances in AI, DNNs have been used to form and implement complex, multiparametric decision algorithms. Machine-driven decisions will improve and optimize approaches in immunohistochemistry, which will provide more rapid and cost-effective diagnoses. Image-based analysis is a cost-effective method that also reduces the workload and eliminates the need for more confirmatory tests.[45]

AI researchers at the AI Precision Health Institute at the University of Hawaii's Cancer Center published two high profile papers demonstrating for the first time that deep learning can distinguish between mammograms of women who'll develop breast cancer and those who won't.[46, 47] In one paper, the researchers confirmed that invasive breast lesions have unique compositional signatures and demonstrated that compositional profiles of the breast combined with CAD predictions can improve the detection of malignant breast cancer (Figure 5.7).[46] In the other, researchers showed that deep learning models performed better than models using clinical risk factors when determining screening-detected cancer risk.[47] The FDA has already approved multiple AI algorithms for the purpose of detecting breast cancer. The best of them has a breast cancer detection sensitivity of 82% and a fixed specificity of 96.6%. When radiologists used the algorithm, it improved sensitivity by 8%.

5.8.3   Tracking Tumor Development

Deep learning has also been used to track and quantify the size of tumors during treatment for the detection of overlooked metastases. The deep learning algorithm becomes more accurate as the number of CT and MRI scans it reads increases.

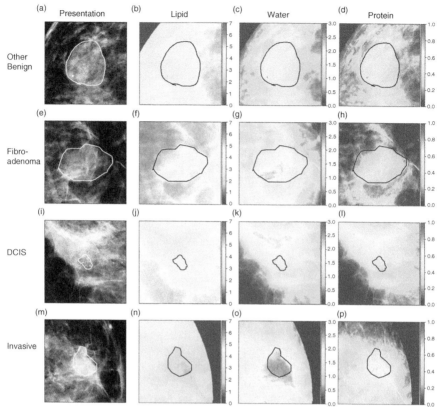

Each row consists of a lesions with a different pathology. a–d contain benign lesions, e–h contain fibroadenomas, i–l contain ductal carcinoma in situ (DCIS), and m-p contain invasive lesions. The first column (a, e, i, m) contains the standard mammogram presentation, the second (b, f, j, n), third (c, g, k, o), and fourth (d, h, l, p) columns contain the corresponding three-compartment breast (3CB) LWP thickness map. Colorbars adjacent to each 3CB map indicate thickness in centimeters where red indicates areas of high thickness and thickness decreases towards the color violet. Thickness ranges are normalized across each column. Yellow lines are radiologist delineations of where biopsies were taken from which lesion pathology was determined.

FIGURE 5.7   AI assists in evaluating the characteristics of breast cancer *(source: Leong et al.[46]/Springer Nature/CC BY 4.0)*

5.8.4   Prognosis Detection

Prognosis establishes the seriousness and the stage of the tumor, which reflects the survival rate of the patient. A model was developed by Lu et al. using deep learning to predict the survival rate of patients who'd undergone a gastrectomy.[48] The deep tool was better at making predictions when compared to the predictions made based on the regular Coz regression. Turkki et al. quantified tumor-infiltrating immune cells in slide analyses of breast cancer samples using an antibody supervised deep learning approach.[49]

There are a number of companies that are pursuing the potential applications of AI in oncology. In addition to helping with image interpretation

Images of a lymph node biopsy with a breast
cancer metastasis
Green areas represent possible tumors according to the algorithm

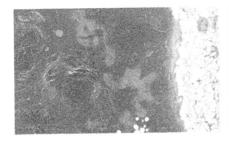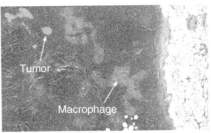

CBINSIGHTS

FIGURE 5.8   *(source: CB Information Services, Inc.)*

such as in mammography and body scanning to find lesions, there's the analysis of genomics and mutations and the process of matching those with the
best treatment combinations and clinical trials. Tempus uses clinical and
biological data to create a digital twin and uses nearest neighbor analysis to
find the best course of management.[37]

Arterys Inc., a medical imaging software provider, has been given 510(k)
clearance for Artyrys Oncology AI suite, which is a web-based tool that helps
clinicians to analyze MRIs and CTs to look for liver and lung cancer. The tool
uses deep learning algorithms to expedite the interpretation of these images
(Figure 5.8).[20]

Meanwhile, start-ups like Freenome are using AI to spot patterns in cell-
free biomarkers in the blood that could be associated with cancer.[37] In 2017,
Freenome released research on tumor identification in which algorithms
were trained on existing images of breast cancer that had metastasized to
adjacent lymph nodes. The algorithms could detect tumors with 92% accuracy, allowing for some false positives (such as macrophages that might look
like tumors).[50] It's Freenome's hope that it will be able to detect cancer earlier
by picking up on the trace amounts of DNA that tumors shed into the blood-
stream, thus circulating tumor DNA.

Google has made significant investments in pursuing AI applications
in healthcare, including in oncology. In 2017, it partnered with the UK's
National Health Service and the Cancer Research UK Centre at Imperial
College London to continue working towards the early detection of breast
cancer. At the same time, DeepMind is working on other cancers, including
head and neck cancer. DeepMind is focused more on treatment design, with
the goal of using AI to speed up the mapping process to determine where to
apply radiotherapy. The current mapping process takes approximately four
hours—DeepMind believes it can shorten it to one.[36]

5.9   GI

The detection of small polyps in real-time to assist gastrointestinal (GI) doctors while performing colonoscopies can improve the diagnosis of these often precancerous lesions. A prospective study showed that AI can be accurate in helping to find small polyps.[51] A team of researchers from Harvard Medical School and Beth Israel Deaconess Medical Center have been working with the Sichuan Academy of Medical Sciences and the Sichuan Provincial People's Hospital in China, and they've been able to use ML to spot adenomatous polyps during colonoscopies.

Announced by Chinese AI vendor Shanghai Wision AI Co, the findings could ultimately lead to "self-driving" during colonoscopy procedures. The model used 5545 images (65.5% of which contained polyps and 34.5% of which didn't) from the de-identified colonoscopy reports of nearly 1300 patients. The algorithm was validated using four independent datasets (two for image analysis and two for video analysis). Researchers have said that this deep learning-based system has a high performance both with colonoscopy images and real-time videos.

Being able to detect and remove precancerous polyps during a colonoscopy is the ideal way to prevent colon cancer. However, the research shows that the "miss rate" for the more than 14 million colonoscopies carried out each year in the US for adenomas is 6%–27%. That's because it's hard for clinicians to visually recognize these polyps. That's where the Wision AI algorithm comes in, acting as a "second set of eyes" and boosting detection rates by as much as 30%.

5.10   COVID-19

AI algorithms have played a key role in diagnosis and treatment planning for COVID-19, and we'll touch on some of these areas later on in the chapter on clinical decision support. In the meantime, it's worth reviewing some of the many ways that AI has played a role in this pandemic. As early as March 2020, researchers were using an AI algorithm that had been trained by data from the 2003 SARS outbreak to predict the number of new infections we could expect to see over time.

Since the beginning of the pandemic, start-ups, universities, and biopharma have used AI to better understand the structure of the novel coronavirus, to identify promising new compounds for treatment, to find existing FDA-approved compounds that could be repurposed, and even to design drug molecules that are structurally stable. To study the structure of SARS-CoV-2, the virus that causes COVID-19, researchers at the University of Texas in Austin and the National Institute of Health used software called cryo-SPARC to create a 3D model of the virus from 2D images captured using cryo-electron microscopy—a technique that can capture molecular structures.[37]

The cryoSPARC software, developed by Structural Biotechnology, uses neural networks to tackle the problem of "particle picking" or detecting and isolating protein structures in the microscopic images.

Recursion has used AI to better understand the virus. In a controlled environment, healthy cells were infected with the SARS-CoV-2 virus, and the microscopic images were analyzed using deep learning to identify the physical changes that occur in these cells as a result of the infection.[37]

During their research, they discovered some DNA that was distinctly different from earlier coronaviruses, mimicking a protein that helps our bodies to regulate the balance of salt and fluid.[52] Through the use of AI, researchers have been able to pinpoint genetic mutations in COVID-19 that can help with both diagnosis and treatment.

Facebook AI Research has created ML tools that can process X-rays to help doctors to make predictions about how a given patient's COVID-19 might progress. One model looked at the amount of supplementary oxygen that a patient might need, while another tried to predict deterioration.

Meanwhile, PhysIQ has been working with an AI-based COVID-19 Decompensation Index, which uses continuous and multiparameter vital sign data from wearables so that healthcare providers can remotely survey patients with high-risk COVID-19 from their homes. They can then step in and intervene if the symptoms start to get worse. Many of the symptoms and characteristics of COVID-19, like the loss of smell and its effects on blood coagulation, were discovered through the use of AI. Algorithms are being used to diagnose, manage, and treat patients, to watch the spread of the pandemic, to understand its characteristics, and to develop new vaccines.

5.11   Genomics

We've already discussed genomics in the context of specific specialties and how AI can be a powerful tool to use genomics to diagnose and treat diseases. Given the amount of data that each human genome contains, analysis of the data and finding relationships to disease is a Herculean task that can only be done with AI. A single human genome sequence generates between 300GB and 1TB of data.[53]

Being able to analyze this data accurately and cost efficiently will mean much better diagnostics for diseases such as cancer where subtyping the tumor will have a material impact on the therapy. Combining AI with genomics can help oncologists to detect cancer earlier and with higher sensitivity than traditional methods such as biopsies. Many companies in the space are using liquid biopsies to analyze cell-free DNA—short fragments of DNA released from tissues into the blood—to create predictive scores.[53]

As we'll discuss in the chapter on AI's applications in life sciences, large language models can be used to build AI-powered tools like ChatGPT to read the codes that make up the building blocks of the human body. Research has found that it's possible to develop a generalizable program—a "genomic language model"—that could be applied to a variety of different tasks, instead of requiring scientists to build fit-for-purpose AIs to chase answers for each major biological question. This power and flexibility, coupled with the fact that these models can be created using unlabeled data, means that they represent the future of AI in genomics.

There are also applications in infectious disease such as the ability to apply AI to a pathogen's genome, which could help to identify the pathogen or predict antibiotic resistance and susceptibility profiles.

5.12   Mental Health

Mental health has always been present in society. However, it's only in recent decades that it's started being properly diagnosed and managed. The taboo around mental health issues has kept people from reporting it and it's traditionally not been fully integrated into the practice of medicine. Fortunately, a lot of that is now changing. There's been a seismic shift in the recognition of mental health as a major cause of human suffering and as a driver of poor outcomes for other diseases. As such, ever-increasing resources are being directed at addressing mental health issues. In 2021, mental health was the number one recipient of venture dollars amongst all medical specialties.

There's increasing evidence that mental health issues can be diagnosed, monitored, and managed using digital technologies such as cell phones, wearables, and AI. Given that there's less reliance on physical exam findings in the diagnosis and management of mental health issues, it's one of the specialties that's well suited for remote management.

Psychiatry researchers are already tapping into AI to better understand mental illnesses, and they're using this newfound knowledge to build more personalized (and thus more effective) treatment plans. Psychiatry is very different than other fields because mental healthcare specialists don't usually have specific biomarkers or clear findings in an imaging scan that they can use to make a diagnosis. Instead, mental health practitioners usually need to rely on a combination of the patient's medical history and the symptoms that they report themselves. As if that wasn't difficult enough, two patients with the same diagnosis could have dramatically different symptoms.

At the moment, AI is being used to help researchers to more fully assess the heterogeneity of psychiatric conditions. Today's models can sift through the huge amounts of data there is about patient behavior, medical, social, and family histories, responses to earlier treatments and information that's acquired from new devices like smartphones and wearable technologies. They can then help medical practitioners to fine-tune the decisions they have to make about patient care.

One of the goals of AI research is to categorize patients' diagnoses into different condition subgroups so that physicians are able to provide personalized treatment. In a study published in Translational Psychiatry, researchers used ML to identify two forms of post-traumatic stress disorder in veterans, a mild form with relatively few symptoms and a chronic, severe form in which patients experienced high levels of depression and anxiety.[54]

Using ML, it may be possible to identify as many as five different subcategories of post-traumatic stress disorder (PTSD), including mild, severe, cognitive functioning impaired, depressed and anxious, and dissociative. Researchers will also focus on molecular and brain circuit markers, genes and the products of genes, such as proteins and metabolites, with the aim of understanding how they're associated with each of the different forms of PTSD. All of this is made possible by using AI to sift through the massive amounts of data and identify patterns and associations. Array Behavioral Care, a mental health provider, is running a pilot where they'll be using an AI program to scan patient intake stories, categorize and highlight significant phrases, recommend certain paths and cadences of treatment, and offer statistical analysis to clinicians about the likelihood of certain diagnoses.[55]

AI is also being used to incorporate sensor data through wearable health technologies to better manage patients. For example, mental health providers have two choices: they can either ask patients to self-report how they've been sleeping or they can access their sleeping data from devices like smartwatches. This is important because there's a big disconnect between how we think we sleep versus how we actually *do* sleep. If we're able to use a combination of smartwatches and AI technology, we might be able to gain a more objective look at how patients are sleeping. Accurately tracking sleep patterns could give providers an indication of which patients with bipolar disorder might be more at risk of experiencing an episode of mania, allowing for adjustments in medication.[56]

5.13   Diagnostic Bots

The intelligent automation of healthcare won't be easy, but once we achieve it, it will be extremely rewarding. In fact, given how much there is to do in healthcare and the limited supply of people, it's essential for us to tap into AI and bots to make it happen. Intelligent bots can help to answer patients' questions, check in with patients and collect information, provide basic cognitive–behavioral therapy (CBT), and help manage chronic diseases.

The recent launch of ChatGPT, which was built using large language models, hints at the potential for intelligent bots to support patients. This could include more effective triage into the right care setting, responding to medical questions, providing general information about diseases, answering care plan management questions, and scheduling appointments. Of course, to enjoy these benefits from the next generation of bots, the models will need full access to patient records. In medical practice, a single piece of data (such as a lab or a medication) can change the picture of a patient's status and the recommendations that need to be provided. "First-generation" bots are already being used by companies like Ada, Buoy, and K Health to help patients. Bots have been shown to improve patient management workflows by collecting and processing data, formulating plans of action and passing them on to providers. That does a lot of the work for the provider and tapping into these technologies is the only way to do this type of care at scale. The proposed benefits include identifying and prioritizing urgent cases, enhancing patient engagement, alleviating pressure on call centers, and increasing the accuracy of care navigation. Diagnostic bots can also help us to reduce the burden on physicians through the use of automated intake summaries, case prioritization, and better matching between patients and providers.

Triage chatbots are much better than leaving patients to Google their symptoms. With a typical chatbot, a patient can enter their details and answer a number of questions based on their symptoms.[57] After the chat is over, the bot can provide some information about the user's condition and make suggestions about what should come next. This may mean funneling patients into video chats or encouraging them to book an appointment, or it may just mean telling people where they can turn for help if their situation isn't serious and can be treated by over-the-counter medication. The route that any given patient takes is less important than ensuring that they find the resources they need or are sent to the best place to receive care. This technology is becoming a key component of patient engagement and "digital front door" solutions and is helping to relieve the burdens that we're placing on doctors and medical teams.

A recent paper in Nature analyzed the studies carried out on the accuracy of digital and online symptom checkers and associated triage advice. The paper concluded that the accuracy of such solutions is low: 19%–38% for the diagnostic accuracy of primary diagnosis and 49%–90% for triage accuracy. Given that there's a push to adopt these technologies in health systems, there's a significant risk to patients from the use of such tools. They recommended large-scale, real-world trials for the systems to document their accuracy and ensure that they don't pose a threat to patients.[58]

Mental health management is a prime area for the use of AI bots to augment clinicians and provide more support to patients. This is an area where there aren't enough providers to address the mental health crisis, especially with the pandemic. This lack of providers is being combined with the high cost of therapy and the appeal of 24/7 availability to lead to a new generation of AI-powered mental health bots. We already have bots that can carry out basic CBT, but most of them aren't powered by AI. The use of bots can provide a touchpoint that's not currently possible and a source of information, triage assistance, and support. Using technologies like computer vision with AI bots can lead to solutions that can detect patient emotions and respond to them.

Researchers are already using deep learning to understand the facial expressions of people in pain and discomfort, which is particularly useful in situations where patients can't talk. Other researchers are using AI to pick up on positive and negative emotions amongst patients with mental health issues. Amazon's health and wellness tracker Halo integrates voice analysis and ML to analyze how positive or energetic users sound based on emotions like happiness, sadness, or excitement in their voice.[59]

Meanwhile, early-stage start-ups are using CBT, an approach which aims to change negative thoughts and behaviors, as a natural extension of the countless digital diary, mood tracking, and health and wellness apps that are out there. One start-up called X2 AI claims that its bot, Tess, has more than four million paid users. The same company has created a faith-based chatbot called Sister Hope, and they're notable for starting their conversations with clear disclaimers and privacy terms.

AI has improved exponentially at carrying out narrow tasks, such as language processing and generation and image recognition. But, as pioneering deep learning researcher Yoshua Bengio said in a podcast on The AI Element, "[AI] is like an idiot savant," with no notion of psychology, what a human being is, or how it all works.[37] Mental health conditions come with a large amount of variability and subjectivity, and we also need to remember that they're a spectrum. But our brains are wired to believe we're interacting with a human when chatting with bots, as one article in Psychology Today explains, without the complexity of having to decipher nonverbal cues.[37]

5.14   At Home Diagnostics/Remote Monitoring

Healthcare will be very different in the future, thanks to technologies like sensors, wearables, cell phones, computers, and AI. The combination of these technologies will allow the remote provision of care for many situations and conditions. This will usher in an era of convenience and, I believe, better care. Why better care? Because people spend more than 99% of their time outside the clinical setting, and being able to monitor and manage them there will improve outcomes for them, as well as being more convenient. This is all very exciting, but it also comes with a challenge. The remote management of conditions will require a lot of heavy lifting and the current healthcare system isn't set up for it. There aren't enough providers to take care of patients in the clinical setting and when they're out in the wild.

That's where AI comes in. As great as it is to have technologies to monitor patients and collect data, the most difficult part of remote patient management won't be data collection. It will be combining that data with other relevant data for that patient, making sense of it and formulating a plan of action. All of this can be done by AI. As such, AI will be a central technology to how medicine will be practiced in the future.

Our smartphones and wearable devices are being turned into powerful at-home diagnostic tools, and it's all thanks to AI. Companies such as Healthy.io use cell phone cameras and AI for urinalysis at home.[37] It has a product called Dip.io which uses a regular urinalysis dipstick to monitor urinary infections. The test strips are analyzed under different lighting conditions and camera quality through computer vision algorithms. Already commercially available in both Europe and Israel, Dip.io has also been cleared by the FDA.

Besides home testing, point-of-care testing at the doctor's office or in other settings (including home visits by concierge services) is another key application of AI. Sight Diagnostics has a portable device that uses computer vision to do complete blood count (CBC) and chem panels in ten minutes at the point of care. This could lead to self-service labs at the office and unlock time savings, faster treatment decisions, and cost savings.

In recent years, smartphone penetration in the United States has continued to grow. At the same time, deep learning has helped to significantly lower the error rate of image recognition tools. The two of these in combination have helped to open up new possibilities for us to use smartphones as diagnostic tools.

One company called SkinVision uses smartphone cameras to assess skin cancer risk and to monitor skin lesions. A number of platforms are offering ML as a service and integrating with FDA-approved home monitoring devices so that they can alert physicians when they spot an abnormality. Biofourmis is using an AI analytics engine that pulls data from FDA-cleared medical wearables and predicts health outcomes for patients.[37] Then there's ContinUse Biometrics, an Israeli company that's developing its own sensing technology using AI to process over 20 bio-parameters—such as glucose levels, blood pressure, and heart rate—and spot abnormalities. In addition to generating a rich source of daily data, AI-IoT has the potential to reduce time and costs associated with preventable hospital visits.[37]

Gauss surgical, an AI diagnostic company, partnered with biotech company Cellex to develop at-home COVID-19 rapid diagnostic kits. To conduct its antigen test, consumers are guided to apply a nasal swab using one of Cellex's at-home test kits. Gauss' AI app then prompts users to scan the test with their smartphones, and then neural networks process the image and display a result within seconds.[37]

Wearables already used in hospital settings are showing success when used outside of clinical settings to monitor patients and facilitate better outcomes. Current Health's device is an upper-arm wearable that taps into AI to track and analyze patients' vital signs at home, tracking temperature, pulse, respiration, oxygen saturation, and movement. This allows it to offer round-the-clock "ICU-level accuracy" and to provide actionable insights so that clinicians can monitor their patients' health and intervene if it spots a problem. It also has a 90% adherence rate in home settings, which is double the national standard, and it's been proven to reduce readmissions and Emergency Department (ED) visits. The company's proprietary algorithms continuously analyze data to derive a patient's health trajectory by detecting potential indicators of patient decline earlier for faster intervention.[60]

AI-powered passive monitoring is taking off and has huge advantages over the traditional way of monitoring patients. The advantage of passive monitoring, as opposed to data collected from wearables, is that it doesn't require patients or seniors to actively wear a device at all times. Used in a hospital setting, the tech reduces healthcare workers' risk of exposure to COVID-19 by limiting their contact with patients and automating data collection for vital signs. Also, camera-based monitoring is unpopular for the simple reason that a lot of people don't like being watched by a camera. As such, passive monitoring represents a nonintrusive way to keep tabs on people's activities without directly watching them or asking them to wear something (Figure 5.9).

A research team at MIT developed a device called Emerald that can be installed in hospital rooms. Emerald emits signals that are then analyzed using ML as they're reflected back. The device differentiates between patients by their movement patterns, can sense people through some walls, and is sensitive enough to capture subtle movements such as the rise and fall of a patient's chest to analyze breathing patterns.[37]

Radar is one of the most promising areas of monitoring technology. There are already passive monitoring technologies using radar that can be deployed at home. Most recently, the industry has coalesced around standards for

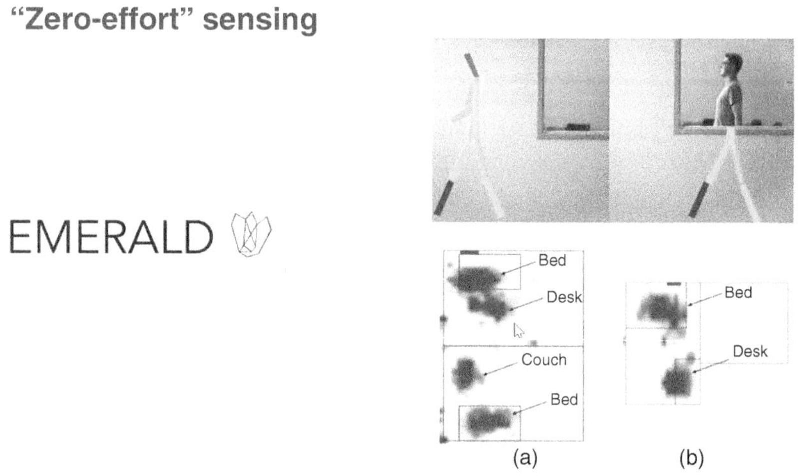

"Zero-effort" sensing

FIGURE 5.9   Passive monitoring allows monitoring of activities without using camera or wearable *(source: CB Information Services, Inc.)*

the use of radar, which has led to the Ripple standard for radar interoperability that's designed to facilitate more rapid adoption for home and hospital monitoring purposes. Radar will be commonplace in consumer and medical applications, and the Ripple standard will help developers to simplify the application creation process so that their software is compatible with radar technologies across different hardware vendors. Companies like Blumio are developing medical applications based on radar to read biomarkers such as blood pressure from outside the body.

Radar sensors could be installed inside a desktop computer or its keyboard to monitor a person's health or to aid pediatric cardiologists when monitoring a baby's heart function. While it might currently take six months to update software to confirm to a new radar standard, Ripple could drastically reduce that time frame.[61]

Caspar.ai has a radar-based passive monitoring system that can create a full report of a senior's activities and monitor them for abnormalities, signs of disease, unsteady gaits, and more. This means that the monitoring will only become obtrusive if something abnormal is detected and the patient requires intervention. Otherwise, it provides reassurance to the operators of long-term care facilities while remaining invisible for the seniors.

Other key applications involve using AI in hardware that can collect key biometric data or enable onsite and remote physical examinations. Companies such as Eko, Tytocare, and Aevice Health allow for the remote examination of heart and lung sounds, eyes, and ears thanks to AI-embedded stethoscopes and other hardware. AI-based smartphone exams are being considered for a number of diagnostic purposes, from skin lesions and rashes to migraine headaches, ear infections, and retinal diseases like diabetic retinopathy and AMD. Then there are apps like AiCure which are using AI to monitor whether patients adhere to their medical treatments. This adds another dimension to the rise of telehealth.

The thinking on telehealth has always been that it can facilitate remote visits for simple conditions but that if the clinician needs to examine the patient or collect labs, the patient will need to do an on-site visit. Well, with these emerging AI-enabled technologies to remotely examine the patient, plus the potential to carry out testing using AI on our cell phones, much more can be done remotely. This means more access to timely care and convenience for patients.

Another way of remotely managing patients is remote monitoring using sensors with the transmission of data to the healthcare providers. This is also an area where the traditional sensor technologies are being enhanced by the use of AI. Clairlab has an AI-based biosensor which is able to remotely monitor patients' physiological markers (such as respiratory rate, heart rate, temperature, and oxygen saturation) with no need for physical contact. It does this by tracking the light particles that are reflected off patients' skin. Clairlab can also monitor behavioral markers like sleep patterns and stress to provide an assessment of a patient's wellbeing. And we've already discussed how PhysIQ uses AI to turn sensor data into digital biomarkers to monitor COVID-19 patients at home.

Remote monitoring devices like insertable cardiac monitors (ICMs) have already provided a huge reduction on the amount of time that clinicians need to spend tracking patients' conditions. French start-up Implicity was recently granted 510(k) clearance by the FDA for its AI software, which is designed to analyze ECG data from ICMs (which are sometimes called implantable loop recorders or ILRs).[62] Their ILR ECG Analyzer sorts through heart rhythm data in search of atrial fibrillation and arrhythmias, and the company says it's more accurate than the implanted monitors themselves. Part of that is due to the fact that ICMs have a reputation for throwing up false-positive alerts of arrhythmia, each of which has to be reviewed and confirmed or rejected by clinicians.

One 2020 study estimated that between 46% and 86% of instances flagged by Medtronic's Reveal Linq device were misdiagnoses.[63] A study of Implicity's technology found that by applying the ML algorithm to ECG data collected by Medtronic's ICMs, they were able to decrease false positives by nearly 80%.[64]

5.15   Sound AI

Given how we're increasingly engaged in the digital world using our smart phones, joining Zoom meetings, exchanging voice messages and interacting with home assistants like Alexa, a huge number of sound files are being created. These sound files are digital and contain structured data. This is a great resource for AI algorithms to mine for health clues. Indeed, we're seeing that AI can analyze all kinds of helpful data to diagnose and track disease. This means that as smart speakers become more ubiquitous and as smartphones expand their use cases, they can be used to improve patients' health.

At the moment, smart speakers are known for playing our favorite music, telling us the weather or reminding us when to get up and take a walk. However, they could also be an important tool for patient management. Researchers from the University of Washington have pioneered a system that allows smart speakers to monitor heartbeats using sonar. ML makes this technology possible.[65] They were even able to detect irregular heart rhythms, which is more challenging than just detecting normal rhythms since those have a regular pattern. The speaker works by emitting a high frequency sound that's inaudible to the human ear and which gets reflected back by the user's chest to be picked up by the microphone array. The researchers then developed a self-supervised learning algorithm to process the signal and to pick up the tiny vibrations in the skin that are caused by the heartbeat. It can even do this against a backdrop of other sounds.

It's able to do this because of the technologies that smart speakers use to pick out a person's voice even when a TV is on or there are multiple different people in the room. The algorithm learns the spatial locations of their heartbeat while simultaneously learning to minimize interferences like environmental noise and respiration. It can then focus specifically on the heartbeat to calculate the intervals between beats.

This is hardly the first time that smart speakers have received attention from the healthcare industry. For example, an insurer called Anthem launched an enhanced version of its Alexa Skills that's available in 13 different commercial insurance markets.[66, 67] The Skills is designed to allow customers to contact an Anthem customer service employee or to order refills on their prescriptions, and it's available to anyone with an Alexa-compatible device or the Alexa mobile app. Google is also using its smart devices for health monitoring, as is shown by the fact that they updated their Nest Hub with a sleep tracking feature. It uses the combination of radar and an algorithm to track sleep and to detect snoring and coughing.[67, 68] In the future, we can expect researchers to build on this work and to detect sleep apnea and cardiac arrests.

Meanwhile, researchers are trying to analyze the sound of coughing to create a cheap tool that could help us to diagnose and stop respiratory diseases like tuberculosis and COVID-19.[69] Delaware's Hyfe has two free smartphone apps (one for researchers and one for consumers) which use AI to track how often people cough, as well as to analyze the sound of it. To do this, they're assembling a database of millions of recordings of people coughing using smartphones and other devices. They're also training AI algorithms to spot patterns and to identify the type and the severity of diseases from the sound of the symptomatic coughing.[70, 71]

In other words, tuberculosis and COVID-19 may have distinctive cough sounds that the AI algorithm can recognize and use to tip off clinicians to the patient's diagnosis before they even see the patient.

ResApp Health Ltd. has an app-based test for cough sounds that helps doctors to diagnose diseases, including COPD, pneumonia, asthma, and bronchitis.[70] Patients are asked to hold their smartphone out and to record five coughs so that the app can analyze the sound and send the results to a doctor.

5.16 AI in Democratizing Care

AI may be able to make certain types of tests and therapeutics more available to a larger swath of the population because it could help frontline clinicians, like primary care doctors and nurse practitioners, to perform specialized testing like ultrasounds. That's because AI can provide real-time guidance and feedback that will enable them to perform these tests in a primary care setting. AI could also help them to interpret those results.

Handheld point-of-care ultrasounds (POCUS) machines can help to change the imaging paradigm because they're sometimes cheap enough for physicians to own them, as opposed to the hospitals. They're also portable, which means that physicians can take them to any care setting that they're working in, including their clinics. This development has important implications for patients in rural healthcare settings who are often referred to distant facilities to get these types of examinations done.[72]

Physicians are now using POCUS to help with diagnostic testing, making it easier for them to rule in or out specific diagnoses. This stops them from being forced to transfer patients to hospitals that are miles away from where they live, only for them to have normal imaging and to be immediately discharged. AI can make this possible. A robust AI on POCUS machines can give the user immediate actionable feedback to improve the image, such as, "Tilt the probe toward the patient's head to acquire the proper apical four chamber image of the heart that includes both atria and both ventricles." This would be a marked improvement over an image which only had the left and right ventricle.[72]

This type of AI feedback has immediate benefits for diagnoses, because it allows physicians to acquire a more standardized and easily interpretable POCUS image. But this is just a short-term benefit, and the long-term impact of immediate AI feedback could be even greater. If AI is built into our POCUS systems, it can perform a role like an expert practitioner at the bedside, but with a lower pressure environment that makes it easier for new POCUS users to gradually improve their skills over time.

It is clear that given the explosion of data in healthcare, successfully analyzing all of this data will be key to better diagnosing many health conditions. AI is the most powerful technology on the horizon to do this. As such, diagnostics will probably be the initial frontier where AI will have its most powerful impact.

References

1. Osman, H. (2019, January 2). New AI imaging tool to accelerate critical patient diagnoses. Healthcare IT News. Retrieved September 11, 2022, from https://www.healthcareitnews.com/news/asia/new-ai-imaging-tool-accelerate-critical-patient-diagnoses
2. Machine Learning in Medical Imaging. (2018, November 14). Signify Research. Retrieved September 11, 2022.
3. Siwicki, B. (2021, May 10). Mass General Brigham and the future of AI in radiology. Healthcare IT News. Retrieved September 11, 2022, from https://www.healthcare-itnews.com/news/mass-general-brigham-and-future-ai-radiology

4. Moor, M., Banerjee, O., Abad, Z. S. H., Krumholz, H. M., Leskovec, J., Topol, E. J., & Rajpurkar, P. (2023). Foundation models for generalist medical artificial intelligence. Nature, 616(7956), 259–265. https://doi.org/10.1038/s41586-023-05881-4

5. Jin, C., Chen, W., Cao, Y., Xu, Z., Tan, Z., Zhang, X., Deng, L., Zheng, C., Zhou, J., Shi, H., & Feng, J. (2020, October 9). Development and evaluation of an artificial intelligence system for COVID-19 diagnosis. Nature Communications, 11(1).

6. Sara Mageit (2020). AstraZeneca partners with Qure.ai for early stage diagnoses of lung cancer. MobiHealthNews

7. Hipolito Canario, D. A., Fromke, E., Patetta, M. A., Eltilib, M. T., Reyes-Gonzalez, J. P., Rodriguez, G. C., Fusco Cornejo, V. A., Duncker, S., & Stewart, J. K. (2022). Using artificial intelligence to risk stratify COVID-19 patients based on chest X-ray findings. Intelligence-Based Medicine, 6, 100049.

8. Shah, F. M., Joy, S. K. S., Ahmed, F., Hossain, T., Humaira, M., Ami, A. S., Paul, S., Jim, M. A. R. K., & Ahmed, S. (2021). A comprehensive survey of COVID-19 detection using medical images. SN Computer Science, 2(6).

9. AI Impact on the Teleradiology Market: The Signify View. 2020, March 26). Signify Research. Retrieved September 12, 2022, from https://www.signifyresearch.net/digital-health/impact-ai-teleradiology-market-signify-view/

10. CB Insights. (2022, June 22). The Big Tech In Healthcare Report: How Facebook, Apple, Microsoft, Google, & Amazon Are Battling For The $8.3T Market. CB Insights Research. Retrieved September 12, 2022, from https://www.cbinsights.com/research/report/famga-big-tech-healthcare/

11. Bejnordi, B., Veta, M., Van Diest, P., et al. (2017). Diagnostic assessment of deep learning algorithms for detection of lymph node metastases in women with breast cancer. JAMA, 318(22), 2199–2210. https://pubmed.ncbi.nlm.nih.gov/29234806/

12. FDA clears Paige's AI as first program to spot prostate cancer in tissue slides. (2021). Fierce Biotech. https://www.fiercebiotech.com/medtech/fda-clears-paige-s-ai-as-first-program-to-spot-prostate-cancer-amid-tissue-slides

13. Liu, Y., Jain, A., & Eng, C. (2020, June). A deep learning system for differential diagnosis of skin diseases. Nature Medicine, 26(6), 900–908.

14. Esteva, A., Kuprel, B., Novoa, R. A., Ko, J., Swetter, S. M., & Blau, H. M. (2017). Dermatologist-level classification of skin cancer with deep neural networks. Nature, 542(7639), 115–118

15. Jain, A., Way, D., & Gupta, V. (2021). Development and Assessment of an Artificial Intelligence–Based Tool for Skin Condition Diagnosis by Primary Care Physicians and Nurse Practitioners in Teledermatology Practices. JAMA Network Open.

16. Google debuts AI-powered app to help consumers identify common skin conditions. (2021). Fierce Healthare. https://www.fiercehealthcare.com/tech/google-previews-ai-dermatology-tool-to-help-consumers-identify-skin-conditions

17. Bui, P. (2021, May 18). Using AI to help find answers to common skin conditions. Google. Retrieved September 13, 2022.

18. Siwicki, B. (2022, February 25). How augmented intelligence can promote health equity. Healthcare IT News. Retrieved September 13, 2022, from https://www.healthcareitnews.com/news/how-augmented-intelligence-can-promote-health-equity

19. Abràmoff, M. D., Lavin, P. T., Birch, M., Shah, N., & Folk, J. C. (2018, August 28). Pivotal trial of an autonomous AI-based diagnostic system for detection of diabetic retinopathy in primary care offices. Npj Digital Medicine, 1(1).

20. Muoio, D. (2018, December 19). Roundup: 12 healthcare algorithms cleared by the FDA. MobiHealthNews. Retrieved September 13, 2022.

21. Gulshan, V., Peng, L., & Coram, M. (2016). Development and validation of a deep learning algorithm for detection of diabetic retinopathy in retinal fundus photographs. JAMA, 316(22), 2402–2410. https://pubmed.ncbi.nlm.nih.gov/27898976/

22. CB Insights. (2020, February 3). How Google Plans To Use AI To Reinvent The $3 Trillion US Healthcare Industry. CB Insights Research. Retrieved September 13, 2022, from https://www.cbinsights.com/research/report/google-strategy-healthcare/

23. Govindaiah, A., Theodore Smith, R., & Bhuiyan, A. (2018). Conference proceedings: Annual International Conference of the IEEE Engineering in Medicine and Biology Society. IEEE Engineering in Medicine and Biology Society, 702–705

24. Schmidt-Erfurth, U, Waldstein, S. M., Klimscha, S., Sadeghipour, A., Hu, X., Gerendas, B.S., Osborne, A., & Bogunović, H. (2018). Prediction of individual disease conversion in early AMD using artificial intelligence. Investigative Ophthalmology & Visual Science, 59, 3199–3208.

25. Peng, Y., Dharssi, S., Chen, Q., et al. (2019). DeepSeeNet: a deep learning model for automated classification of patient-based age-related macular degeneration severity from color fundus photographs. Ophthalmology 126(4), 565–575

26. Johnson, K. W., Soto, J. T., Glicksberg, B. S., Shameer, K., Miotto, R., Ali, M., Ashley, E., & Dudley, J. T. (2018). Artificial intelligence in cardiology. Journal of the American College of Cardiology, 71(23), 2668–2679. https://pubmed.ncbi.nlm.nih.gov/29880128/

27. Comstock, J. (2015, December 1). AliveCor ECG gets FDA clearance for two more algorithms. MobiHealthNews. Retrieved September 13, 2022, from https://www.mobihealthnews.com/40089/alivecor-ecg-gets-fda-clearance-for-two-more-algorithms

28. Giudicessi, J. R., Schram, M., Bos, J. M., Galloway, C. D., Shreibati, J. B., Johnson, P. W., Carter, R. E., Disrud, L. W., Kleiman, R., Attia, Z. I., Noseworthy, P. A., Friedman, P. A., Albert, D. E., & Ackerman, M. J. (2021, March 30). Artificial intelligence–enabled assessment of the heart rate corrected QT interval using a mobile electrocardiogram device. Circulation, 143(13), 1274–1286.

29. Hale, C. (2022). AI researchers at Mayo Clinic use the Apple Watch to detect silent, weakening heart disease. Fierce Biotech. https://www.fiercebiotech.com/medtech/ai-researchers-mayo-clinic-use-apple-watch-detect-silent-weakening-heart-disease

30. Slomka, P. J., Dey, D., Sitek, A., Motwani, M., Berman, D. S., & Germano, G. (2017, March 4). Cardiac imaging: working towards fully-automated machine analysis & interpretation. Expert Review of Medical Devices, 14(3), 197–212.

31. CB Insights (2018). The AI Industry Series: Top Healthcare AI Trends To Watch

32. Poplin, R., Varadarajan, A. V., & Blumer, K. (2018). Prediction of cardiovascular risk factors from retinal fundus photographs via deep learning. Nature Biomedical Engineering, 2, 158–164.

33. Rousset, A., Dellamonica, D., Menuet, R., Lira Pineda, A., Sabatine, M. S., Giugliano, R. P., Trichelair, P., Zaslavskiy, M., & Ricci, L. (2021, November 15). Can machine learning bring cardiovascular risk assessment to the next level? A methodological study using FOURIER trial data. European Heart Journal – Digital Health, 3(1), 38–48.

34. Duffy, G., Cheng, P. P., Yuan, N., He, B., Kwan, A. C., Shun-Shin, M. J., Alexander, K. M., Ebinger, J., Lungren, M. P., Rader, F., Liang, D. H., Schnittger, I., Ashley,

E. A., Zou, J. Y., Patel, J., Witteles, R., Cheng, S., & Ouyang, D. (2022, April 1). High-throughput precision phenotyping of left ventricular hypertrophy with cardiovascular deep learning. JAMA Cardiology, 7(4), 386.

35. Khan, J. (2018). The AI that spots a stopped heart. Bloomberg. https://www.bloomberg.com/news/articles/2018-06-20/the-ai-that-spots-heart-attacks

36. Krishnan, N. (2018, April 26). How google plans to use AI To reinvent the $3 trillion US healthcare industry. Retrieved September 13, 2022, from https://www.linkedin.com/pulse/how-google-plans-use-ai-reinvent-3-trillion-us-nikhil-krishnan

37. CB Insights. (2021, January 5). Healthcare AI Trends To Watch. CB Insights Research. https://www.cbinsights.com/research/report/ai-trends-healthcare/

38. A.I. Tool Promises Faster, More Accurate Alzheimer's Diagnosis 2020, August). Stevens Institute of Technology. https://www.stevens.edu/news/ai-tool-promises-faster-more-accurate-alzheimers-diagnosis

39. Bresnick, J. (2018). Top 12 Ways Artificial Intelligence Will Impact Healthcare. Health IT Analytics. https://healthitanalytics.com/news/top-12-ways-artificial-intelligence-will-impact-healthcare

40. Bresnick, J. (2016). What Is the Role of Natural Language Processing in Healthcare? Health IT Analytics. https://healthitanalytics.com/features/what-is-the-role-of-natural-language-processing-in-healthcare

41. Elias, H. (2020, September 21). AI diagnoses Alzheimer's with more than 95% accuracy. TechHQ. Retrieved September 13, 2022, from https://techhq.com/2020/09/ai-diagnoses-alzheimers-with-more-than-95-accuracy/

42. Siwicki, B. (2022, May 18). AI-enabled app evaluates MRI data to help analyze dementia. Healthcare IT News. Retrieved September 13, 2022, from https://www.healthcareitnews.com/news/ai-enabled-app-evaluates-mri-data-help-analyze-dementia

43. Office of the Commissioner. 2018, May 24). FDA permits marketing of artificial intelligence algorithm for aiding providers in detecting wrist fractures. U.S. Food and Drug Administration. Retrieved September 14, 2022, from https://www.fda.gov/news-events/press-announcements/fda-permits-marketing-artificial-intelligence-algorithm-aiding-providers-detecting-wrist-fractures

44. Guermazi, A., Tannoury, C., Kompel, A. J., Murakami, A. M., Ducarouge, A., Gillibert, A., Li, X., Tournier, A., Lahoud, Y., Jarraya, M., Lacave, E., Rahimi, H., Pourchot, A., Parisien, R. L., Merritt, A. C., Comeau, D., Regnard, N. E., & Hayashi, D. (2022, March). Improving radiographic fracture recognition performance and efficiency using artificial intelligence. Radiology, 302(3), 627–636.

45. Londhe, V. Y., & Bhasin, B. (2019, January). Artificial intelligence and its potential in oncology. Drug Discovery Today, 24(1), 228–232.

46. Leong, L. T., Malkov, S., Drukker, K., Niell, B. L., Sadowski, P., Wolfgruber, T., Greenwood, H. I., Joe, B. N., Kerlikowske, K., Giger, M. L., & Shepherd, J. A. (2021, August 31). Dual-energy three-compartment breast imaging for compositional biomarkers to improve detection of malignant lesions. Communications Medicine, 1(1).

47. Hinton, B., Ma, L., Mahmoudzadeh, A. P., Malkov, S., Fan, B., Greenwood, H., Joe, B., Lee, V., Kerlikowske, K., & Shepherd, J. (2019, June 22). Deep learning networks find unique mammographic differences in previous negative mammograms between interval and screen-detected cancers: a case-case study. Cancer Imaging, 19(1).

48. Lu, S., Yan, M., Li, C., Yan, C., Zhu, Z., & Lu, W. (2019). Machine-learning-assisted prediction of surgical outcomes in patients undergoing gastrectomy. Chinese Journal of Cancer Research, 31(5), 797–805.

49. Turkki, R., Linder, N., Kovanen, P. E., Pellinen, T., & Lundin, J. (2016, January). Antibody-supervised deep learning for quantification of tumor-infiltrating immune cells in hematoxylin and eosin stained breast cancer samples. Journal of Pathology Informatics, 7(1), 38.

50. Stumpe, M., Peng, L. (2017, March3). Assisting Pathologists in Detecting Cancer with Deep Learning. Google AI Blog. Retrieved September 14, 2022, from https://ai.googleblog.com/2017/03/assisting-pathologists-in-detecting.html

51. Miliard, M. (2018, November 5). AI algorithms show promise for colonoscopy screenings. Healthcare IT News. Retrieved September 14, 2022, from https://www.healthcareitnews.com/news/ai-algorithms-show-promise-colonoscopy-screenings

52. Miliard, M. (2020, December 1). Mayo Clinic CIO says AI has been key to understanding COVID-19. Healthcare IT News. https://www.healthcareitnews.com/news/mayo-clinic-cio-says-ai-has-been-key-understanding-covid-19

53. CB Insights. (2020, December 22). Can Applying AI To Genomics Improve Healthcare? CB Insights Research. https://www.cbinsights.com/research/ai-genomics-healthcare/

54. Siegel, C. E., Laska, E. M., Lin, Z., Xu, M., Abu-Amara, D., Jeffers, M. K., Qian, M., Milton, N., Flory, J. D., Hammamieh, R., Diagle Jr., B. J., Gautam, A., Dean, K. R., Reus, V. I., Wolkowitz, O. M., Mellon, S. H., Ressler, K. J., Yehuda, R., Wang, K., … Marmar, C. R. (2021). Utilization of machine learning for identifying symptom severity military-related PTSD subtypes and their biological correlates. Nature. https://www.nature.com/articles/s41398-021-01324-8

55. Siwicki, B. (2023, June 14). AI, licensing and remote prescribing among key issues facing telepsychiatry. Healthcare IT News. https://www.healthcareitnews.com/news/ai-licensing-and-remote-prescribing-among-key-issues-facing-telepsychiatry

56. Lindsey, H. (2021, September 30). AI's push to understand psychiatry research has the potential to tackle mental illness. Business Insider. Retrieved September 14, 2022, from https://www.businessinsider.in/science/health/news/ais-push-to-understand-psychiatry-research-has-the-potential-to-tackle-mental-illness/articleshow/86651895.cms

57. HIMSS Insights Ebook Series: Artificial Intelligence. (2018). HIMSS (Health Information Management Systems Society.

58. Wallace, W. J., Chan, C. K., Chidambaram, S., Hanna, L., Iqbal, F. M., Acharya, A., Normahani, P., Ashrafian, H., Hanna, G. B., Sounderajah, V., & Darzi, A. (2022). The diagnostic and triage accuracy of digital and online symptom checker tools: a systematic review. Npj Digital Medicine, 5(1).

59. CB Insights. (2022a, January 28). 12 Tech Trends To Watch Closely In 2021. CB Insights Research. Retrieved September 14, 2022, from https://www.cbinsights.com/research/report/top-tech-trends-2021/

60. Landi, H. (2019). Current Health's AI wearable for keeping chronically ill patients out of the hospital gets FDA clearance. Fierce Healthcare. https://www.fierce-healthcare.com/tech/ai-wearable-device-for-home-care-gets-fda-clearance

61. Hamblen, M. (2022). Ripple spec to boost radar sensing for years to come, proponents say. Fierce Electronics. https://www.fierceelectronics.com/sensors/ripple-spec-boost-radar-sensing-years-come-proponents-say

62. Park, A. (2021, December 17). FDA clears implicity's AI heart algorithm to improve Medtronic monitors' afib detection. Andrea Pak, Fierce Biotech. Retrieved

December 11, 2022, from https://www.fiercebiotech.com/medtech/fda-clears-implicity-s-ai-algorithm-to-improve-medtronic-heart-monitors-afib-detection

63. Afzal, M. R., Mease, J., Koppert, T., Okabe, T., Tyler, J., Houmsse, M., Augostini, R. S., Weiss, R., Hummel, J. D., Kalbfleisch, S. J., & Daoud, E. G. (2020). Incidence of false-positive transmissions during remote rhythm monitoring with implantable loop recorders. Heart Rhythm, 17(1), 75–80. https://pubmed.ncbi.nlm.nih.gov/31323348/

64. Rosier, A., Crespin, E., Lazarus, A., & Laurent, G. (2021). A novel machine learning algorithm has the potential to reduce by 1/3 the quantity of ILR episodes needing review. European Heart Journal, 42(Supplement_1), ehab724.0316.

65. Wang, A. (2021). Using smart speakers to contactlessly monitor heart rhythms. Communications Biology, 4(1), 1–12.

66. Minemyer, P. (2020). Anthem launching enhanced version of its Alexa skill in 13 commercial markets. Fierce Healthcare. https://www.fiercehealthcare.com/payer/anthem-launching-enhanced-version-its-alexa-skill-13-commercial-markets

67. Horowitz, B. (2021). Alexa, do I have an abnormal heart rhythm? UW researchers use AI and smart speakers to monitor irregular heartbeats. Fierce Healthcare. https://www.fiercehealthcare.com/tech/alexa-do-i-have-an-abnormal-heart-rhythm-uw-researchers-use-ai-and-smart-speakers-to-monitor

68. Landi, H. (2021). Google moves further into health and wellness monitoring with updated Nest Hub that tracks sleep. Fierce Healthcare. https://www.fiercehealthcare.com/tech/google-moves-further-into-health-and-wellness-monitoring-new-nest-hub-tracks-sleep

69. Dizik, A. 2020, September 14). Flu vs. Covid: Ways to Identify Symptoms and Differences. WSJ. Retrieved September 16, 2022, from https://www.wsj.com/articles/flu-vs-covid-ways-to-identify-symptoms-and-differences-11600088401?mod=article_inline

70. Loten, A., & Hand, K. 2021, July 8). How Computers With Humanlike Senses Will Change Our Lives. WSJ. Retrieved September 16, 2022, from https://www.wsj.com/articles/how-computers-with-humanlike-senses-will-change-our-lives-11625760066?mod=article_inline

71. McKay, B. 2021, September 8). Coughs Say a Lot About Your Health, if Your Smartphone Is Listening. WSJ. Retrieved September 16, 2022, from https://www.wsj.com/articles/diagnose-respiratory-illness-smartphone-11631041761

72. Jercich, K. (2022, May 2). How AI can increase the effectiveness of point-of-care ultrasounds. Healthcare IT News. Retrieved September 16, 2022, from https://www.healthcareitnews.com/news/how-ai-can-increase-effectiveness-point-care-ultrasounds

CHAPTER 6

Therapeutics

DIGITAL THERAPEUTICS have gained momentum in recent years. What was once thought to be an adjunctive form of treatment at best and a toy at worst is now headed toward mainstream clinical practice. There are FDA-approved solutions for a number of conditions, including addiction, depression, and post-traumatic stress disorder (PTSD). Some of these are prescription treatments and are becoming part of the treatment guidelines for certain conditions. Digital therapeutics that are powered by behavioral science, patient data, and artificial intelligence (AI) are able to help patients to adopt and sustain healthier behaviors through engagement-based functionality like gamification.

There're also expanding applications to areas like musculoskeletal disease and chronic disease management. We hear about other potential applications of AI in therapeutics almost every day. These now include the use of machine vision in surgeries and with robotics, assistance in microsurgery such as in eye radiation therapy improvement, and more.

Juniper Research, a UK-based analyst, found that the number of people using wellness apps and digital therapeutics is set to grow from 627 million in 2020 to more than 1.4 billion in 2025, a rise of 123.3%.[1] And that's not all. Over the same period of time, the value of this market is expected to grow by nearly ten times, from $5.8 billion to over $56 billion. This robust growth will be driven by the myriad of applications many of which are still in the research stage.

My feeling on digital therapeutics is that the current use cases in healthcare are just the tip of the iceberg. We're barely scratching the surface, and in the near future, we'll be relying on it for many different therapeutic applications. The large language models that underpin ChatGPT suggest that a new generation of AI models could be developed using more complete clinical datasets. These can result in surprisingly effective applications that can do a better job of diagnostics, therapeutics, and patient management. Some of these tools could include more intelligent bots to help with chronic disease management, more effective CBT for mental health, and real-time assistance in surgical suites. Although some of these are already being used, their capabilities are far more limited than what's promised by new models trained on the vast amounts of historic medical literature and data that are available to us.

6.1   Robotics

The use of robotics in healthcare isn't new. The Davinci system has been used for various types of surgeries and the use cases have been expanding for some time now. Recently, with the introduction of AI in healthcare and its expanding use cases, some interesting overlaps between these two areas are emerging.

One of the first areas where we're seeing interesting synergies is in the operating room. Although this is still in its early stages, the use cases being discussed involve improving surgeons' decision-making, increasing the precision of procedures, improving the economics and workflow of the operating room and surgery, and using predictive analytics to see which patients have the highest risk of complications (Figure 6.1).

Certain algorithms are being piloted that guide imaging that helps surgeons make their surgery more precise. This could be an intermediate step before we reach full robotics use guided by AI. Intuitive Surgical is one of the companies that's currently experimenting with such systems. Harrison AI is an Australian company that uses AI to read pathology slides for better and faster pattern recognition, which is a critical and time-consuming step in the OR during surgery.[2]

Cognitive robotics can integrate information from pre-operation medical records with real-time operating metrics to guide and enhance the precision of physicians' instruments. By processing data from genuine surgical experiences, they're able to provide new and improved insights and techniques. These kinds of improvements can improve patient outcomes and boost trust in AI throughout the surgery. Robotics can lead to a 21% reduction in length of stay.[3]

AI in healthcare: assisted robotics surgery

- These robots are well-suited for procedures that require the same, repetitive movements as they are able to work without fatigue
- AI can identify patterns within surgical procedures to improve best practices and to improve a surgical robot's control accuracy to sub-millimeter precision

FIGURE 6.1   *(source: Original Research)*

This is also one of the most promising areas for the new General Medical AI (GMAI) models that are trained using large language models. These models can take different inputs (e.g. text, images, and video) and act as an assistant in the OR. They can be asked questions and be expected to respond in real time with rapid analysis of the available data. Moor et al. have discussed a GMAI model that can assist surgical teams with procedures, carrying out visualization tasks and even annotating video streams of procedures in real time.[4] They can also reason through findings that they've not been trained on but arrive at a reasonable answer based on their overall training on vast amounts of data.

Verily has partnered with Johnson & Johnson to create Verb Surgical, a robotic surgery company that "involves machine learning, robotic surgery, instrumentation, advanced visualization and data analytics".[5] Meanwhile, human-like robots with humanoid features and temperaments are already being made, especially in Japan. These robots can be powered by AI software and perform a multitude of tasks including providing assistance and even companionship for the elderly. They can make eye contact and track humans, using sensors to detect moods and respond appropriately.

Intuition Robotics has created a robot, ElliQ, that will be used to help seniors with a variety of tasks including by providing medication reminders, wellness suggestions, and friendly conversations in a "proactive and empathetic" manner.[6] This is an in-home, AI-enabled companion robot that's designed to increase seniors' independence and keep them socially active. Through voice commands, emotive gestures, or its paired tablet screen, seniors can use the device to initiate video calls, send messages, schedule appointments, and receive medication reminders. ElliQ is designed to proactively initiate conversations with its users or to suggest activities like physical exercises, trivia games, sleep relaxation exercises, or informational discussions on nutrition.

6.2   Mental Health

We've already discussed how AI and mobile devices can be a powerful combination to remotely diagnose and monitor mental health conditions. The emerging digital biomarkers that can detect mood based on voice, activity, and interaction with smart devices will be vital for the better diagnosis and management of mental health. It turns out that this same combination can also be effective in treating mental health issues.

The high costs of mental health therapy and the appeal of round-the-clock availability are giving rise to a new era of AI-based mental health bots. Mindstrong Health, now part of Sondermind, uses AI to diagnose and treat neuropsychiatric disorders. The company's patient-facing app provides healthcare providers with real-time tracking of cognition and mood and also offers CBT.[7]

Mental health is a spectrum, with high variability in symptoms and sub-jectivity in analysis. But our brains are wired to believe we're interacting with a human when chatting with bots, and this can be powerful when providing the companionship and guidance that the current healthcare system could never offer. This on-demand support for the large number of patients suffering from mental health conditions isn't possible at present due to resource shortages and a lack of providers.

During a time when healthcare providers face unprecedented demand, internet-based CBT provides accessible, effective, clinically proven support for people with mild-to-moderate symptoms. This in turn alleviates wait times, frees up capacity, and addresses other potential barriers to care such as stigma and transportation issues. In a randomized controlled trial, published in Nature's *npj Digital Medicine*, internet-based CBT programs were both effective and potentially cost-effective in treating depression and anxiety.[8]

As mentioned in the previous chapter, most modern CBT applications aren't AI-based. Traditional training for AI-based CBT applications takes time, as the underlying data is challenging to collect or access and is often unstructured. This is where emerging large language models could represent a breakthrough in enabling the more effective training of models that allow for better CBT based on unstructured data.

The fact that generative AI models like ChatGPT, trained on large amounts of general data, have the power to respond to patient questions with reason-able accuracy, could suggest that models trained on therapeutic area-specific literature could be even more accurate. As they're trained on vast amounts of clinical literature, they can tap into most of the body of evidence that's avail-able to engage in meaningful patient interactions.

This is especially relevant in mental health, as the data needed to mean-ingfully interact with the individual can be supplied by the patient. This includes their current mood, new thoughts and feelings, and their previous diagnoses and medications. There's far less reliance on lab or imaging data for patients with mental health conditions, which means that the mental health bots that don't already have access to the totality of the patients' medical records can still help to address acute situations.

Emotional AI is the attempt to use AI to recognize and respond to emo-tion, and it's not a new concept. The idea is largely associated with American scholar and inventor Rosalind Picard and her early research on the topic, which is also known as affective computing and is defined as "computing that relates to, arises from or deliberately influences emotions". Today, the $87 billion global market for affective computing has far-reaching potential, and interest in the space has been gradually building. Machines employing emotional AI attempt to interpret human emotion from text, voice patterns, facial expressions, and other non-verbal cues. In many cases, they'll simu-late those emotions in response. By tapping into unspoken behaviors and reactions, AI can leverage this "emotional data" to increase gains and better cater to patients. This can be an important aspect of addressing the growing mental health crisis.

6.3   Precision Medicine

Genomics is enabling more individualized treatment by providing insights into which genes contribute to various medical conditions. For example, scientists are currently using genomics to understand how COVID-19 spreads and affects the immune system. This information could help with vaccine development.

A single human genome sequence generates between 300 GB to 1 TB of data. Technological improvements have driven down the costs of sequencing—a historically expensive process—and caused an explosion in genomic data over the past decade. This has created multiple opportunities for AI in the space. Companies are working to commercialize AI-based genomics solutions to develop better pharmaceuticals, power more accurate disease diagnosis, and help physicians to identify the most effective treatments.

In many big data applications, data loses its value over time, but the opposite is true for genomics. As genomics datasets grow, they can be reanalyzed to discover new mutations or biomarkers. Further, AI can improve treatment recommendations for patients using population-level data.

By analyzing massive amounts of genomic and clinical data, AI-based solutions can help physicians determine the right treatment for each patient. Precision medicine is projected to be a $217 billion market by 2028. Use cases here can include identifying the various mutations that can further subtype a disease and spotting the best candidates from the different available therapies. It also includes dosing optimization based on genotypic or phenotypic characteristics, as well as biomarker analysis and linkage to disease and therapy selection.

AI can have a big impact in oncology through the analysis of genomics and mutations and matching those with the best treatment combinations and the right clinical trials (Figures 6.2 and 6.3). Tempus taps into clinical and biological data to create a digital twin and uses nearest neighbor analysis to find the best course of management. Another start-up developing AI-driven genomic solutions is South Korea-based Syntekabio, which analyzes an individual's unique genetic map to provide personalized medical treatments. SOPHiA Genetics's technology is used by around 1,000 hospitals to detect genomic variants and determine the proper course of treatment for cancer, hereditary disorders, and COVID-19.[7] Also, using AI algorithms on radiology images can improve radiation treatment in cancer. Varian Medical Systems trains algorithms on diagnostic images to automate radiotherapy treatment planning.

Imagene, an AI start-up, directs cancer patients to the proper targeted therapies using only digital images of biopsied tissue, instead of relying on

TREATMENT: EMR- and claims-based AI model identified patients likely to benefit

Challenge

Recently approved asset for an advanced cancer with **low incidence combined with low diagnosis** and **underdiagnosis**

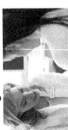

Unclear burden and clinical definition of disease in different stages

Needed to **identify risk factors** that **increase the likelihood to progress** to an **advanced cancer**

Approach

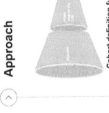

Cohort definition funnel

Data

RWE EMR- and claims-based cohort definitions were built while overcoming:

- Real world **patient behavior** and **visibility** skewed observations

- **Lack of a standardized treatment approach** complicated ability to identify patients

Analytics

More than 100 features identified in EMR and claims data as potential risk factors were **defined and programmed**

Trained 3 classes of advanced analytics models to predict risk at the patient level

Impact

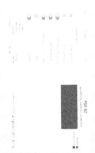

The final model improved on the baseline model by:

26%

as measured by the C-Index[1]

16x

Improved **identification of potential patients** likely to benefit from treatment

1. Concordance index

FIGURE 6.2   *(source: McKinsey & Company)*

ECOSYSTEM: Understanding treatment adoption and variation

Challenge

Dozens of **imperfect, incomplete data sources**
- Low resolution sales
- Partial visibility claims
- Blinded EMR data
- Affiliations
- Epidemiology

Approach

Features and modeling

100s of nuanced clinical journey features defined with expert input

Bayesian statistical modeling and ML to integrate cross-data insights

Care visibility and variability

Significant variability across HCPs and institutions
- Molecular testing rates
- Regimen selection
- Dosing
- Duration

Impact

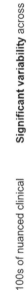

Shift outreach to redress gaps in

~25%

of providers

FIGURE 6.3   *(source: McKinsey & Company)*

full molecular sequencing and analysis. Imagene says its deep learning algorithms can pick out the biomarkers needed to guide treatments within just two minutes by visualizing the patterns put forward by tumor cells that carry different mutations.[9] AI is also being applied to other omics data to guide treatment recommendations. For example, Cofactor Genomics uses "Predictive Immune Modeling" based on transcriptomic data to create multi-dimensional biomarkers that can predict a patient's therapeutic response.[10]

Much of what is discussed in this section and the chapter can also be considered Decision Support. There is another chapter that goes deeper into some of these topics. However, given the impact of AI in the selection of therapeutics, it is worth to discuss some of that in this chapter also.

6.4 Chronic Disease Management

Chronic disease management is complicated and onerous, both for the care team and for the patients. Most chronic disease management programs haven't shown significant ROI. It's a daily process that requires attention, follow-through, follow-ups, and ongoing communication. Most patients don't have the time or patience for it and most care teams don't have enough resources to do it well. A lot of chronic disease management comes down to figuring out how the patient is doing with their diseases and addressing their issues. This is laborious and time-consuming, but if you dissect it carefully enough, you can see that we're increasingly using tools that can automate much of it.

Data collection is getting much more streamlined thanks to sensors, cell phones, wearables, interactive questionnaires, and other tools. Basic decision-support software is now being used for both patients and providers. These decision-support software applications are currently mostly rules-based and limited in what they can do, but they're good for first-line support and can obviate the need for the care team to get involved with basic tasks. The next generation of decision-support software could be powered by AI, trained on large sets of data, use emerging language models, and analyze similar scenarios for it to learn from. This means that it will be much more dynamic in its assessments. It's not as though this will be available to us tomorrow, but some versions of it are already being rolled out.

One example of this is in diabetes. Due to the explosion of obesity in the United States (and the rest of the world), this is now a disease that's consuming major resources and dollars in our healthcare system. Diabetes management requires monitoring blood glucose on a daily basis and adjusting the patient's treatment, sometimes daily if they're taking insulin. This is perfect for AI: identifying patterns in long-term data and making recommendations on what should be done next to optimize for the defined outcomes. AI solutions can make treatment recommendations based on the analysis of how thousands and millions of patients have responded to different treatments.

Recently, the University of Utah Health, the Regenstrief Institute, and Hitachi announced the development of a new AI approach that could improve treatment for patients with Type 2 diabetes mellitus.[11] Researchers from all three organizations collaborated to develop and test a new AI approach to analyzing EHR data across Utah and Indiana. As they did so, they uncovered some patterns for Type 2 diabetes patients with similar characteristics. The hope is that those patterns can now be used to help determine optimal drug regimens for specific patients.

Pooling data from different institutions enabled an AI-based approach that groups patients with similar disease states and then analyzes treatment patterns and clinical outcomes. The model then matches specific patients to the disease state groups and predicts a range of potential outcomes depending on different treatment options.

Researchers assessed how well this method worked for predicting successful outcomes for drug regimens administered to patients with diabetes in Utah and Indiana. Their findings showed that the algorithm was able to support medication selection for more than 83% of patients, even when two or more medications were used together.[12]

Part of the thinking behind this effort was that while 10% of adults throughout the world have been diagnosed with Type 2 diabetes, a smaller percentage requires multiple medications to control blood glucose levels and avoid serious complications, such as the loss of vision and kidney disease. For this group of patients, physicians may have limited clinical decision-making experience or evidence-based guidance for choosing drug combinations. It's hoped that this new AI-enabled clinical approach can help patients who require complex treatment by checking the efficacy of various drug combinations.

Still on the subject of diabetes, Twin Health's Whole Body Digital Twin platform collects thousands of data points each day from wearable sensors, then combines those readings with the results of blood tests and self-reported questionnaires to build a computer model of each patient. The AI continuously updates and analyzes the model to spot problem areas in a patient's individual metabolism and suggest potential changes and improvements for their nutrition, activity, sleep, and breathing, all with the ultimate goal of reversing diabetes symptoms. In a clinical trial, they showed impressive results using this approach to reverse diabetes.[13]

The company's clinical trial analyzed 199 patients who'd been diagnosed with diabetes for an average of almost four years and who began the study with an average A1C of 9%. After six months, researchers found that with the sustained use of the digital twin technology, almost 95% saw A1C levels drop below 6.5%. They reported an average drop of 3.3 points compared to improvements of just 0.39 in the trial's control group, which received the current standard of care for Type 2 diabetes. The digital twin group was able to achieve that drop without relying on any medications besides metformin. In addition, all nine of the patients who'd been using insulin were able to stop injections before the 90-day point.

Chronic pain is another area that's a source of significant morbidity for patients, leading to a high amount of use for healthcare resources. Its treatment often involves a variety of procedures and can lead to long-term narcotic addiction. Interesting areas that are being explored for the management of chronic pain include immersive experiences with virtual reality (VR). AI could help here, too.

One example of that is neurostimulation, a powerful tool that's already being used to treat chronic pain, anxious depression, overactive bladder, and more by sending electrical pulses to areas of the brain linked to each condition. Despite the technology's proven success, it only works if the correct areas of the brain are stimulated, which is often easier said than done. To provide a map showing the way forward, the Mayo Clinic and Google Research's Brain Team are developing a new type of AI algorithm to chart out the neural connections spanning each region of the brain.[14, 15]

Using a technique dubbed "basis profile curve identification," the algorithm goes deeper than traditional methods to see the interactions between different parts of the brain. Their findings show that this new type of algorithm may help us to understand which brain regions directly interact with one another, which in turn may help guide the placement of electrodes for stimulation devices to treat network brain diseases. As new technology emerges, this type of algorithm may help us to better treat patients with epilepsy, movement disorders like Parkinson's disease, and psychiatric illnesses like obsessive-compulsive disorder and depression.[14]

One of the main causes of chronic pain is musculoskeletal issues, such as back pain, joint pain, and injuries from long-term repetitive movements as part of one's job or in athletic activities. As well as managing the pain from these conditions, we also need to manage the underlying issues. That typically involves physical therapy, injections, and surgery. In most cases, the management of these conditions starts with physical or occupational therapy, which is done in-person by the patient going to a facility and working with a therapist. AI has shown some promise at being able to facilitate this remotely. Using computer vision to analyze movements and then providing feedback based on any identified problems, AI can enable remote physical therapy with the assistance of an AI-based therapist.

Kaia Health, a German start-up, has developed an AI-enabled digital therapist that is, by many measures, as good as a human. One trial, which involved 552 exercises by osteoarthritis patients, found that human therapists agreed with the corrections suggested by Kaia's app as often as they agreed with corrections suggested by other human therapists. In clinical trials, patients with back pain who used the app improved more than those who got in-person physiotherapy. Making people with injuries bend and twist carries some risks, but Kaia's app is just as safe as working with a human expert. Less than 0.1% of nearly 140,000 app users reported adverse events.[16]

Hinge Health delivers a digital care program to manage chronic back and joint pain. The company focuses on employee recovery programs for large enterprises and has over 100 corporate customers. Its platform uses sensors to collect real-time insights about a patient's progress and, based on those insights, it can build a recovery program including exercise therapy, health coaching, and education. It acquired computer vision technology provider Wrench to further develop its AI-enabled offering for remote physical therapy.

6.5   Medication Supply and Adherence

Making sure that people take their prescribed treatment is an important aspect of chronic disease management. Nonadherence is a major issue leading to poor outcomes in healthcare. There are plenty of causes for nonadherence including lack of motivation, financial issues, lack of transportation, health literacy issues, memory issues, and dementia. Improving adherence is vital for chronic disease management programs and involves identifying the specific barriers for patients and addressing them.

AI can be a powerful tool for ensuring adherence. Patients with chronic diseases could use voice-enabled AI to more easily track symptoms, prescriptions, diet, exercise, and questions just by speaking. Voice can also be used for tutorials and instructions, as well as serving as another way for patients and caregivers to connect to healthcare providers.

Pharma companies are experimenting with voice as a new channel to communicate with patients, caregivers, and physicians. With 25% of households already owning smart speakers, pharma companies are experimenting with ways to use voice-enabled AI to improve treatment adherence.[17] By identifying patients at risk of nonadherence using clinical, pharmacy, claims, and other data, providers can proactively intervene to remove barriers and improve adherence rates. Provider organizations and retail pharmacies can optimize their interventions by using prescriptive, rank-ordered, preferred, and recommended intervention lists. Longitudinal and large datasets can evaluate whether these algorithms and models are effective and successful. The goal is to measure the outcomes over time for large populations.[18]

Another major issue is the availability of drugs. Every year, almost half a trillion dollars are spent on medications in the United States. This includes costs for prescription drugs (and their supply chain), pharmacy benefit managers, pharmacies, distributors, and providers to dispense and administer the medications. One out of every seven dollars we spend on healthcare is related to medications. However, about 20–30% of prescriptions are never filled. Many patients aren't retrieving or using their pharmacy medications. The overall cost of medication nonadherence is $300 billion, according to the New England Healthcare Institute. A million emergency department visits each year occur from adverse drug effects in outpatient settings. Of those, about one in every eight results in hospitalization.[18]

AI could help to address drug shortages, both those that are ongoing and those that occur intermittently. This results in hard dollar and soft dollar costs. A hard dollar cost comes from buying more expensive substitutes. Brand names cost more than generics. Soft dollar costs include solutions research and involve a good deal of coding, analysis, and planning, not to mention a risk to patient safety. AI models can help to address these issues by proactively identifying risk, pre-shortage. This can be done by identifying and applying risk scores to drugs. We can also use AI algorithms to identify therapeutic alternatives. This could all be automated and caregivers could be notified.

Another use case here is drug diversion (aka theft!), which occurs when a drug is diverted away from its intended use and from the patients who need it. According to a Protenus 2019 Drug Diversion Report[19]:

- 47.2 million doses were diverted in 2018, up 126% versus 2017.
- $454 million worth of drugs was lost.
- 94% of diversion incidents involved opioids (in fact, diversion is a major cause of the opioid crisis).
- 15% of pharmacists, 10% of nurses, and 8% of physicians are responsible for diversion.

AI can be effective for diversion monitoring and detection. By using models built on more comprehensive data matching, AI can make it more difficult for diverters to avoid detection. The models can create actionable insights to identify the risk of diversion and provide a clear path to reconcile discrepancies.

6.6   VR

One last area that holds great promise is the combination of VR and AI. Immersive technologies will have a place in the future of medicine in many areas such as physician training, radiology, chronic pain management, and mental health therapy. VR can be thought of as a reality that you need to view through some sort of optics (usually glasses), while augmented reality uses a digital display that's separate from the real physical environment.

The benefits of using VR and machine learning are that they can lead to substantial improvements in immersive technologies, allowing them to achieve their intended outcomes with more intelligence. One example is the work being done at Dalio Institute for Cardiovascular Medicine in using VR and AI to improve the precision of cardiac procedures.[20] When procedures are difficult or have a risk of serious complications, additional preparation and staff are often needed during the procedure. Being able to create three-dimensional models to study and then to use them in real time during the procedure could greatly increase the success of procedures while at the same time decreasing the supporting cast that cardiologists require.

Using this method, an algorithm and model were created with over 99% accuracy that could place a catheter within 1 mm of the true position in three-dimensional space. As hearts are all shaped differently, a flexible algorithm is required so that catheters can be accurately guided into different spaces of the heart.

This area is still in its infancy given the fact that both technologies are still in development and haven't found their footing yet in the practice of medicine. Still, the initial use cases suggest a bright future for their combination.

References

1. Mageit, S. (2020, October 28). Digital therapeutics and wellness app users to reach 1.4 billion by. MobiHealthNews. Retrieved September 16, 2022, from https://www.mobihealthnews.com/news/emea/digital-therapeutics-and-wellness-app-users-reach-14-billion-2025

2. AI in Surgical Suite. (2021, December 7). [Video]. Columbia Business School.

3. AI is the Future of Growth. (2017). Accenture.

4. Moor, M., Banerjee, O., Abad, Z. S. H., Krumholz, H. M., Leskovec, J., Topol, E. J., & Rajpurkar, P. (2023). Foundation models for generalist medical artificial intelligence. Nature, 616(7956), 259–265. https://doi.org/10.1038/s41586-023-05881-4

5. Krishnan, N. (2018). How google plans to use AI to reinvent the $3 trillion US healthcare industry. Retrieved September 13, 2022, from https://www.linkedin.com/pulse/how-google-plans-use-ai-reinvent-3-trillion-us-nikhil-krishnan

6. Muoio, D. 2022, May). New York Program will Provide Companion Robot ElliQ to Hundreds of Isolated Seniors. Fierce Healthcare. Retrieved September 16, 2022, from https://tmgpulse.com/new-york-program-will-provide-companion-robot-elliq-to-hundreds-of-isolated-seniors/

7. From Drug R&D To Diagnostics: 90+ Artificial Intelligence Startups In Healthcare. (2019, September 12). CB Insights. https://www.cbinsights.com/research/artificial-intelligence-startups-healthcare/

8. Richards, D., Enrique, A., Eilert, N., Franklin, M., Palacios, J., Duffy, D., Earley, C., Chapman, J., Jell, G., Sollesse, S., & Timulak, L. (2020). A pragmatic randomized waitlist-controlled effectiveness and cost-effectiveness trial of digital interventions for depression and anxiety. NPJ Digital Medicine, 3, 85. https://www.nature.com/articles/s41746-020-0293-8

9. Hale, C. (2022). Imagene nets $21.5M for cancer biopsy-scanning AI. Fierce Biotech. https://www.fiercebiotech.com/medtech/imagene-nets-215m-cancer-biopsy-scanning-ai

10. CB Insights. (2021, January 5). Healthcare AI Trends To Watch. CB Insights Research. https://www.cbinsights.com/research/report/ai-trends-healthcare/

11. Tarumi, S., Takeuchi, W., Qi, R., Ning, X., Ruppert, L., Ban, H., Robertson, D. H., Schleyer, T., & Kawamoto, K. (2022). Predicting pharmacotherapeutic outcomes for type 2 diabetes: an evaluation of three approaches to leveraging electronic

health record data from multiple sources. Journal of Biomedical Informatics, 129, 104001.

12. Tarumi, S., Takeuchi, W., Qi, R., Ning, X., Ruppert, L., Ban, H., Robertson, D. H., Schleyer, T., & Kawamoto, K. (2022, May). Predicting pharmacotherapeutic outcomes for type 2 diabetes: An evaluation of three approaches to leveraging electronic health record data from multiple sources. Journal of Biomedical Informatics, 129, 104001. https://doi.org/10.1016/j.jbi.2022.104001

13. Twin Health's AI tech leads to Type 2 diabetes remissions, study finds. (2022, June 28). Retrieved September 18, 2022, from https://biotech-insider.com/twin-healths-ai-tech-leads-to-type-2-diabetes-remissions-study-finds/

14. Park, A. (2021). Google, Mayo Clinic build new type of AI algorithm to map interactions between areas of the brain. Fierce Biotech. https://www.fiercebiotech.com/medtech/google-mayo-clinic-build-new-type-ai-algorithm-to-map-interactions-between-areas-brain

15. Miller, K. (2021). Basis profile curve identification to understand electrical stimulation effects in human brain networks. PLOS Computational Biology. https://doi.org/10.1371/journal.pcbi.1008710

16. The Economist. (2022, May 11). Some health apps are able not just to diagnose diseases, but also to treat them. Retrieved September 18, 2022, from https://www.economist.com/technology-quarterly/2022/05/02/some-health-apps-are-able-not-just-to-diagnose-diseases-but-also-to-treat-them

17. Bulik, B. S. (2019). Can you hear me, pharma? Voice-enabled apps are on the rise—and please don't freak out about privacy. Fierce Pharma. https://www.fiercepharma.com/marketing/can-you-hear-me-pharma-voice-enabled-apps-rise-and-please-don-t-freak-out-about-privacy

18. Perez, K. (2020, October 19). The autonomous pharmacy: applying AI and ML to medication management across the care continuum. Ai4. Retrieved September 18, 2022, from https://ai4.io/blog/2020/02/27/the-autonomous-pharmacy-applying-ai-and-ml-to-medication-management-across-the-care-continuum/

19. Protenus Drug Diversion Digest. (2020). $183M lost due to healthcare workforce diverting drugs from patient care in 2019.

20. Jang, S. (2021, May 12). Augmented reality guidance for structural heart disease interventions using deep learning-based catheter segmentation. Ai4. Retrieved September 18, 2022, from https://ai4.io/blog/2020/02/27/augmented-reality-guidance-for-structural-heart-disease-interventions-using-deep-learning-based-catheter-segmentation/

CHAPTER 7

Clinical Decision Support

IF THERE'S ONE AREA that artificial intelligence (AI) won't be a luxury for in the future of medicine, it's decision support. But how do we define decision support? Well, it has many definitions. If an algorithm helps a radiologist to read a CT scan, that's a form of decision support. If an algorithm helps to interpret a home urine sample to diagnose a urinary tract infection, that's also a form of decision support. Both of these involve an algorithm that uses a single data file to arrive at its output. The CT scan is a single data file that feeds into the algorithm to diagnose tumors or hemorrhages. This is an important point: the algorithm can do its job of timely decision support because it has all the data it needs to do its job. That's why these types of applications have formed the bulk of the Food and Drug Administration (FDA)-approved algorithms so far.

There is significant overlap between what we discussed in the Diagnostics, Therapeutics and the discussion in this chapter. One can argue that some of these topics belong in the other chapters, or vice versa. Since decision support has always been one of the ambitions for analytics and AI, I think it's worth deovting a chapter to this topic. Also, decision support that involves analyzing data from different sources and arriving at the best decision goes beyond analyzing one data file to make a diagnosis.

In the course of clinical workflows, a clinician often makes decisions based on different types of data: clinical notes, labs, radiology, pathology, and more. The clinician reviews all of this data, sometimes in different places like in the electronic health record (EHR), on a radiology system, or in a report that the patient brings in on paper. This critical distinction between the decision support of an algorithm helping a radiologist with a CT scan and the decision support of an algorithm helping a clinician make decisions about patient diagnosis or treatment is important. Given the fragmented nature of

AI Doctor: The Rise of Artificial Intelligence in Healthcare: A Guide for Users, Buyers, Builders, and Investors, First Edition. Ronald M. Razmi.

the data and that much of it is still unstructured, the applications of clinical decision support at the point of care are challenging.

We're a long way from a world where all of the data needed for an algorithm to help a clinician to make the best decision is available in one place and in usable formats. We talked about this when we tackled the data issues that currently keep algorithms from being developed, validated, or deployed. Radiology reports are in an unstructured format. Pathology reports are often in an unstructured format. When a clinician is visiting with a patient, he's reviewing the information in real time and integrating it all into his decision-making.

For an algorithm to augment physician decision-making, it will need to ingest all of that information in real time and provide its recommendations to the physician while they're visiting with the patient. That's the most common setting for making decisions about patient management and having the output of a decision support tool at the right moment and in the right setting can help to decide whether it gains traction. That's what the current state of data is preventing: the data is often not available or is in a format that can't be used in a timely manner to provide decision support to clinicians. Because of this, decision support using AI will initially focus on applications that require a single data source and where the output doesn't need to be provided in real time to a clinician while visiting with a patient.

Dr. Kang Zhang, Professor of the Faculty of Medicine at Macau University of Science and Technology, is a global expert on the applications of AI in healthcare, and he told me that many of the same issues plague the health system in China, the world's second most populated country and the second largest economy. He talked about how there's no standard format for generating clinical, radiology, and pathology data. It's therefore been difficult to apply natural language processing (NLP) techniques to accurately extract important clinical data out of this information and to feed it into the structured data models that deep learning applications use for decision support. He also thinks that although NLP has made rapid progress in extracting information from unstructured EHR systems, it may take considerable time to achieve complete and accurate identification of multidimensional health data and thus to generate effective clinical decisions with AI. Dr. Zhang also mentioned that current AI clinical application scenarios are basically post-hoc analyses and the improvement of order sets, such as guiding the treatment of severe pneumonia in a hospital.

This is also true of the decision support systems that are based on large language model (LLM)-based generative AI systems. Although these systems hold great promise for clinical decision support, it's important to remember that even if they're trained on large amounts of historic structured and unstructured data, they'll need complete patient data to provide accurate decision support. So, although these powerful models will be transformative in building effective decision support systems, these systems will still need timely access to complete patient data to reach their true potential.

The foundation models that ingest large amounts of information and synthesize it for clinicians can prove to be a game changer here. Clinicians are challenged with absorbing incredibly large amounts of clinical literature in the form of publications and scientific studies about their specialty. If foundation models are used to consume and summarize scientifically validated data, it could help physicians to stay up-to-date. For maximum effectiveness, these models would need to be fed the most current publications on an ongoing basis. This practical application of the tool would benefit the clinician and healthcare in general without AI making definitive clinical decisions. This is important given the ongoing issues about having access to timely and complete patient data at the point of care.

Further into the future, the technology could play a valuable role by working alongside clinicians and helping them to improve the accuracy of diagnoses and the quality of treatment plans. Only a few months after the release of ChatGPT, foundation models were already being used to create a medical version of this. I've been testing two different versions and found them to be accurate and impressive. The use case here is that the clinician could enter prompts and receive responses. Ideally, the model would have access to patient data and proactively provide suggestions to the clinician based on its training in valid medical literature. The bottleneck here would be the limited access to complete and accurate patient data.

Several EHR vendors are already rolling out initial versions of medically trained GPT models inside their systems to help physicians and patients. Epic's initial rollout of this includes support for answering medical questions from patients and is being tested with customers like UC San Diego Health, UW Health in Madison, Wisconsin, and Stanford Health Care.[1]

If a patient asks for an update on their thyroid medication, the automation could decipher which of the patient's prescribed medications is for the thyroid and how many refills are remaining, as well as providing options about what the patient could do. Another use case is for clinicians to research patients' charts or to prompt for instructions, such as for colonoscopy prep. Epic's integration allows the user to apply results, to resubmit the query to get a different result, to summarize the result, and to adjust the language's grade level or translate it into another language.

The opportunities to improve how medicine is practiced, improve quality, and lower costs are enormous and AI could play a big part in realizing them. Here are some of the categories where the current setup and practice of medicine is wasting dollars[2]:

- **Administrative complexity:** $265.6 billion
- **Pricing failure:** $230.7 billion–$240.5 billion
- **Overtreatment:** $75.7 billion–$101.2 billion
- **Fraud and abuse:** $58.5 billion–$83.9 billion
- **Failure of care coordination:** $27.2 billion–$78.2 billion
- **Failure of care:** $102.4 billion–$165.7 billion

AI could offer concrete solutions for many of these categories. The more that AI techniques are integrated into overdiagnosis, overtreatment, and misdiagnosis solutions, the more likely it will be to minimize waste.[2]

Ultimately, there will be a much better way to manage people's health in the future. EHR data is biased and data is sparse as there may be occasional blood pressure readings, ECGs every six months, and infrequent collection of data on chronic diseases. Coupling algorithms with ongoing data collection during the course of patients' daily lives will make precision medicine possible, better match patients to treatments, predict disease, and recommend interventions. We'll ultimately get to a place where we'll be able to predict disease using data and AI decades ahead of time. Symptom-based illness will disappear because we'll be able to predict them based on data from multiple sources and head them off at the pass.

Given the explosion in healthcare data through genomics, microbiomes, wearable data, social data, labs, and much more, AI will be needed to integrate it all and to create the best management decisions for patients. This will be beyond the capabilities of the human mind given the massive nature of this data. Advanced analytics tools such as AI will be used every day to handle all of this data and to better manage patients. This is a future worth looking forward to: using different types of data from a patient to better diagnose their issues and personalizing their management to a degree that we've never done before.

The FDA released new guidance in 2022 about AI tools where they explained that they should be regulated as medical devices as part of the agency's oversight of clinical decision support (CDS) software (Figure 7.1). The new guidance includes a list of AI tools that should be regulated as medical devices, including devices to predict sepsis, identify patient deterioration, forecast heart failure hospitalizations and flag patients who might be addicted to opioids. This is a significant move as it clearly aims to prevent poorly developed models from being deployed in the clinical setting and potentially harming patients.

The FDA's Center for Devices and Radiological Health (CDRH) explained, "A total product lifecycle-based regulatory framework for these technologies would allow for modifications to be made from real-world learning and adaptation while ensuring that the safety and effectiveness of the software as a medical device is maintained." There's been severe backlash from the industry to this new guidance, and many in the field have been stunned by this development. It remains to be seen whether this backlash will lead to changes to the guidance, but it definitely raises the bar in how these models will be developed and approved and will therefore mean less of them in the near future. Ultimately, given their output, ensuring that they won't cause harm, propagate biases, or worsen equity issues will be for the good of the industry in the long term.[3]

The FDA issued a guidance, Clinical Decision Support Software, to describe the FDA's regulatory approach to Clinical Decision Support (CDS) software functions. This graphic gives a general and summary overview of the guidance and is for illustrative purposes only. Consult the guidance for the complete discussion and examples. Other software functions that are not listed may also be device software functions. *

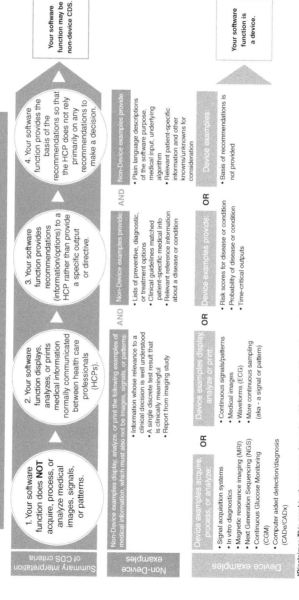

FIGURE 7.1 *(source: FDA)³/U.S. Food and Drug Administration/Public domain*

7.1   AI in Decision Support

One of the key developments of the last decade is the digitization of clinical and personal data. EHRs, where most of the clinical information resides, have become commonplace due to policy changes and the incentives created for providers. This is a positive development for the future of AI, even if the data there is currently incomplete and often messy. There's also much more data that's increasingly being created and used in clinical care, including genetics, proteomics, RNA, metabolites, immunome, microbiome, epigenome, sensor data, environmental data, social data, and behavioral data (Figure 7.2).

Although all of this data holds great promise for better managing patients and doing so in a more personalized way, most of it isn't being taken into account by clinicians as they diagnose patients and create management plans. AI can help us to fix this. Figure 7.3 shows how all of this data could be fed into an AI algorithm, with modern AI algorithms having the ability to ingest large, multimodal data, and to carry out pattern recognition and make predictions.

Medical information has become increasingly complex over time. The range of disease entities, diagnostic testing, biomarkers, and treatment

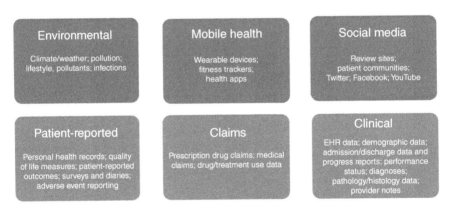

FIGURE 7.2   **The Different Types of Patient Date** *(source: Adapted from[4])*

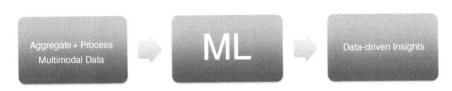

FIGURE 7.3   **Using AI for Decision Support Insights** *(source: Adapted from[4])*

modalities has increased exponentially in recent years. Subsequently, clinical decision-making has become more complex and demands the synthesis of numerous data points. In the current digital age, EHRs represent a massive repository of electronic data points covering a diverse array of clinical information. AI methods have emerged as potentially powerful tools to mine EHR data to aid in disease diagnosis and management, mimicking and perhaps even augmenting the clinical decision-making of human physicians.

Being able to extract the right information from the EHR and feed it into the AI algorithms is one of the foundational tasks that needs to be mastered to make these algorithms useful. The main issues with the data these days are twofold: the data resides in different systems and much of it is unstructured. Clinical decision support is difficult using EHR data because of the vast quantity of data, high dimensionality, data sparsity, and deviations or systematic errors in medical data. These challenges have made it difficult to use AI to perform accurate pattern recognition and to generate predictive clinical models. Additional issues with real-time, multimodal machine learning (ML) include scalability and reproducibility, cost, and translating model outputs to practice decisions (Figure 7.4).

As for fragmented data, we'll need to come up with data infrastructure that aggregates all of the data and makes it available to other applications. Processing data across different domains is messy and building those pipelines can be complex. We might need different algorithms for differently structured data from different contexts. Building data pipelines comes with major issues such as API limitations, complex dependencies leading to failure cascades, and pipeline/data engineering issues.[4]

We've already discussed the issue of bias in the context of AI. Bias can be a major factor once we build pipelines and ingest data. Missing elements as a result of the abovementioned issues could lead to a lack of robustness in the predictions. The distribution of missing data is a critical factor and there's evidence that specific combinations of missing variables can affect AI mortality predictions.[4]

Clinical Decision Making Using AI Has Serious Challenges:

- Techniques that work in papers or in small data do not translate to real-time, messy data systems

- Out-of-the-box, commodity systems often fall short

- Dependencies are not always obvious

- Technical debt accumulates rapidly and inhibits progress

FIGURE 7.4   *(source: Adapted from[4])*

In the context of clinical decision support, where real-time processing of information and delivering the model output is critical to provider workflows, opportunities for exacerbating bias abound. Some of these include[4]:

- **Unknown unknowns**: implicit bias.
- Multiple splitting decisions of training/validation data across disparate data sources.
- **Portability issues**: algorithms don't account for differing contexts.
- Defining notions of fairness is hard.
- Defining fairness across disparate data sources is even harder.

As for the unstructured nature of data in the EHR, this could be tackled using AI itself. Given that GPT models are already being put inside EHRs, one of their first use cases will be to synthesize key insights about patients for the clinicians. Users could enter questions and prompts and access patient information or retrieve summaries of patient data. Models for bedside decision support could leverage clinical knowledge and provide free-text explanations and data summaries. They could also provide links to the sources of recommendations to give clinicians more confidence about the decision support tools. The training datasets for these systems would be text sources (such as academic publications, educational textbooks, international guidelines, and local policies) and EHR time series data with eventual patient outcomes, which can be collected from discharge reports and ICD (International Classification of Diseases) codes. Also, the model must be able to compare potential treatments and estimate their effects, all while adhering to therapeutic guidelines and other relevant policies.[5]

To date, the performance of NLP on clinical notes has been underwhelming. Although NLP is making great progress in various areas (including healthcare), clinical notes still represent a challenge. There's no standard for creating clinical, radiology, pathology, and other unstructured notes. Therefore, it's been difficult to train NLP techniques to accurately extract important clinical data and concepts out of these notes and to feed them into the structured data models that deep learning applications use for decision support. The emergence of LLMs that can be trained on large amounts of unlabeled data means that these models will most likely become more effective at extracting key features about patient conditions from clinical notes.

In a recent study, researchers used an ML-based NLP model that could process free text from physicians' notes in the EHR to accurately predict the primary diagnosis in a pediatric population.[6] The model was initially trained using a set of notes that were manually annotated by an expert team of physicians and informatics researchers. Once trained, the NLP information extraction model used deep learning techniques to automate the annotation process for notes from over 1.4 million patient encounters from a single institution in

China. With the clinical features extracted and annotated by the deep learning NLP model, logistic regression classifiers were used to predict the primary diagnosis for each encounter. This system achieved excellent performance across all organ systems and subsystems, demonstrating a high level of accuracy for its predicted diagnoses compared with the initial diagnoses determined by an examining physician.

The authors stipulate that this type of AI-assisted diagnostic system could be integrated into clinical practice in several ways. First, it could assist with triage procedures. For example, when patients come to the emergency department or to an urgent care setting, their vital signs, basic history, and notes from a physical examination could be entered into the framework, allowing the algorithm to generate a predicted diagnosis. These predicted diagnoses could help to prioritize which patients should be seen first by a physician. Some patients with relatively benign or nonurgent conditions may even be able to bypass the physician evaluation altogether and be referred for routine outpatient follow-up in lieu of urgent evaluation. This diagnostic prediction would help to ensure that physicians' time is dedicated to the patients with the highest and/or most urgent needs. By triaging patients more effectively, waiting times for emergency or urgent care could decrease, allowing improved access to care within a healthcare system that's struggling with limited resources.[6]

Another potential application of this framework is to assist physicians with the diagnosis of patients with complex or rare conditions. While formulating a differential diagnosis, physicians often draw upon their own experiences, and therefore the differential may be biased toward conditions that they've recently seen or that they've commonly encountered in the past. However, for patients presenting with complex or rare conditions, a physician might not have extensive experience with that particular condition. Misdiagnosis is a distinct possibility in these cases. Using this AI-based diagnostic framework would allow us to harness the power generated by the data from millions of patients and would be less prone to the biases of individual physicians. In this way, a physician could use the AI-generated diagnosis to help broaden his or her differential diagnosis and think of diagnostic possibilities that might not have been immediately obvious.

As mentioned earlier, great progress is being made in this area with LLMs that can train on structured and unstructured data in a self-supervised fashion. This minimizes the need for annotation and human manual work to train these models. Like ChatGPT, the same models can be trained on medical literature to create systems that can respond to clinical and research questions. But to reiterate, to provide point-of-care decision support for physicians, access to complete and accurate patient data is a must. So regardless of the model's capabilities, solving the data issues is the first step to successful decision support.

Also, generative AI applications like ChatGPT aren't currently suited to helping clinicians treat patients because they pull from existing medical and popular literature to answer clinical questions and therefore aren't as accurate as they should be for medical use cases. As such, medical versions of Chat-GPT are being developed and as I mentioned earlier, they're already showing good results.

7.2 Initial Use Cases

Flagler Hospital in Saint Augustine, Florida, is using AI tools to improve the treatment of pneumonia, sepsis, and a dozen other high-cost, high-mortality conditions. They've partnered with Ayasadi, an AI company, to use a form of AI to better manage patients in the hospital.[7]

Ayasadi uses a branch of mathematics called topological data analysis to group patients together that have been treated similarly and to find relationships between those groups. They load relevant clinical data into the application and use an unsupervised learning AI algorithm to generate treatment groups. For the pneumonia patients, Ayasadi produced nine treatment groups. Flagler analyzes the treatment groups and selects a "Goldilocks" group. This is the group with the lowest cost, the lowest length of stay (LOS), and the lowest readmission rate, making it "just right."

Then the AI tools generate a care path, showing all the events which should occur in the emergency department, at admission, and throughout the hospital stay. These events include all medications, diagnostic tests, vital signs, IVs, procedures and meals, along with the ideal timing for each occurrence.[7]

The next step is to use AI to adjust Flagler's order sets both on the inpatient side and in the emergency department. Flagler has a physician IT crew called the PIT Crew which uses the model's output to make recommendations for set adjustments and to obtain department approval. As part of their oversight, the hospital administration reviews changes. Through 2300 lines of SQL code, Flagler is able to extract the data that the AI tools use from its CPM analytics platform, its enterprise data warehouse, its Allscripts EHR, and its financial system.

Flagler's leadership team has said that while the process could be replicated in a manual or semi-manual environment, it would take years to achieve even a fraction of these insights. AI tools allow them to do it in just a few days. Flager is set to implement the new pneumonia pathway by changing the order set in its EHR, and it expects to save over $1350 per patient in direct variable costs while simultaneously reducing the average stay length by two days. As if that wasn't enough, it will also reduce the readmission rate from 2.9% to 0.4%.

This is an example of how AI can be used to improve patient care and provide decision support in spite of the data issues that are keeping it from receiving and processing real-time data to provide point-of-care decision support.

In another example, clinicians at Northwell Health, which is New York State's largest healthcare provider, have used AI to augment their post-discharge workflows, reducing the readmission rate by 23.6%. The clinicians studied clinical AI-stratified patients for their risk of readmissions, identified the clinical and nonclinical factors driving their risk, and recommended targeted outreach and interventions to reduce patient risk.[8] Their tech is able to provide a highly informed recommendation that's determined by a complex matrix of data points and which aims to improve patient outcomes.

Indiana's Regenstrief Institute, which is a key research partner for the Indiana University School of Medicine, is also making huge investments when it comes to advancing AI in healthcare. As part of this, they've created a ML system called Uppstroms which incorporates social determinants of health (SDOH), such as the availability of affordable housing and the accessibility of food, to address patients' socioeconomic, financial, and behavioral needs.[9] The information that Uppstroms uses is added to EHRs and then the algorithm identifies which patients might need wraparound services, such as those that are provided by counselors and social workers. This allows care providers to make referrals before the situation becomes a crisis, because crises lead to higher costs and worse outcomes.

Uppstroms is being used in nine clinics throughout Indianapolis and could be integrated into EHRs and used in a number of different healthcare settings to address SDOH. AI can also be used to sort through the plethora of available data and to display only the most relevant to help with clinical decision support. For example, there's an app called Health Dart which has been developed by Regenstrief and its partners and which is being used in a university health system's emergency departments. It sorts through EHRs and identifies the most relevant tests and diagnostic information required for seven of the most common emergency department patient complaints: abdominal pain, chest pain, weakness and dizziness, headaches, back pain, pregnancy and heartbeat irregularities, and trouble breathing. This novel search algorithm saves clinicians several minutes of clicks and searching, allowing them to spend more time with patients.[9]

A study at NYU using NLP on clinical notes from their EHRs to train LLMs showed that an LLM-based decision support system can integrate in real-time with clinical workflows and show improvement in both clinical and operational metrics.[10] Their LLM-based decision support system, NYUTron, was trained on 7.25 million clinical notes (e.g. radiographic reads, history, and physicals) from 387,144 patients across four hospitals, resulting in a 4.1 billion-word corpus curated from January 2011 to May 2020. The study showed that such a model can deliver better results than the traditional predictive models that are harder to train and incorporate into existing workflows.

They assessed NYUTron on a battery of five tasks, including three clinical and two operational tasks (30-day all-cause readmission prediction, in-hospital mortality prediction, comorbidity index prediction, LOS prediction, and insurance denial prediction). NYUTron had an area under the curve (AUC) of 78.7%–94.9%, with an improvement of 5.36%–14.7% in AUC from traditional clinical predictive models. This means that the advances in NLP and LLMs are now opening the door for workflow-integrated decision support systems that can work alongside clinicians.

In 2022, the Washington Post highlighted the use of AI to improve clinical decision-making in combat as an area of active research for the Defense Advanced Research Projects Agency (DARPA).[11] DARPA is going to create and evaluate AI-based algorithms to help military decision-makers to deal with small unit injuries (such as those faced by special ops in combat situations) and mass casualty events (like terrorist attacks). In the future, we could create similar algorithms to help with disaster relief in the aftermath of natural disasters. For example, AI tools could identify available resources (like blood supplies, medical staff, and drug availability) and use this data to help with decision-making. Like DARPA, NATO is working with Johns Hopkins University to create a digital triage assistant that can be used by NATO member countries.[12]

The triage assistant NATO is developing will use NATO injury datasets, casualty scoring systems, predictive modeling, and inputs about a patient's condition to create a model to decide who should get care first in a situation where resources are limited.[12]

7.3   Primary Care

In a paper in the *Journal of Internal Medicine,* Steven Lin and his colleagues discuss the key areas where AI can improve primary care (Figure 7.5).[13] Some of these areas include population health management, risk prediction, intervention, and patient triage using AI bots, determining the complexity of practices' patient populations, better resourcing of support staff, remote patient management, digital coaching for chronic conditions, augmenting primary care physicians' knowledge to help them diagnose complex conditions where specialists aren't easily available, and clinical decision support.

The authors argue that with over 500 million visits per year in the United States—51% of all physician office visits, more than any other medical specialty—primary care is where the power, opportunity, and future of AI are most likely to be realized in the broadest and most ambitious scale.[14]

Many of the following applications involve decision support:

- Helping primary physicians to diagnose and manage complex conditions
- Helping patients to get answers to their questions and decide where to seek care

From: Ten Ways Artificial Intelligence Will Transform Primary Care

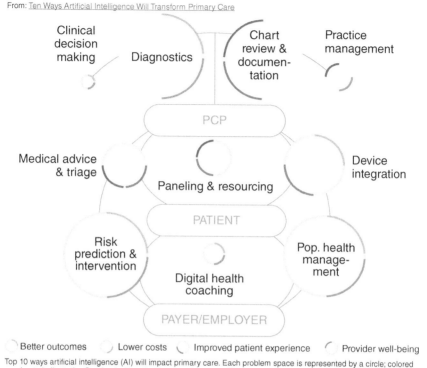

Top 10 ways artificial intelligence (AI) will impact primary care. Each problem space is represented by a circle; colored quadrants indicate the Quadruple Aims that are most impacted. Size of the circles is the estimate of the market value of each problem space in billions of dollars (USD)/year in the USA: risk prediction and intervention, $100B; population health management, $89B; medical advice/triage; $27B; risk-adjusted paneling/resourcing, $17B; device integration, $52B; digital health coaching, $6B; chart review and documentation, $90B; diagnostics, $100B; clinical decision making, $1-2B; practice management, $10B. PCP = primary care physician.

FIGURE 7.5   Ten Ways Artificial Intelligence Will Transform Primary Care
(source: Adapted from[14])

- Digital coaching of patients so they make better decisions about their health and specific conditions
- Resource allocation decisions
- Remotely managing chronic disease patients
- More!

While AI could augment our current decision-making process in these areas, it's important to remember that the barriers we previously discussed (e.g. fragmented and unstructured data, outdated IT infrastructures, incomplete EHR data, talent shortage, and the need for upfront investments) will keep many of these applications from reaching their potential in the near future. However, taking tangible steps in the right direction will mean that we'll get there eventually.

If we want to investigate these areas within the practice of medicine while examining the barriers and their expected benefits, we need to understand that even with the best information and intentions, changing outcomes and lowering costs is difficult.

In risk prediction and management, the promise has always been that by identifying high-risk patients and proactively addressing those risks, we can prevent the need for institutional care, improving patient outcomes and lowering costs.[15-17] AI-driven predictive modeling with EHR data can now outperform traditional predictive models at forecasting in-hospital mortality, 30-day unplanned readmission, prolonged LOS, and patients' final discharge diagnoses.[18] Ochsner Health System and Epic have created an AI using over 1 billion clinical data points to predict patient deterioration with 98% accuracy.[19]

All of this is fantastic news, and it's expected that if we start using clinical data (rather than claims data), we can create more accurate risk models. AI is perfect for using this large, multidimensional data to predict risk. The idea behind using AI for risk assessments is to build a prospective predictive algorithm without relying on claims data, which will always be retrospective. So, are we going to see a rapid decline in costs or improved patient outcomes? Well, if history is any indication, no!

There's a big difference between identifying risk and mitigating it. Managing risk will involve making an organized effort to engage patients to address those risks on an ongoing basis. This has proven to be far more difficult than expected, because patients have other things to do that usually take priority over their health. Also, population health management is difficult and most payers and providers haven't created the right organization to effectively address those risks.

A prime area for AI is decision support for patients, in the form of responding to medical questions, helping with triage to the right care setting and providing ongoing coaching for chronic conditions. Historically, individuals decide where to seek care based on their own assessment of what might be wrong with them and the severity of those issues. However, there's an opportunity to significantly improve this using AI. Intelligent systems that can answer questions and figure out the ideal setting for patients to get care could improve efficiency, provide intelligence, reduce costs, and free up medical staff to focus on higher priority tasks. The initial results from the implementation of such systems by a number of companies like Babylon, Ada, Buoy, and others have been encouraging, but the accuracy of these systems has been inconsistent.[16, 17] This is poised to change with the new foundation models that have training on the large body of medical literature. Also, if these systems are within the EHR or have access to that data, they can be far more personalized in their interactions with patients.

Also, in digital coaching where we can provide long-term engagement for patients managing costly chronic conditions, there's emerging evidence that AI could augment the human touch. Companies such as Lark and Nutrino are using AI-powered, text-based health coaching to engage patients in lifestyle changes that will result in better health outcomes. The initial results show that these interventions can be quite effective and stack up well against human coaching.[20] We discussed diagnostics in an earlier chapter, but it's worth mentioning here that AI can help clinicians, especially primary care physicians, to perform and interpret tests like ultrasounds, eye examinations, and skin inspections, meaning that more physicians can better diagnose these conditions. This will mean that conditions that are under-diagnosed or undertreated due to a shortage of specialists or insufficient skills will be easier to diagnose and manage. This could cut down on unnecessary referrals and allow specialists to focus on those with the highest needs.

In the near future, this will mostly be for conditions where we need limited data for the AI solutions to provide decision support. For example, the algorithms will use fundus photos, skin photos, ultrasounds, and X-rays, rather than data from multiple sources such as clinical notes, radiology reports, and outside data.[21–23]

7.4 Specialty Care

7.4.1 Cancer Care

Oncology is one of the key areas where AI can have a large impact. Given the many different types of cancer, the genetic and environmental causes of cancer, the interactions between these drivers, and the opportunity to personalize treatments based on a variety of factors (e.g. genetic markers and labs), AI can provide huge benefits in decision support.

There's clearly a need for being able to predict who will develop cancer so that we can help them to avoid it, as well as to identify the best treatments once a diagnosis has been made. The increasing use of multimodal information— such as phenotype, genotype, and exposure information—almost necessitates the use of AI algorithms. It would be difficult for any physician to integrate all of this information into their brains to manage the patient.

Also, AI can help with radiation oncology. Radiology treatments typically require a lot of work to prevent nerve or artery damage. The Mayo Clinic has developed a series of algorithms that can reduce the time required to build the three-dimensional model needed to administer the radiation.[24]

7.4.2 Neurology

Strokes remain one of the main courses of mortality and morbidity throughout the world and so they're a major concern for public health. AI presents exciting opportunities to improve stroke care delivery. In the coming years, part of early-career stroke neurologists' roles will be to integrate AI and smart technology into stroke research and practice.[25]

Previous research has shown that AI algorithms can be used for the early diagnosis of atrial fibrillation using normal sinus rhythm electrocardiographs, which allows for early intervention to reduce stroke risk.[26] Mayo Clinic studies have shown that AI algorithms can predict atrial fibrillation that's associated with cerebral stroke and cognitive decline.[27] According to researchers, this could be a result of the algorithm detecting non-atrial fibrillation (AF) cardiac pathology, which can also cause cognitive decline and small vessel cerebrovascular disease. This provides an opportunity to initiate anticoagulation therapy before a stroke happens.

At the moment, AI algorithms are being used to screen populations that are at high risk of strokes. Lekadir et al. have shown that there's potential for using deep learning algorithms for the automatic characterization of carotid plaque composition (lipid core, fibrous cap, and calcium) in ultrasound, which is correlated with risk stratification in ischemic stroke.[28] ML has already been used to predict the outcomes of patients that have suffered from an acute ischemic stroke. A deep neural network model trained with six variables from the Acute Stroke Registry and Analysis of Lausanne score was able to predict three-month modified Rankin Scale scores better than the traditional Acute Stroke Registry and Analysis of Lausanne score (AUC 0.888 versus 0.839; $P < 0.001$).[29]

Deep learning-based systems could detect acute neurological events in cranial imaging 150 times faster than radiologists (1.2 versus 177s). As such, applying deep learning algorithms to medical imaging for computer-assisted diagnosis could have positive effects on workflow efficiency and the quality of stroke care.[30] AI tools could also help neurologists to identify patients who've had an acute ischemic stroke due to large vessel occlusions. On top of that, they could help neurologists to spot patients with anterior circulation large vessel occlusions and determine in real time which candidates should be selected for revascularization.

7.4.3   Cardiology

Cardiology-based AI applications hold great promise for improving patient care. In the section on neurology, we discussed the application of AI in remotely detecting atrial fibrillation using rhythm detection tools such as cell phone–based solutions like the one offered by cardiogram. The Mayo Clinic spun out an AI company, Anumana, which uses cardiology algorithms that can measure ejection fractions to diagnose diseases based on data from remote monitoring devices.[24] Anumana taps into neural network algorithms that are based on billions of pieces of heart health data in Mayo's Clinical Data Analytics Platform for this early detection capability.

This powerful combination of remote data collection and ingestion into a data infrastructure that has AI on top of it can help provide access to specialty care for more people in more places.

7.4.4   Infectious Diseases

Sepsis is a major cause of hospital mortality. It's been shown that detecting it earlier and implementing the right interventions can significantly lower mortality. We've already discussed how Flagler Hospital is using a form of AI to find a Goldilocks group for the management of sepsis. There's evidence that using AI for the earlier detection of sepsis could result in faster life-saving treatment. According to Suchi Saria, Founder and CEO of AI-based clinical decision support platform Bayesian Health, and John C. Malone, Endowed Chair and Director of the Machine Learning and Healthcare Lab at Johns Hopkins University, AI could reduce time to treatment by an average of 1.85 h.[24]

In a study that used the Bayesian Health AI system at Hopkins for the early detection of patients at risk of sepsis, researchers applied it in the ED and the ICU across clinical floors in five different hospitals. They were able to show high sensitivity, precision, and significant early detection rates. When the tool was applied prospectively, patients received antibiotics significantly earlier, which led to associated reductions in LOS and mortality rates. The most interesting part of the study was that although it was implemented as a passive flag and its use wasn't mandatory, they saw provider adoption rates of around 90% sustained over two years.[24]

7.4.5   COVID-19

AI-powered decision support tools are being used in a variety of settings and medical centers to manage COVID-19. It's being used to more quickly diagnose or risk stratify patients using findings on chest X-rays and CT scans. Physicians are also using a combination of clinical data from EHRs and AI algorithms to monitor COVID patients and to anticipate clinical deterioration. There are also AI tools that have been trained using ML to offer clinical decision support in managing patients and to help with decisions about how to ration care.

Some medical centers are repurposing existing AI systems that are meant to predict the course of patients' illnesses, retooling them to predict COVID-19 outcomes like intubation.[31] These AI systems have ingested data from thousands of patient records and used it to learn illness patterns. By using around 100 variables, they found that the amount of supplementary oxygen required to keep a patient's blood oxygen level up was the best signal for predicting whether their condition was deteriorating. This is particularly true for COVID-19, where an increased oxygen requirement is a key signal that the patient's lungs are failing.

If doctors have an eight-hour warning that a patient will need to be intubated or transferred to the ICU, they can try different treatments like using nasal cannulas that deliver supplemental oxygen through the nose. Also, the Bayesian Health tool can help hospital management to predict caseloads and resources. For example, if the algorithm predicts a surge of demand for ventilators in the next 24 h, they can call in reserve staff, acquire ventilators from strategic stockpiles, and plan to send patients to other hospitals.[32]

7.5   Devices

The realm of devices is one of the key areas where AI could have a huge impact in the medium term. Patients are increasingly wearing devices to manage their conditions. These devices collect information and, in the near future, might provide recommendations to patients based on that information without needing to pass it back to a clinician who can review it and decide what needs to be done. To the extent that devices have been used to date, the workflows have involved data collection and transferring that data to clinicians. It's been their job to figure out what the data means in the larger context of the patient and to make a decision about the next steps. Given how busy clinicians are with their day jobs, the data rarely makes its way back to them and few recommendations are generated or passed on to the patients. This has been a big drawback for these devices to date: the infrastructure to receive the data, to understand what it means in the wider context of the patient and to make treatment decisions doesn't exist.

New devices that incorporate decision support could overcome this lack of infrastructure and free up medical resources that would otherwise be involved in processing and acting on this information. But this approach has risks of its own. What if the AI recommendation leads to an action that harms the patient? Do we have enough experience with these algorithms to cut them loose on their own? Who bears the responsibility in that situation? Can the algorithm make accurate recommendations without knowing the full context of patients' situations? Well, in some cases, that might be possible. In fact, that's probably where the medical community will start using them: in focused applications where all of the required information is available.

One such application is DreaMed Advisor Pro, a cloud-based diabetes treatment decision support tool which takes data from glucose monitors, insulin pumps, and self-monitoring to make recommendations for insulin delivery. By using event learning, the software processes data points like basal rate, carbohydrate ratio, and correction factor to make its recommendations.

It provides dosage recommendations to the monitoring clinician, who can make adjustments to the patients' diabetes management devices with just the click of a button. The algorithm was granted a De Novo approval by the FDA in 2018.[33, 34]

Although this doesn't cut the clinician entirely out of the loop, it does a lot of the heavy lifting so that the clinician can just review it and push the recommendation to the patient. This is a safe place to start using devices and AI to build experience and monitor the recommendations. Over time, we'll probably reach a place where the device can directly communicate with the patient—or better yet, program the amount of insulin that will be released into the patient with the same device.

7.6   End-of-Life AI

In recent months, there have been reports of AI algorithms predicting mortality in patients. The researchers and clinicians who are using these systems say that the early data suggests that they're leading to important conversations that would otherwise have happened either too late or not at all. This is badly needed in a healthcare system where doctors are stretched too thin and don't have the training they need to prioritize talking to patients with serious illnesses about end-of-life care.

The algorithms are usually built using ML to process data that's stored in EHRs. They're trained and tested on thousands of data points from previous patients, and this includes their diagnoses, the medications they took and whether they recovered or whether they deteriorated and died. Some of these models also use socioeconomic data and information from insurance claims.

Then there are tools like the commercial model developed by Georgia's Jvion which measures patients against their peers and flags those in need of review. When it's rolled out in an oncology practice, Jvion's model compares all of the clinic's patients and then flags those it deems to have the highest chance of dying in the next month.[35]

In a recent study, researchers looked at how more than 25,000 cancer patients fared after the AI system predicted their risk of dying in the next six months.[36] Of the patients that the algorithm identified were at risk of death, 45% died, compared to just 3% of the patients that the algorithm said were at low risk. Even when models flag the wrong patients, the data shows that they can also lead to conversations about end-of-life care and increase the quality of the care that they receive along the way.

In another study of the algorithm, researchers found that when the health system's oncology clinics started using the algorithm, 4% of patient visits involved a documented conversation about a patient's wishes and goals, compared to 1.2% of visits in the weeks before the algorithm was rolled out.[37] Meanwhile, a study that looked into Jvion's rollout at Northwest found that palliative care consults increased by 168% in the 17 months after it was deployed when compared to the 5 months beforehand. The rate at which Northwest patients were referred to a hospice also jumped eightfold.[38]

7.7   Patient Decision Support

Patients at home could receive decision support via AI bots with the ability to answer medical questions, help them to decide the best setting to receive care, or provide text-based coaching for chronic diseases. Voice technology is also helping to support patients' decision-making. This is all the more likely now due to the breakthroughs in generative AI and the self-supervised learning of LLMs. Systems can be trained on historic clinical data and appropriate medical literature to respond to patient inquiries, support disease management efforts by patients, and identify the right resources based on the patients' issues and questions.

As mentioned earlier, the current version of ChatGPT is trained on both clinical and popular literature and thus it might not be accurate in responding to patient inquiries. What makes it even riskier is that ChatGPT presents information in a way that appears to be relevant and authoritative. However, early experience shows that it can present the wrong information—that is, information that appears relevant but isn't. Worse, it can fabricate sources. As such, the current versions of these systems need to be treated with caution, but the underlying methodology is promising for training future versions with the appropriate medical literature.

There's reason to believe that AI chatbots could provide significant value once these risks are accounted for. That's because AI chatbots can be more available and faster to respond, which are both important to ensure patient treatment adherence, higher satisfaction, and better outcomes. In a study in JAMA, when comparing physician and AI chatbot responses (based on ChatGPT) to a set of medical questions posted on a public social media forum (Reddit's r/AskDocs), the evaluators preferred AI chatbot responses for both quality and empathy. This study is significant in that it's one of the first well-designed studies comparing AI chatbots (rather than programmed chatbots) with humans.[39]

KidsMD, a tool that's available through Amazon's Alexa, allows parents to talk to their device about common illnesses, such as colds, fevers, and ear infections, and to receive bespoke guidance and information from Boston Children's Hospital. This includes suggestions about whether they should visit the doctor and how they can care for their child at home. KidsMD has logged 100,000 interactions to date, and IDHA plans to bring other kinds of wellness and disease-specific education to home voice assistants that consumers can access even more easily and intuitively.[40]

This optimism surrounding the use of voice technologies in healthcare is being bolstered by research and surveys among clinicians. One survey of pediatricians found that 48% would deploy the technology in their clinics, while only 16% said that they wouldn't try voice. A further 36% were undecided, mostly due to a lack of familiarity around how the technology could help patient care.

Many physicians have said that they'd be happy to use voice assistants for clinical decision support both at work and at home. They can also imagine patients using an interactive voice system before their visit to fill out medical questionnaires and save on time and frustration. It seems that everyone agrees that voice assistants could be a useful way to educate and engage with patients at the clinic and to have it continue once they're sent home.

References

1. Fox, A. (2023, April 19). EHR vendors demo new GPT features at HIMSS23. Healthcare IT News. https://www.healthcareitnews.com/news/ehr-vendors-demo-gpt-himss23
2. Ai4. (2020, January 28). Convergent AI in reducing overdiagnosis, overtreatment and misdiagnosis (Houston Methodist) [Video]. YouTube. Retrieved September 18, 2022, from https://www.youtube.com/watch?v=_9MLcYLpHVY
3. Clinical decision support software: guidance for industry and Food and Drug Administration Staff. (2022). Food and Drug Administration (FDA). Retrieved March 11, 2023, from https://www.fda.gov/media/109618/download
4. HIMSS. (2019). Building a real-time community insights: engine for a Healthcare system: challenges and opportunities. https://365.himss.org/sites/himss365/files/365/handouts/552672016/handout-MLAI13.pdf
5. Moor, M., Banerjee, O., Abad, Z. S. H., Krumholz, H. M., Leskovec, J., Topol, E. J., & Rajpurkar, P. (2023). Foundation models for generalist medical artificial intelligence. Nature, 616(7956), 259–265. https://doi.org/10.1038/s41586-023-05881-4
6. Liang, H., Tsui, B., & Ni, H. (2019). Evaluation and accurate diagnoses of pediatric diseases using artificial intelligence. Nature Medicine, 25, 433–438.
7. Siwicki, B. (2018, November 7). Flagler hospital uses AI to create clinical pathways that enhance. Healthcare IT News. Retrieved September 18, 2022, from https://www.healthcareitnews.com/news/flagler-hospital-uses-ai-create-clinical-pathways-enhance-care-and-slash-costs
8. Siwicki, B. (2021, July 23). Northwell health uses machine learning to reduce readmissions by. Healthcare IT News. Retrieved September 18, 2022, from https://www.healthcareitnews.com/news/northwell-health-uses-machine-learning-reduce-readmissions-nearly-24
9. Siwicki, B. 2021, October 18). How CIOs are prioritizing AI investments for the next 5 years, Healthcare IT News
10. Jiang, L. Y., Liu, X. C., Nejatian, N. P., Nasir-Moin, M., Wang, D., Abidin, A. Z., Eaton, K., Riina, H. A., Laufer, I., Punjabi, P., Miceli, M., Kim, N. C., Orillac, C.,

Schnurman, Z., Livia, C., Weiss, H., Kurland, D. B., Neifert, S., Dastagirzada, Y., Kondziolka, D., Cheung, A. T. M., Yang, G., Cao, M., Flores, M., Costa, A. B., Aphinyanaphongs, Y., Cho, K., & Oermann, E. K. (2023). Health system-scale language models are all-purpose prediction engines. Nature. https://doi.org/10.1038/s41586-023-06160-y

11. Verma, P. (2022). The military wants AI to replace human decision-making in battle. The Washington Post. https://www.washingtonpost.com/technology/2022/03/29/darpa-artificial-intelligence-battlefield-medical-decisions

12. Graham, C. (2021, August 20). Undergrads partner with NATO to reduce combat casualties. The Hub. Retrieved September 18, 2022, from https://hub.jhu.edu/2021/08/20/wearable-device-for-combat-triage

13. Lin, S. Y., Mahoney, M. R., & Sinsky, C. A. (2019). Ten ways artificial intelligence will transform primary care. Journal of General Internal Medicine, 34, 1626–1630.

14. National Ambulatory Medical Care Survey (NAMCS) – Health, United States, 2020-2021. Retrieved September 18, 2022, from https://www.cdc.gov/nchs/hus/sources-definitions/namcs.htm

15. Japsen, B. (2016, October 11). IBM Watson, Siemens Partner to tap population health industry. Forbes. Retrieved September 19, 2022, from https://www.forbes.com/sites/brucejapsen/2016/10/11/ibm-watson-siemens-partner-to-tap-population-health-industry

16. Mukherjee, S. (2021, June 10). You can now download an artificial intelligence doctor. Fortune. Retrieved September 19, 2022.

17. Razzaki, S., Baker, A., Perov, Y., & Middleton, K. (2018). A comparative study of artificial intelligence and human doctors for the purpose of triage and diagnosis. Research Gate https://www.researchgate.net/publication/326056790_A_comparative_study_of_artificial_intelligence_and_human_doctors_for_the_purpose_of_triage_and_diagnosis

18. Rajkomar, A., Oren, E., & Chen, K., Dai, A.M., Hajaj, N., Hardt, M., Liu, P.J., Liu, X., Marcus, J., Sun, M., & Sundberg, P. (2018). Scalable and accurate deep learning with electronic health records. NPJ Digital Medicine, 1(1), 18. https://www.nature.com/articles/s41746-018-0029-1

19. Winners of the 2018 Microsoft Health Innovation Awards. (2018, March 7). Microsoft Industry Blogs. Retrieved March 7, 2019.

20. Stein, N., & Brooks, K. (2017). A Fully Automated Conversational Artificial Intelligence for Weight Loss: Longitudinal Observational Study Among Overweight and Obese Adults. JMIR Diabetes.

21. Haenssle, H. A., Fink, C., & Schneiderbauer, R., Toberer, F., Buhl, T., Blum, A., Kalloo, A., Hassen, A. B. H., Thomas, L., Enk, A., & Uhlmann, L. (2018). Man against machine: diagnostic performance of a deep learning convolutional neural network for dermoscopic melanoma recognition in comparison to 58 dermatologists. Annals of Oncology, 29(8), 1836–1842

22. University of Iowa Health care first to adopt IDx-DR in a diabetes care setting. (2018, June 28). Retrieved September 19, 2022, from https://www.prnewswire.com/news-releases/university-of-iowa-health-care-first-to-adopt-idx-dr-in-a-diabetes-care-setting-300672070.html

23. VisualDx to launch AI-enabled smart symptom checker: beta testing of Aysa, an AI-driven app, begins and revolutionizes the public's understanding of skin

conditions. (2018). VisualDx. https://www.prnewswire.com/news-releases/visualdx-to-launch-ai-enabled-smart-symptom-checker-300697148.html

24. Health Evolution. (2021, November 11). Promising AI clinical use cases beyond imaging. Retrieved September 19, 2022, from https://www.healthevolution.com/insider/promising-ai-clinical-use-cases-beyond-imaging

25. Ding, L., Liu, C., Li, Z., & Wang, Y. (2020). Incorporating artificial intelligence into stroke care and research. Stroke, 51(12):e351–e354

26. Attia, Z. I., Noseworthy, P. A., Lopez-Jiminez, F., Asirvatham, S. J., Deshmukh, A. J., Gersh, B. J., Carter, R. E., Yao, X., Rabinstein, A. A., & Erickson, B. J. (2019). An artificial intelligence-enabled ECG algorithm for the identification of patients with atrial fibrillation during sinus rhythm: a retrospective analysis of outcome prediction. Lancet, 394(10201), 861–867

27. Weil, W. L., Noseworthy, P. A., & Lopez, C. L. (2022). Artificial intelligence enabled electrocardiogram for atrial fibrillation identifies cognitive decline risk and cerebral infarcts. Mayo Clinic Proceedings, 97(5), 871–880

28. Lekadir, K., Galimzianova, A., Betriu, A., Del Mar Vila, M., Igual, L., Rubin, D. L., Fernandez, E., Radeva, P., & Napel, S. (2017). A convolutional neural network for automatic characterization of plaque composition in carotid ultrasound. IEEE Journal of Biomedical and Health Informatics, 21(1), 48–55

29. Heo, J., Yoon, J. G., Park, H., Kim, Y. D., Nam, H. S., & Heo, J. H. (2019, May). Machine learning–based model for prediction of outcomes in acute stroke. Stroke, 50(5), 1263–1265. https://doi.org/10.1161/strokeaha.118.024293

30. Titano, J. J., Badgeley, M., Schefflein, J., Pain, M., Su, A., Cai, M., Swinburne, N., Zech, J., Kim, J., & Bederson, J. (2018). Automated deep-neural-network surveillance of cranial images for acute neurologic events. Nature Medicine, 24(9), 1337–1341

31. Chaffim, M.AI may help hospitals decide which COVID-19 patients live or die – Marcus Chaffim. Retrieved September 20, 2022, from https://fga.unb.br/marcus.chaffim/blog/ai-may-help-hospitals-decide-which-covid-19-patients-live-or-die

32. Siwicki, B. (2021, May 19). How AI can truly advance healthcare and research, and where it's gone. Healthcare IT News. Retrieved September 20, 2022, from https://www.healthcareitnews.com/news/how-ai-can-truly-advance-healthcare-and-research-and-where-its-gone-wrong

33. Muoio, D. (2018, June 18). FDA grants DreaMed's de novo request for device-friendly diabetes. MobiHealthNews. Retrieved September 21, 2022, from https://www.mobihealthnews.com/content/fda-grants-dreameds-de-novo-request-device-friendly-diabetes-software

34. Muoio, D. (2018, December 19). Roundup: 12 healthcare algorithms cleared by the FDA. MobiHealthNews. Retrieved September 13, 2022, from https://www.mobi-healthnews.com/content/roundup-12-healthcare-algorithms-cleared-fda

35. Robbins, R. (2020, July 15). An experiment in end-of-life care: tapping AI's cold calculus to nudge the most human of conversations. STAT. Retrieved September 21, 2022, from https://www.statnews.com/2020/07/01/end-of-life-artificial-intelligence

36. Manz, C., Chivers, C., Liu, M., Regli, S. B., Changolkar, S., Evans, C. N., Rareshide, C. A. L., Draugelis, M., Braun, J., Navathe, A. S., Kumar, P., Bekelman, J. E., Patel, M. S., O'Connor, N., Schuchter, L. M., Schulman, L. N., & Parikh, R. B. (2020). prospective validation of a machine learning algorithm to predict short-term mortality among outpatients with cancer. ASCO.

37. Manz, C., Parikh, R. B., Evans, C. N., Chivers, C., Regli, S. B., Changolkar, S., Bekelman, J. E., Small, D., Rareshide, C. A. L., O'Connor, N., Schuchter, L. M., Shulman, L. N., & Patel, M. S. (2020). Effect of integrating machine learning mortality estimates with behavioral nudges to increase serious illness conversions among patients with cancer: a stepped-wedge cluster randomized trial. ASCO.

38. Gajra, A., Zettler, M., Kish, J., Miller, K., Frownfelter, J., Valley, A. W., & Blau, S. (2020). Impact of augmented intelligence (AI) on utilization of palliative care (PC) services in oncology. Journal of Clinical Oncology, 38(15_suppl), 12015–12015. https://doi.org/10.1200/jco.2020.38.15_suppl.12015

39. Ayers, J. W., Poliak, A., Dredze, M., Leas, E. C., Zhu, Z., Kelley, J. B., Faix, D. J., Goodman, A. M., Longhurst, C. A., Hogarth, M., & Smith, D. M. (2023). Comparing physician and artificial intelligence chatbot responses to patient questions posted to a public social media forum. JAMA Internal Medicine, 183(6), 589–596. https://doi.org/10.1001/jamainternmed.2023.1838

40. Small, C. E., Nigrin, D., Churchwell, K., Brownstein, J. (2020, October 24). What will health care look like once smart speakers are everywhere?. Harvard Business Review. https://hbr.org/2018/03/what-will-health-care-look-like-once-smart-speakers-are-everywhere

CHAPTER 8

Population Health and Wellness

HEALTH AND WELLNESS PROMISES to be a huge area for artificial intelligence (AI) in healthcare. Doing good public health, keeping people healthy at scale, and carrying out preventive health have been difficult, to say the least. People have different types of diseases, different barriers to being healthy, and different habits and styles of learning and communication. If we want to reach them, we need to engage them in a way that appeals to them about their health concerns and issues, and in a way that they like and understand. This isn't easy, which is why so many attempts have failed to date.

The promise of data, digital technologies, and AI is that we can personalize at scale. We can apply AI to each individual's data to figure out what issues they have, what barriers are keeping them from addressing those issues, and to offer solutions that are tailored to how they like to consume information or feedback that motivates them to take action. There's hope that using AI tools to figure out what to do with data collected through passive methods will allow us to shift the playing field to improve patient health using technology and innovation.

Due to the COVID-19 pandemic, consumers have been increasingly buying connected monitoring devices, and that trend is expected to gather pace in the future. Deloitte projected there to be strong demand for wearable wellness tech this decade, with 320 million health and wellness wearables shipped to consumers throughout the world in 2020.[1] The figure is due to hit 440 million by 2024. Meanwhile, CCS Insight says that over 1.2 billion devices will be in use by the end of 2025.[1] It's believed that new product launches and more demand from healthcare providers is helping to drive this growth.

AI Doctor: The Rise of Artificial Intelligence in Healthcare: A Guide for Users, Buyers, Builders, and Investors, First Edition. Ronald M. Razmi.
© 2024 Ronald M. Razmi. Published 2024 by John Wiley & Sons, Inc.

People from all over the world are increasingly using smartwatches to monitor everything from their running pace to their health, with new hardware and software turning their watches into personalized health clinics. Innovation in the field is rapidly accelerating through advances in semiconductors, sensors, and AI. These increasingly sophisticated devices mean that consumer wearables could become a screening tool to flag potential medical issues much earlier than ever before.

It's becoming increasingly possible to use real-time data analysis with advanced AI algorithms to process the data coming from sensors about sleep, nutrition, exercise, blood pressure, weight, and mood to provide real-time advice and coaching to patients. Ultimately, AI-powered digital health coaches could someday become a reality, incorporating various types of data and designing personalized plans for each individual before working with them over time to implement those plans. Using deep learning, we could build predictive models to determine patients' biological ages. We could then use AI to develop different phenotypes that are more precise and which correlate with accelerated biological aging and even cognitive decline. More advanced phenotypes will allow for more personalized analysis of diet, lifestyle choices, and glucose responses and have a huge impact on individuals.[2]

8.1   Nutrition

Nutrition is an area of great interest with lots of investment and a huge amount of promise but where little progress has been made so far. Although a number of companies are already touting personalized nutrition, supplements, and vitamins, there's little evidence that it's making people healthier in the long term. But that's okay because we need to start with less-than-perfect options and keep on building our collective experience and evidence to find the best solutions.

AI seems well-suited for this as our response to food involves many factors such as our genes, our environment, our microbiome, and other factors that we don't even understand right now. As such, we need to analyze massive amounts of data to identify patterns and relationships to our health. One key area to focus on is the analysis of our gut microbiome as one way to determine our response to different foods. Machine learning (ML) is showing incredible promise, but studies are hard to carry out because we can't construct blind studies for nutrition.

The first major development here happened a couple of years back when Eran Elinav, Eran Segal, and their team at Israel's Weizmann Institute of Science published a paper titled "Personalized Nutrition for Prediabetes by Prediction of Glycemic Responses."[3] In their study, which appeared in the journal Cell, they continuously monitored glucose levels in 800 patients, measuring their responses to 46,898 meals and finding a high amount of variability in the way that they responded to identical meals. This suggests that universal dietary recommendations are of limited use. They also used a machine-learning algorithm to factor in dietary habits, anthropometrics, blood parameters, physical activity, and gut microbiota, showing that it accurately predicted patients' postprandial glycemic response to their meals. They were also able to validate their predictions in an independent 100-person cohort. On top of that, a blinded, randomized, and controlled dietary intervention based on their algorithm led to significantly lower postprandial responses and consistent alterations to the configuration of gut microbiota. When put together, all of these results suggest that personalized diets could successfully modify elevated postprandial blood glucose levels and mitigate its consequences on the metabolism.

There are now a host of companies that offer personalized diets based on the analysis of genomes, microbiomes, and other factors. This is an emerging science with a lot of promise and scientific sense behind it, but we don't yet have enough evidence to know if it's better than eating a healthy and balanced diet full of fruits and vegetables.

The Academy of Nutrition and Dietetics is just one of many bodies that's calling for caution here, saying, "The practical application of nutritional genomics for complex chronic disease is an emerging science and the use of nutrigenetic testing to provide dietary advice is not ready for routine dietetics practice."[4] But that still hasn't put investors off from investing millions in the space.

One such company is Whole Biome, which is pioneering the use of gut-assisting microbes to create medical food to treat diabetes. This company is working with the likes of the Mayo Clinic to generate the required evidence for such an approach.[5] Other companies include Wellness FX, Pure Genomics, Cell, and DayTwo. They use a range of approaches including genetic testing, epigenetics testing, labs, microbiomes, and prediction of glycemic responses to recommend a personalized nutrition approach.

Another example is 23andMe, which provides its customers with gene-based food recommendations. Customers submit a sample of their saliva to the personal genetics startup via an at-home kit. They can then choose to receive high-level dietary recommendations, such as how many vegetables they should eat and how often they should eat red meat. These recommendations are based upon health information that's reported by other customers with a similar genetic makeup.

Gut microbiome tests are gathering momentum as nutritional tools. They work by analyzing the makeup of the bacteria and microorganisms that live in our digestive tracts, many of them playing a vital role in our bodily functions by allowing us to break down food.

Viome is one of the most prominent companies in the space. Its at-home tests assess users' microbes to suggest foods and supplements that could complement them. This includes identifying specific foods amongst wider categories, such as by telling users to skip bell peppers if they find a virus that specifically interferes with the peppers' digestion. The company has also partnered with the Mayo Clinic to study the microbiome's role in chronic conditions, with an initial focus on sleep-related disorders like sleep apnea and obesity. Together, they'll track measures of obesity, metabolism, and sleep and analyze how they respond to nutritional modifications. Ultimately, they seek to assess the effectiveness of personalized nutrition as a disease management strategy.[6]

In Japan, Nestlé's Wellness Ambassador program provides personalized nutrition by allowing users to upload photos of the food they're eating. Its app then uses AI to analyze the photos and combines that with personal data from DNA and blood tests to recommend nutrient-infused teas, smoothies, and snacks. The program had picked up around 100,000 users.[7]

Then there's Care/Of, which invites its customers to complete a quiz that details key factors like their gender, lifestyle habits, age, diet, and existing health problems. It can then use an algorithm to create a personalized pack of vitamins, saving users the time and effort of looking for suitable products themselves. Their vitamins are then delivered once per month through a subscription service.

A similar company called Rootine offers up microbeads that can provide a personalized dose of vitamins throughout the day. They say that this mimics the way that real food is absorbed. Rootine uses an algorithm that analyzes data from genetic testing, a lifestyle questionnaire, and bloodwork to create tailored microbead combinations for users.[7]

One of the challenges of this approach is that online questionnaires have been criticized for being reductionist. The critics argue that any nutritional advice that's based on a questionnaire is almost certainly less accurate and less beneficial than tests that are overseen by healthcare providers. However, it's important to remember that there's not a lot of evidence for the more extensive testing, either.

Wearables can provide us with hard data, but their use cases are limited and several nutrition-recommendation tools are still asking their users to self-report their activity levels and what they're eating. Even if we assume that the nutrition platform is giving good advice, there's a risk of its accuracy being undermined due to missing data or personal biases. This challenge is unlikely to be resolved any time soon, but wearables can at least help to provide us with a larger amount of data as the technology improves, taking some of the burden to report away from users.

AI can help by analyzing what people eat, understanding its nutritional content and providing feedback and guidance based on the patient's goals. Some nutrition studies are asking participants to photograph their meals so that the images can be processed by deep learning tools to accurately determine what they're eating. This avoids the hassle of manually logging the data and the use of unreliable food diaries.[8] Other companies are playing with novel approaches that might pay off in the future, such as by analyzing the sound of chewing. Other companies like Vessyl track and analyze what you drink.

Many of the most common wearable devices, including those by Apple and Fitbit, can be used to log meals and track diets, usually through manual entry or by the user scanning barcodes. They're then able to provide an estimated calorie intake along with a breakdown of micronutrients. The Georgia Institute of Technology was able to create a mouth wearable that monitors salt intake and uses sensors to wirelessly report back to an app to help its users to manage the sodium in their diet. Similarly, Tufts University researchers developed a tooth-mounted sensor that detects glucose, salt, and alcohol intake.[7]

Tel-Aviv's Nutrino uses AI to recommend diet plans based on signals like stress and activity levels. Medical device giant Medtronic acquired Nutrino at the end of 2018, with the stated aim of using its technology to help patients with diabetes.[7]

Buoyed by the broader wellness trend, the personalized nutrition market is expected to continue to grow in the coming years as more and more people expect the same amount of personalization that they get from other industries like fashion and entertainment. From 3D-printed pills to DNA-driven dietary recommendations and nutrient-tracking mouth wearables, the idea is to achieve better health through wellness offerings which are tailored to each user's individual circumstances.

With that said, we need to remember that the current generation of personalized nutrition platforms can't replace advice from qualified professionals. Many wellness wearables still aren't ready to go to market, while up-and-coming fields like nutrient genomics are being subjected to ever-increasing skepticism and scrutiny. We'll need to make significant advancements if we want to establish public trust and to maintain it over the longer term. We've already seen a number of high-profile failures in this space for well-funded companies like Arrivale, Ubiome, and Driver, all of which had high price tags and niche customer segments. Each of their business models relied on consumers spending a large amount of money to buy a product with uncertain benefits.

The National Institutes of Health have been carrying out new research that centers on precision nutrition and which should be instrumental to the growth of the field. One study, announced at the start of 2022, is nested in the organization's All of Us research program, which aims to enroll a million people in healthcare research to promote precision medicine and to speed up the pace of medical discoveries.[9, 10] The goal is to gather data that we can use to create healthy and effective diet plans that are grounded in human diversity and which are tailored to each individual patient.

Research into precision nutrition will allow us to build on the advances we've already made in biomedical science, much of which comes from the fields of AI, genetics, and microbiomes. All of this research will contribute additional data on people's dietary habits, and we'll be able to use a combination of AI processing and data mining to create and validate algorithms that can be used in clinics.

We're seeing ever-increasing demand for better wellness and more personalized nutrition, and we can hope that this will eventually encourage mainstream consumers to improve their health. It all depends whether technology and its real-life applications can fulfill their full potential. The next step is to do prospective studies to see if personalized nutrition really does help with better weight loss, improved blood lipids, and other areas.

8.2   Fitness

As a result of the pandemic, many fitness tech startups are capitalizing on people being home more and avoiding going to the gym. As people were temporarily unable to seek wellness experiences from physical businesses like spas and studios, digital products and services are finding new audiences. This may lead to more people finding that these are viable wellness options and sticking with them over the longer term. It also can facilitate a fitness experience that's characterized by wearables, interactive services, personalization, and on-demand availability.

These efforts include AI-based wellness applications that are designed to allow consumers to track their fitness over time, providing feedback and guidance and enabling personalized exercise plans. One emerging trend is fusing biosensors with AI. To do so, some startups are creating sensors and monitoring devices, as well as machine-learning algorithms that they can use to interpret the data. Then there are those companies that do one or the other, such as those that are only developing the software and which are then integrating it with devices from third-party providers. This allows them to design personalized exercise programs while simultaneously providing monitoring and feedback.

Tokyo-based FiNC, for example, uses an AI-driven chatbot to provide personalized recommendations to help users achieve their exercise, sleep, and nutrition goals.[5] AI is increasingly being used to design exercise programs to promote weight loss, control blood pressure, boost cardio fitness, increase muscle mass, and improve core strength and flexibility. The goal is to individualize based on genetics, clinical data, activity data, preferences, motivation, lifestyle, work schedule, child care, past history with programs, and more.

To see this in action, we can look at companies like AthGene, which provides genetic analysis for fitness buffs so that they can better optimize their workouts and diet. Companies are also experimenting with other types of equipment and training formats. Tonal, an at-home connected fitness device equipped with an AI-enabled personal trainer, uses electromagnetic resistance to adjust the difficulty of exercises in real time.[11] It adjusts the resistance to power upper and lower-body weight lifting programs. Tonal's device also offers personalized coaching and uses AI to adapt weights to each user.

Another company, Tempo, has a connected device that streams fitness classes and uses AI-enabled computer vision to offer real-time form and technique corrections.[11] The company Vi offers a set of headphones and an app that comes with an AI trainer to motivate and coach runners of varying experience levels. Its biosensing headphones give users live feedback during cardio workouts, like step rate coaching and heart rate training. Individuals can also compete against other runners in real time.[11]

There are also companies producing connected apparel and athleisure gear that collects data, and they're increasingly adding AI layers to make sense of that data and provide actionable feedback. For example, Athos Works produces sensor-laden performance apparel and an accompanying fitness tracker app that helps users to monitor their fitness progress.[11]

As consumers are increasingly interested in on-demand, personalized, and mobile exercise programs, more solutions featuring at-home health monitoring with AI-enabled guidance are entering the market. If evidence is created that the AI-powered personalization of exercise recommendations results in improved metabolism, better fitness, fewer injuries, and more engaging programs, the use of such solutions will become more and more commonplace.

8.3   Stress and Sleep

More than half of adults globally suffer from insufficient sleep, according to a study by Wakefield Research.[6] This is bad news, because the lack of sleep can contribute to a number of major health issues like heart disease, and all of this places our society (and our healthcare systems) under a huge amount of financial strain. One 2016 study by RAND found that insufficient sleep costs the United States $411 billion per year due to lost productivity. Prior to the COVID-19 outbreak, insufficient sleep was already a prevalent and global phenomenon.

For many individuals, recent events have caused stress and anxiety, which are exacerbating current sleep disorders or creating new issues. For instance, one study found that 34% of healthcare workers in China were experiencing insomnia related to the pandemic. Further, many studies state the importance of a proper night's rest for the body to fight infection and recover from illness. Due to sleep issues caused by heightened stress, as well as a societal move toward prioritizing rest and achieving a healthier work/life balance, sleep technologies are likely to continue to gain attention in the years to come. Across the spectrum, consumers spending more time at home may see the need to upgrade their sleep routines to increase comfort, protect immune function, or tackle sleep disorders.

AI promises to play a role in addressing this issue, with new technologies enabling us to better treat sleep disorders. Companies across a wide range of different specialisms are all coming together to try to push the sleep tech industry forward. Just as with nutrition and exercise, the technology-enabled management of sleep starts with sensors to collect data and then algorithms can make sense of that data to provide personalized feedback and guidance. The same is true for stress management. The initial steps are about using modern devices such as cell phones to remotely and passively evaluate people's moods and stress levels. Once large enough datasets are built, AI will find patterns to diagnose and hopefully start recommending helpful and timely interventions.

Sleep-tracking devices are gaining popularity as individuals look to measure a number of sleep-based data points (such as duration, sleep quality, and the percentage of time spent in light/deep/REM sleep) so that they can turn them into therapeutic insights. These come in a variety of forms, such as wristbands (Whoop and Polar), rings (Oura and Motiv), headbands (Dreem and Muse), headphones (Kokoon), under-the-mattress sensors (EarlySense, Emfit, and SleepScore Labs), and more. Headbands, headphones, and under-the-mattress devices generally only track sleep, while wristbands and rings tend to be multifunctional. Right now, these companies mostly collect data and make rudimentary assessments and recommendations.[11]

There are also smart bed startups that adjust sleep conditions based on data. Companies like Eight, ReST, and Sleepace use mattress-embedded bio-sensors to adjust factors such as mattress temperature and firmness. Somnox has developed a sleep robot that acts as a sleep companion that's designed to improve breathing and help calm the mind.

Mattress giant Tempur Sealy partnered with Fullpower Technologies, a sleep tracker company, to enhance its product line. Together, the companies developed the Tempur-Ergo Smart Base, which features contactless sleep/snore-monitoring sensors and an adaptive base. Using that data, Fullpower's AI platform generates automated snoring interventions and personalized coaching modules (displayed in an accompanying mobile app) to promote better sleep.[6]

Meanwhile, companies are taking steps to integrate sleep wearables into the smart home. For example, Chinese sleep wearable manufacturer, Sleepace, has added smart bedrooms to its sleep suite of products. The sleep module features a connected sleeping routine with bedroom temperature monitoring, smart pillows, alarm and light activation upon waking up, and more.[6]

We talked earlier about Viome and its partnership with the Mayo Clinic for personalized nutrition. The company has also partnered with the Mayo Clinic to study the microbiome's role in chronic conditions, with an initial focus on sleep-related disorders like sleep apnea and obesity. Together, they'll track measures of obesity, metabolism, and sleep and analyze how they respond to nutritional modifications.[6] A similar collaboration between microbiome startup Holobiome and Johnson & Johnson focused on developing microbiome therapeutics for sleep disorders and related comorbidities.[12] A number of companies, including tech giants Amazon and Google, are developing wearables that they hope will eventually gain Food and Drug Administration (FDA) clearance and allow users to detect sleep apnea.

Improving sleep through devices like these could also unlock mental health benefits, including everything from more mindfulness and reduced stress to better clarity and even the ability to unlock lucid dreaming. For stress management, companies are increasingly using digital biomarkers to monitor physical and mental health. Companies like Thymia and Ksana Health are using cell phones to collect information about mood for the detection and diagnosis of stress. The data can be used by AI to assess stress based on voice, activity, and movement. Dreem is developing a headband that uses audio to promote relaxation and improve sleep. The device also tracks brain activity, heart rate, breathing, and movement via embedded sensors to provide insights into users' sleep quality.[11]

Mood trackers such as Woebot use app-based interactions with users to drive the content and frequency of their interactions with them and also use AI to provide interactive first-line, chat-based therapy. Wearables are also becoming more prevalent in mental health and wellness. Some of these products use electroencephalogram sensors to measure the brain's electrical activity and create a personalized approach to achieving relaxation and mindfulness. Muse's wearable device uses brainwaves to create sounds that help users relax and focus during guided meditation sessions. Other startups, such as Kokoon and Dream, also use this technology to bring more tailored approaches to relaxation.[11]

Some companies are developing AI-powered software and chatbots to support mental well-being by engaging with consumers. For example, Shine sends daily tips and content to its users through text to help boost confidence, happiness, and productivity. Wysa offers self-care exercises and can connect people to live therapists.[11]

AI-based algorithms are already working on understanding human emotions by analyzing data points on nonverbal cues like voice patterns and facial expressions. In some cases, these algorithms can even simulate emotions themselves. Called emotion AI or affective computing, this approach is a promising area of research and one that could have huge implications for the future of AI in managing stress and mental health.

8.4   Population Health and Management

One of the most discussed topics in the delivery of healthcare over the last ten years has been population health management. The idea is that we can manage everyone's health in a way that keeps them healthier and in less need of medical care. This is as opposed to the traditional way of providing care to people when they don't feel well and seek medical attention. The thinking behind this approach is that if we find and address health risks in individuals, we can prevent more costly downstream medical care. People will live healthier lives and we'll lower the cost of care. Everyone wins!

Even with the upstream investment of screening the population and carrying out risk assessments and management, this would be a massive cost saver overall. Why? Because most healthcare dollars are spent dealing with the complications of chronic diseases. If we can prevent those, the savings will be massive and the upfront investment will be minuscule in comparison. For example, elevated blood pressure causes kidney disease and cerebrovascular issues in the long term. Those are costly because chronic kidney disease care (such as dialysis) costs the system a lot of money every year. However, with a generic $10 per month blood pressure pill, all of that could be avoided. A person with high blood pressure who takes blood pressure medication won't develop any of those complications. But for that to happen, we need to find those individuals, convince them to be screened, and ensure that they take their prescribed medication. We'll also need them to follow the recommended behavioral changes such as lowering their salt intake, losing weight and exercising, following up with their doctor on a regular basis, and continuing to be checked for complications.

There are a number of barriers that can stop this approach from being successful. People often prioritize things other than their health unless they're not feeling well. They find it hard to change their diet and exercise habits, might not have the time, money, or transportation to show up for appointments, don't always understand instructions from their providers, and can have preexisting beliefs about medication that keep them from taking it on a long-term basis. They also often forget to take their meds.

Many historical attempts by payers to control the cost of care through "case management" didn't show any appreciable benefits. Around ten years ago, when the Affordable Care Act passed, the thinking shifted toward providers being expected to do this instead of payers. This was due to a couple of reasons. First, much of the data needed to manage patients is clinical data and not the claims data that the payers have access to. As such, providers should theoretically be more effective at identifying people at risk and understanding what those risks are for each individual. Second, providers have relationships with their patients and are trusted by them to provide advice and care. As such, they should be able to succeed where payers can't.

Although progress is being made here, it's also difficult and has led to mixed results so far. I built one of the first companies in this space. Acupera built software to allow for the intelligent automation of the ongoing care management process for health systems. Given the number of activities that need to be performed beyond what's traditionally been done, providers simply can't do all of this. Technology has to be used to scale these programs to touch enough patients. What we found is that medical institutions and healthcare providers are already busy managing the patients who are presenting for care, and so it's not easy for them to take on the additional job of managing population health. It requires a rethinking of their entire business model and a redesign of processes, staffing, and the technological infrastructure. That takes time, planning, and execution, along with realigned incentives. That's why progress toward true population health management has been slow and why we haven't seen the expected payoffs just yet.

At the core of all this is that by asking providers to carry out population health management, we're asking them to take on activities that are outside their traditional role, training, and daily workflow. It requires checking in with patients outside of the clinical setting and addressing barriers such as financial issues, transportation issues, mental health problems, health literacy issues, and abnormal readings from home devices. How can they do this when their clinic is already full of patients? Well, technology will be a big part of the answer, but as we saw at Acupera, it won't be enough. However, the better the technology gets in off-loading more and more from the providers' to-do list, the more likely it will be that providers will be able to successfully execute these programs.

What if a lot of the checking-in, numerical analysis, and education could be done automatically? What if the data could be collected passively or with minimal effort? Algorithms could then analyze the data and figure out what needs to be done, address basic issues, create plans, and assign activities to the appropriate resources.

This is where sensors, wearables, AI, and telehealth come in. As these technologies mature and their use cases become better formulated, they can become the cornerstone of population health management. They can take on the extra work that the providers are unable to do at scale. This means that in the near future, we should be able to identify and manage health risk much better and at scale, improving people's health at a fraction of what we're spending today.

One of the reasons why AI-based digital health tools have the potential to be so valuable to us is that they have the potential to remove the access barriers that are stopping us from reaching more people. Better still, AI can help to reduce the day-to-day load of managing chronic conditions, both for the provider and the patient. In my opinion, the key reason for the mixed results of population health programs so far is the fact that ongoing care management requires many activities to be performed by the patient and the care team, and there's just not enough people or time to do it all. Providing intelligent automation that takes care of a lot of these tasks would go a long way toward ensuring the success of these programs.

This is one of the areas where I'm the most optimistic about generative AI (e.g. ChatGPT) in healthcare, because it could eventually power meaningful interactions with patients. If responding to patient questions can be handled by generative AI, that removes the burden of the care team having to respond to every patient issue. And if generative AI can create discharge summaries and make patient care plans more personalized, it will improve the odds of patients adhering to those plans. When a telephone encounter is created, the assigned nurse will be able to use generative AI to create a response based on the patient's message. The tool will provide recommendations based on what the patient is calling for, the nurse will review the choices, select the response, and add it to the record with a single click.[13]

For people with chronic conditions to achieve optimum health outcomes, it's essential for them to use digital solutions that are built on behavioral data science. These integrated solutions are also critical for digital health companies, because uptake and ongoing engagement will be higher for tools that can adjust to the patients' situation.[14] But to do this, digital tools will need to go way further than just providing people with data or basic instructions. They'll need to motivate people to proactively improve their health, encouraging engagement and retention to push people to become motivated to stay healthy.

8.5   Risk Assessment

At the heart of good population health management is figuring out who's at risk and what those risks are. This is a lot easier if you have good data about people. We talked in the chapter on clinical decision support about how the amount of data available for each person has increased dramatically and how this data holds valuable insights about their health. In the long term, we'll be able to use that data to successfully manage people's health and keep them healthy. In the short term, we need to figure out how to handle the data and figure out what it means.

Traditionally, providers and health systems have relied on claims-based risk models, such as the Center for Medicare and Medicaid Services-Hierarchical Condition Category (CMS-HCC), Adjusted Clinical Group (ACG), and Diagnostic Cost Group (DxCG). Models like these are pretty good at estimating population risk, but they're less than satisfactory when used to predict risks at an individual level. Using the increasing amount of clinical, behavioral, environmental, and other types of data (Figure 8.1), we can now assess risk at an individual level and be more predictive.

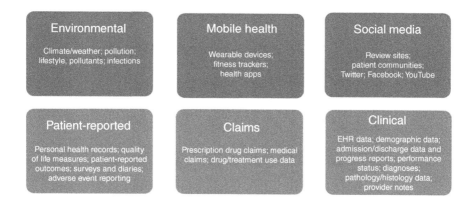

FIGURE 8.1   **Different Types of Patient Data** *(source: Adapted from[15])*

The emergence of cloud computing to store all of this data, interoperability standards and tools to pool each person's data, AI to clean up the data and identify patterns and relationships, and mobile technologies to engage and communicate with the population about risks and interventions are all great steps forward. Much heavy lifting remains to be done in all of these areas, but we're on our way. AI helps with the analysis of all of that data and figuring out what to with those insights. I'm of the belief that deploying AI is the only way that this could work, because there's so much more data than before and the human mind isn't very good at integrating all of this data into its decision-making.

Predictive analytics and risk scoring will be at the heart of this foundational piece of population health management. There are a number of AI-based solutions that are tackling this challenging task using the expanded amount of data that's increasingly available. These solutions use natural language processing (NLP) and machine learning to process and collate data from a number of disparate sources, ranging from medical images to genomics data and electronic health records (EHRs), to identify the patients that are the most at risk. This in turn will give clinicians much better data that can be used to make diagnoses. It will also give insurers a more realistic view of the potential medical costs that any given patient could be facing.

Machine-learning approaches to managing high-risk individuals using patient risk models based on EHRs, labs, claims, pharmacy data, and social determinants of health (SDOH) can yield significant improvements in patient outcomes and costs. When not managed correctly, nearly 18% of patients with rising risk end up in the high-risk category each and every year. Machine learning can help us to detect these rising risks at a minute scale from the huge pool of training data.[16]

These high-value risk models can be applied to different settings. In an inpatient setting, the models can help to identify those at the highest risk of pressure ulcers and/or falls. Transitioning to outpatient settings, the AI models can identify those at the highest risk of readmission and high usage of healthcare resources. Not only is AI capable of identifying those at the highest risk but also it highlights the drivers of that risk and can create personalized management plans.

Tempus, a technology company, is already using AI to assess and help manage risk. The company has harnessed AI for the purposes of analyzing clinical and molecular data to assess the risk of patients with cancer and to create personalized cancer treatment plans for patients. Then there's Welltok, a SaaS-based consumer health platform which uses AI to connect pharmacies and Pharmacy Benefit Managers (PBMs) to healthcare providers and employees. The goal is to create personalized health plans which are tailored to each individual patient based upon their medical history.[17]

8.6   Use of Real World Data

If we want to improve population health, we need to gather huge amounts of real world data based on people's day-to-day behavior. The good news is that consumers are growing more and more used to using wearables, smartphone apps, and virtual assistants to track their health data. These days, human activity is one of the biggest sources of healthcare information, and this data can help healthcare organizations to assess behavior and biometrics in the wild, as opposed to within the clinic. I'd always rather have a home blood pressure reading than reading taken in the doctor's office. I'd also always prefer to see the actual steps taken in a week over a manual log.

AI can help us to extract and segment the data we need, and it can also be used to power data analysis and community-based health campaigns. That will put it at the heart of successful population health management, enabling researchers to study clinical interventions, as well as interventions addressing social determinants and measuring the success of population health initiatives. Tools like big data and NLP are already being used to screen for potentially fatal diseases like cancer, as well as for developing customized treatments.[18]

8.7   Medication Adherence

Ensuring that patients follow through with recommended treatments is challenging and many issues can act as barriers. People might not understand their treatment plan and why they're being given a certain medication. They might not be able to afford transportation to pick up the medication. They might experience side effects and not know how to deal with it, leading to them stopping the medication. Here, AI can use data like patients' past behavior (e.g. not showing up to their appointments) or other data such as their zip code, education level, and indications of their mood and mental health to identify those most at risk of nonadherence, meaning the patients who are most likely to either not use their medication or to fail to collect it in the first place. This can prompt healthcare providers to intervene proactively. Pharmacies and healthcare providers will then be able to optimize their interventions by using rank-ordered, prescriptive, recommended, and preferred intervention lists. Large, longitudinal datasets could be used to determine whether the models are successful and/or effective. The goal is to measure the outcomes over time for large populations.[19]

8.8 Remote Engagement and Automation

Ongoing engagement with patients at risk is one of the cornerstones of population health management. This is to ensure that patients under-stand and follow their care plan and that if things take a turn for the worse, immediate intervention can prevent a debilitating and costly exacerbation of their chronic issues. Of course, it's easier said than done. We're talking about millions of patients and limited healthcare resources. How can we ensure the success of a population health program? Enter digital technologies, mobile phones, and AI.

AI is increasingly showing the capability to engage in basic interac-tions with individuals to check in with them, answer basic questions, send information, triage them to the appropriate care settings, and escalate their issues to the right care providers when appropriate. In short, AI is starting to facilitate scaled up, ongoing engagement.

One of the most promising areas for generative AI is the potential for more sophisticated chatbots that can engage with patients and perform many of the activities that are currently performed by the care team. These include checking in with patients about their chronic disease symptoms, asking them about social issues that could keep them from fully following their care plan, ensuring medication and lifestyle adherence, answering their questions, and helping to create patient communication material. This is where technologies like ChatGPT can have a huge impact. This may turn out to be the key to the success of these population health programs, since it provides scale to teams that are often short-staffed.

A company called MyndYou is selling an AI-based virtual care assistant called MyEleanor, an effective and automated tool that can help care teams to more efficiently engage with their patients. With a diverse patient population and the need for high engagement to achieve that population's desired health outcomes, Essen Healthcare in New York has used MyEleanor to engage with their patient population.[20]

MyEleanor conducts automated calls to high-risk patients and collects information from them. This information helps with planning the right interventions for each person and with the prioritization of caseloads. It also allows Essen's clinical staff to focus only on those patients that are getting worse. This wouldn't otherwise be possible due to the limited number of people on the care management team.

MyEleanor works by contacting patients by phones and using AI, NLP, and proprietary algorithms to listen to both what they say and how they say it. The system engages the patients, collects the right information, identifies key insights, and passes it on to the care team. Essen reports that its patients often tell Eleanor things that they wouldn't tell their doctor, while the system can detect worsening conditions based on what they're *not* saying, too. This includes everything from behavioral and mental health issues to their risk of falls. The vast majority of Eleanor's patients are underprivileged, and a lot of them can only speak Spanish. Because of that, it's designed to reduce the need for translators by carrying out calls in both English and Spanish and by providing care coordinators with a Health Insurance Portability and Accountability Act (HIPAA)-compliant transcript of every call it makes.[20]

Eleanor can even provide customized health questionnaires which offer real-time feedback to coordinators based upon patients' responses. This feedback tackles concerns about patients and highlights every patient's unique needs as well as any support that they might need, providing coordinators with customized alerts based on MyEleanor's findings. This is a form of triage, allowing care teams to focus on the high-risk patients and to provide a more intensive level of engagement. I tested this system and found it be impressive. It maintained an appropriate conversation with me based on my issues. I even threw some curveballs at it, but the system was able to navigate the conversation effectively. Essen reports that by using this AI-enabled virtual assistant, they've reduced hospitalizations and Emergency Department (ED) overuse while simultaneously supplying patients with more personalized care and treatment.[20]

Also, MyEleanor was able to clean up the patient contact lists, such as by identifying when phone numbers were outdated or no longer in service. This is a great example of an AI-enabled virtual assistant doing some of the heavy lifting of a care management program. We've already discussed how difficult it is to carry out population health management and how the providers haven't had much success, partly due to the sheer number of additional activities that have to be completed to manage a patient population.

All told, advances in AI, software, and mobile technology have enabled people to command machines to take desired actions, ushering in a new level of engagement through intelligent automation.

8.9 SDOH

In recent years, population health management strategies have started incorporating SDOH, as well as interventions addressing these needs. This is critical as many of the issues that keep patients from succeeding in managing their health aren't directly health-related. These include factors like health literacy, financial issues, transportation issues, mental health problems, and more. Determining the right interventions for these issues will require organizations to accurately assess patients' individual social needs and to provide timely responses. Done well, this will enable us to improve clinical outcomes across the board.

In short, placing organization-level and provider-level emphasis on including SDOH alongside traditional diagnosis data is helping us to create more complete pictures both of individual patients and patient populations as a whole. This will enable us to better target care management interventions, and so identifying and removing these barriers is often more important than the actual medical issues.

In the past, care management services have largely focused on patient education, clinical disease management, pharmaceutical adherence and appointment navigation, issues which chronically ill patients have to deal with each and every day. Now, we're starting to see the next stage of an evolution in care management services that also address social needs. These social issues can be identified partly by analyzing the various available data (Figure 8.1) and also by conducing assessments by asking the patient about these issues. By combining the available data from both clinical and social data sources, AI tools will help us to risk-stratify patient populations. We'll be able to identify those who are at a higher risk of social factors impacting their health access and place those at the top, with those facing less of a burden at the bottom. Once again, this will remove work from the to-do lists of providers and care teams, enhancing the success rates of these programs.[21]

As organizations and provider networks intervene on identified social needs, the resulting changes in clinical outcomes can be used in a feedback loop to retrain the machine-learning algorithm, helping the model to become more precise in determining which social need intervention is most likely to produce the greatest positive impact, improving efficiency for the intervening organization.[21] It might be best to train these models on data from the local patient population for accuracy and ensure that they're using data that will be available once they're operationalized, since not all of the clinical and social data will be available in different situations.

One key issue about SDOH is that they're rarely captured in structured formats in EHRs or other databases. Instead, the information is usually captured in a narrative format, and for large-scale analysis to take place for the purposes of population health management, it needs to be extracted and put into a machine-readable format. AI can help here through the use NLP.

An example of this was provided in a 2012 article in Healthcare IT News.[21] Bill Siwicki explained, *"Let's take a very straightforward example. A clinician documents the following for an elderly patient at admission: 'This gentleman was brought in by ambulance having been found lying outside his home. He lives alone, his wife having passed away three years ago. He normally uses a Z frame and can't drive.' This kind of documentation is standard in healthcare, and nine times out of ten, it remains hidden in the notes section of the EHR. With NLP, this statement can be transformed into structured data that reads: 'Social isolation; widowed; walks with assistive device; no transportation.' Having this information in a structured format against not just one patient, but an entire population, means providers can better identify those patients at higher need and higher risk."*

I've already written extensively about the limitations of NLP for extracting the desired insights out of clinical notes, but all of that could be changing with the emergence of large language models that can be trained on unstructured and unlabeled data and generate appropriate output based on that data. That means that these new models can identify key SDOH out of EHRs and other databases and summarize them for the care team. They can also help to create personalized care plans based on those issues. That takes a lot of heavy lifting away from the care team and allow them to focus on higher level activities.

8.10   Aging in Place

As baby boomers age and are increasingly reaching their later years, many are interested in staying in their own homes and living independently. An array of technologies is making it possible for older individuals with reduced functional abilities to age in place. Innovators are building health intelligence into existing caregiving products, such as voice-activated home assistants, virtual nurse avatars for routine checkups, and even sophisticated robotic home companions.[22, 23] AI technologies are playing a key role in this. Combined with sensors, cameras, wearables, and other technologies, they can monitor patients, send alerts if there's an adverse event, provide companionship for those who are lonely and help people to access medical care. Sensors and algorithms can monitor gait, speech, cognition, mood, and other factors. AI tools will sit at the center of all of this, improving safety and independence.

Human-like robots with humanoid features and temperaments are already being made, especially in Japan. These are companion robots that can become socially aware when combined with AI, making eye contact and tracking humans. Companies like Google, Amazon, and Apple are working on health elements for their home solutions with voice interfaces that can help the aging adults (Figure 8.2).

Americans older than 50 have 70% of the buying power in the United States. Given their desire to stay in their homes and age in place, this means

Alexa brings voice AI to healthcare

Created with features that provide assurance for you and independence for them

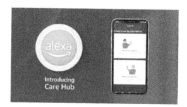

Alexa, Amazon's HIPAA-compliant virtual assistant, brings conversational AI to consumers and healthcare organizations through a variety of smart devices.

Notable enterprise adoption of Alexa:

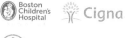

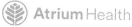

In 2020, Amazon launched Alexa Care Hub, a free virtual assistant designed specifically to support independent seniors and their family caregivers.

FIGURE 8.2   *(source: CB Information Services, Inc)*

that companies see these types of products and services as a major priority with the potential for a large return on investment.[24, 25] Consumers aged 65+ commanded about $8.4 trillion in spending power in 2020—a number that's expected to grow to $14 trillion over the next ten years per World Data Lab, signaling a key opportunity for aging-focused tech solutions.[25] This also includes products and services that help families and caregivers. Technologies that provide peace of mind to these groups have a high chance of adoption. These include tools which[26]:

- Monitor and alert them when their loved one requires urgent care. These tools need to be barely visible and easy to set up with little upkeep.
- Ensure home safety.
- Check on their loved ones.
- Monitor daily patterns such as movement around the house, bathroom usage, opening/closing doors, and sleep.
- Provide ambient intelligence for safety, health maintenance, and disease management.
- Provide medication management for refills and pickups and monitor consumption.
- Provide personalized information on the resources needed to provide care.
- Provide personalized guidance specific to the health conditions of their loved ones, including guidance on how best to care for them.
- Monitor nutrition and exercise and provide advice.
- Manage chronic conditions and provide disease-specific care instructions (such as what the patient needs to do and when they need to do it), as well as clear, automated prompts from trusted sources.

AI is having an impact on all of these categories by making existing products more engaging and intuitive, but significant unmet needs remain in many market opportunity areas, such as social innovation, respite care, and caregiver training. Some of the current work in this area includes designing systems to collect data that allows for the analysis and prediction of needs so that we can proactively intervene, personalize solutions, and monetize the data and insights.[27]

Some of the key barriers to the adoption of these technologies include lack of awareness, cost, fragmented solutions that don't manage all aspects of needs, lack of interoperability with pharmacies, insurers, other caregiving tools, the time constraints of finding and setting up technology, and more.

A prime application of AI in healthcare is fall detection and alerting others in case of a fall. The company SafelyYou uses AI technology to prevent falls amongst the elderly. A camera is installed in a resident's room and runs video that only saves a recording when the AI detects a fall. It's consensual, there's no audio or live streaming, and there are no wearables. We previously discussed passive monitoring technologies like the one developed by caspar.ai that use radar or infrared to monitor seniors' activity without using cameras or wearables. Companies like Caspar.ai are already using these technologies in long-term care facilities and improving the safety of residents. These technologies can also predict looming issues such as falls by detecting increasingly unsteady gaits using their AI algorithms. Also, they can detect patterns that can be predictive of deteriorating health. These patterns could involve patient activity level, number of visits to the bathroom, and time spent in bed. All of this can help proactively keep seniors safe and healthy at home or in long-term facilities.

Another prime area for innovation with AI is social companionship and ways to fight loneliness in the elderly. Companies like Revel and Element3 Health are creating communities for seniors with shared interests. While some of these companies focus on AI connection or virtual communities—a necessity during the pandemic—in the long-term, hybrid solutions that offer some element of in-person connection while enabling scale through digital platforms will be best positioned to succeed. Element3 Health uses matching algorithms to connect seniors who share hobbies and similar interests.[28]

References

1. Landi, H. (2021). Fueled by the pandemic, the growth trend in the market for smart, wearable devices is expected to continue this year and beyond. Fierce Healthcare. https://www.fiercehealthcare.com/tech/ai-wearable-device-for-home-care-gets-fda-clearance
2. Day, S., & Kaganoff, S. (2021). Healthcare's middle children: Potential disruptors flying under the radar, Rock Health

3. Ben-Yacov, O., Godneva, A., & Segal, E. (2020). 230-OR: personalized nutrition for prediabetes by prediction of glycemic responses. Diabetes, 69(Supplement_1). https://doi.org/10.2337/db20-230-or

4. Camp, K. M., & Trujillo, E. (2014). Position of the academy of nutrition and dietetics: nutritional genomics. Journal of the Academy of Nutrition and Dietetics, 114(2), 299–312. https://doi.org/10.1016/j.jand.2013.12.001

5. CB Insights. (2021, January 5). Healthcare AI trends to watch. CB Insights Research. https://www.cbinsights.com/research/report/ai-trends-healthcare/

6. CB Insights. (2020, August 17). Reinventing sleep: what 10 partnerships tell us about where sleep tech is going next. CB Insights Research. Retrieved September 22, 2022, from https://www.cbinsights.com/research/sleep-tech-partnerships/

7. CB Insights. (2020, July 13). Nutrition is moving beyond 'one size fits all.' Here's how tech is personalizing your diet. CB Insights Research. Retrieved September 22, 2022, from https://www.cbinsights.com/research/personalized-nutrition-wellness/

8. Topol, E. (2017). The A.I. Diet. The New York Times. https://www.nytimes.com/2019/03/02/opinion/sunday/diet-artificial-intelligence-diabetes.html

9. Nutrition for Precision Health, powered by the All of Us Research Program. 2022, September 14). NIH Common Fund. Retrieved September 22, 2022, from https://commonfund.nih.gov/nutritionforprecisionhealth

10. Siwicki, B. (2022, May 20). NIH All of Us Research Program puts focus on precision nutrition. Healthcare IT News. Retrieved September 22, 2022, from https://www.healthcareitnews.com/news/nih-all-us-research-program-puts-focus-precision-nutrition

11. CB Insights. (2020, June 29). 8 Trends redefining consumer wellness for 2020 and beyond. CB Insights Research. Retrieved September 23, 2022, from https://www.cbinsights.com/research/trends-redefining-consumer-wellness/

12. Holobiome, Inc. (2019, April 1). Holobiome Announces Second Collaboration with Johnson & Johnson innovation to create novel microbiome therapeutics. Retrieved September 23, 2022, from https://www.prnewswire.com/news-releases/holobiome-announces-second-collaboration-with-johnson--johnson-innovation-to-create-novel-microbiome-therapeutics-300822007.html

13. EHR vendors demo new GPT features at HIMSS23. (2023, April 19). Healthcare IT News. https://www.healthcareitnews.com/news/ehr-vendors-demo-gpt-himss23

14. Goldner, D., & Nagra, H. (2021, November 19). Contributed: The biggest merger in digital health should be between behavioral and data sciences. MobiHealthNews. Retrieved September 23, 2022, from https://www.mobihealthnews.com/news/contributed-why-biggest-merger-digital-health-should-be-between-behavioral-and-data-sciences

15. HIMSS. (2019). Building a real-time community insights: engine for a health-care system: challenges and opportunities. https://365.himss.org/sites/himss365/files/365/handouts/552672016/handout-MLAI13.pdf

16. Addressing the needs of your rising-risk patients, Advisory Board, Population Health Advisor. Advisory.com.

17. CB Insights. (2020, August 14). From drug R&D to diagnostics: 90+ artificial intelligence startups in healthcare. CB Insights Research. Retrieved September 26, 2022, from https://www.cbinsights.com/research/artificial-intelligence-startups-healthcare/

18. O'Sullivan, D., & Thomas, B. (2018). Is Artificial Intelligence (AI) Really Smart Enough to Transform Healthcare? | TripleTree. Retrieved September 23, 2022, from https://www.triple-tree.com/strategic-insights/2018/september/is-artificial-intelligence-ai-smart-enough/

19. Perez, K. (2020, October 19). The autonomous pharmacy: applying AI and ML to medication management across the care continuum. Ai4. Retrieved September 18, 2022, from https://ai4.io/blog/2020/02/27/the-autonomous-pharmacy-applying-ai-and-ml-to-medication-management-across-the-care-continuum/

20. Siwicki, B. (2021, November 30). How Essen Health Care used an AI virtual care assistant to make. Healthcare IT News. Retrieved September 23, 2022, from https://www.healthcareitnews.com/news/how-essen-health-care-used-ai-virtual-care-assistant-make-thousands-patient-calls-just-days

21. Siwicki, B. (2022, May 12). How NLP can help with at-risk patients, SDOH and pop health. Healthcare IT News. Retrieved September 23, 2022, from https://www.healthcareitnews.com/news/how-nlp-can-help-risk-patients-sdoh-and-pop-health

22. Caregivers & Technology: what they want and need. (2016, April 30). AARP & HIT Lab. https://doi.org/10.26419/res.00191.002

23. Project Catalyst, Parks Associates. (2017, June 1). Can 40 million caregivers count on you? AARP. Retrieved September 23, 2022, from https://www.aarp.org/research/topics/care/info-2019/caregiving-innovation-frontiers.html

24. Markets, R. A. (2020, December 16). Global health caregiving industry (2020 to 2027) - market trends and drivers. Research and Markets. Retrieved September 25, 2022, from https://www.globenewswire.com/news-release/2020/12/16/2145930/28124/en/Global-Health-Caregiving-Industry-2020-to-2027-Market-Trends-and-Drivers.html

25. Global Health Caregiving Market: Industry Analysis & Forecast | Persistence Market Research (PMR). (n.d.). Persistence Market Research. Retrieved September 25, 2022, from https://www.persistencemarketresearch.com/market-research/health-caregiving-market.asp

26. Dives, D., Hanss, K., Stotz, C., Zweig, M., With help from:, Evans, B., & Cassels, T. (2020, September 9). We've entered an unprecedented market for aging in place | Rock Health. Rock Health

27. CB Insights. (2021, March 24). How consumer health tech could improve aging in place for seniors. CB Insights Research. Retrieved September 25, 2022, from https://www.cbinsights.com/research/consumer-health-tech-aging-in-place-senior-care/

28. Hall, C. (2020, October 13). Living their best life at home: senior-focused start-ups and VCs reevaluate elder care. Crunchbase News. Retrieved September 25, 2022, from https://news.crunchbase.com/startups/living-their-best-life-at-home-senior-focused-startups-vcs-reevaluate-elder-care/

CHAPTER 9

Clinical Workflows

ONE OF THE GREAT DISAPPOINTMENTS of the last decade has been that most of the promises about implementing digital information systems to document clinical care never materialized. Electronic health records (EHRs), electronic reporting systems for radiology and pathology, data warehouses, and other information systems couldn't show that they improved care or made patients' lives and clinicians' jobs easier (quite the opposite). Although it's better to have as much of the patient information in one place as possible, usually in an EHR, so that the care team can look up patient information quickly, the entry of that data has been a major issue. This turns physicians, one of the most highly trained and important groups of professionals, into glorified data-entry clerks. It wastes their valuable working time that could and should be spent with patients.

The design of these EHRs hasn't made it easy for healthcare workers to easily find the most important information. Given that a lot of the information is in an unstructured format, it's also difficult to use it for analysis. That means that the promise of point-of-care decision support, analytic-driven workflows, and automation hasn't come to fruition, which is disappointing to everyone who uses them to provide care. Worse, the combination of not seeing any of these benefits and having to do the tedious work of entering the information has led to disillusionment and burnout. There's no question that entering this information has led to additional work hours for the care team.

It's against this backdrop that we view the promise of artificial intelligence (AI) in clinical workflows. The data that gets entered into the EHRs comes from interactions between clinicians and patients, is generated by devices that monitor the patients in the hospital and the clinic, and from the review of radiology scans and pathology slides, as well as a number of other sources. Some of these activities can generate structured data consisting of voice

AI Doctor: The Rise of Artificial Intelligence in Healthcare: A Guide for Users, Buyers, Builders, and Investors, First Edition. Ronald M. Razmi.
© 2024 Ronald M. Razmi. Published 2024 by John Wiley & Sons, Inc.

files, images, numbers from devices and digital text that AI can use to create files inside the EHR. AI can listen to physician–patient interactions and generate notes, place orders for tests, send messages to other providers or care members, create referrals and complete the forms, create testing reports, and more. Also, AI can improve how information is presented to the care team based on the context of the encounter to make their jobs easier and more efficient.

All of this is now much more possible thanks to the recent breakthroughs in generative AI. Much of clinician burnout is due to spending time writing notes, placing orders, generating referrals, writing prior authorization letters, and creating patient communication. In other words, burnout is caused by physicians having to generate output! With the emergence of large language models that are used to train generative AI solutions, these use cases will be at the frontier of AI's applications in healthcare. Given that these language models allow for better training of algorithms on unstructured data without having to annotate so much of the data, it seems that documentation and content generation will be low-risk use cases that could gain traction in the short term. Solutions are already emerging in this space that we'll discuss later in this chapter.

AI can also start to provide first-line support to patients in the form of bots using voice or text. This would be not only helpful to patients but also free up the care team to focus on more important activities and lighten their heavy load. Emerging applications for passively collecting data from patients, analyzing it for insights, and informing providers of the results with a preliminary action plan (rather than just passing numbers to the provider and giving them more to do!) would also improve care and help busy physicians, many of whom are suffering from burnout, especially after COVID.

AI solutions can be involved in a range of clinical and administrative tasks that will benefit the quality of decision-making and reduce the amount of work for everyone involved.

9.1   Documentation Assistants

Figure 9.1 shows some of the promising areas where AI can eventually help patients and providers. We've discussed some of this in other chapters. Areas such as smarter care and top-of-license applications are more futuristic. However, areas like data collection from patients, mining EHRs for relevant information, and improving the experience of the providers and patients are much closer to coming to fruition. Improving the ability to generate documents, extracting insights from them, ordering tests, and generating referrals create a lot of work for the care team but don't have to be done by them.

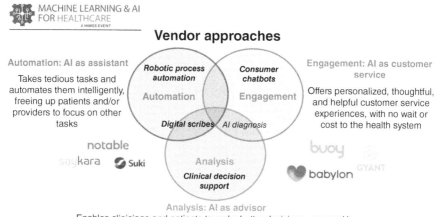

FIGURE 9.1   **AI As Advisor to Patients and Providers** *(source: Adapted from[1])*

Removing this from their to-do list would significantly improve their experience and reduce the pandemic of provider burnout. This would fulfill the promise of AI "augmenting" clinicians.

AI can become a foundational solution for—rather than a contributor to—burnout among physicians and achieving the quadruple aim of improving health, enhancing the experience of care, reducing cost, and attaining joy in work for health professionals (Figure 9.2). Augmented intelligence can be used to increase the capacity of healthcare professionals by combining the power of AI with human perception, empathy, and experience.

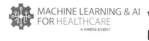
MACHINE LEARNING & AI FOR HEALTHCARE A HIMSS EVENT

Vision for AI and bots to support patients and providers

- **Before the visit:** Collect data from patient and mine EMR information to assist the provider and prepare the visit

- **Smarter care:** Reduce or eliminate unnecessary care that should be algorithmic/self-service

- **Navigate:** Patients to the right care option

- **Top-of-license:** Help direct lower level licensed (or the patients themselves) to conduct low-acuity physical exams where a higher license is not available or not required

- **Seamless experience:** Partner with technology companies and platforms to modularly access many AI/bots while providing a consistent experience and continuity

FIGURE 9.2   *(source: Adapted From[1])*

Common consumer applications of AI are already being used to augment human decision-making. A few examples of this include:

- Automated suggestions for the names of people in photographs to reduce the burden of manually documenting it (e.g. on Facebook).
- Voice-based communication with a virtual assistant (such as Alexa and Google Voice) decreasing the amount of screen time needed to find information.
- Recommended products and services based on your prior selections save time and reduce cognitive effort (e.g. on Netflix and Amazon).

In the context of clinical workflows, this can be helpful for documentation, coding, quality improvement, and more.

Clinical documentation in the EHR is one of the biggest drivers of physician burnout in the USA, causing as much as $90–140 billion in lost physician time per year.[2] Reducing the clinical documentation burden on physicians, which has been exacerbated by the adoption of EHRs, is a priority. A study supported by the American Medical Association (AMA) found that primary care physicians spend almost six hours a day on EHR data entry during a typical 11.4-h workday.[3] By auto-populating structured data fields (for example, allergies and problem lists) from open-ended physician notes, querying relevant data from prior clinical records and transcribing recorded patient encounters, AI has enormous potential to free physicians from their computers and dramatically reduce documentation burden. An example of this is clinical language understanding applications that analyze physician free-text narratives and extract problems and allergies as structured data.

Technology companies with expertise in automatic speech recognition—including Google and Stanford, Microsoft and UPMC, Nuance (Microsoft) and Epic, and NoteSwift and Athenahealth, plus a handful of startups such as Saykara and Suki—are already tackling this task. Their goal is to develop AI-driven digital scribes that can listen in on patient–physician conversations and automatically generate clinical notes.[4, 5] Only a few months after the release of ChatGPT by OpenAI, Microsoft's Nuance added the second version of ChatGPT, GPT4, to its medical note-taking tool. It's integrating GPT-4 into its Dragon Ambient Intelligence platform, which is used by hospitals around the country to ease doctor workloads by using AI to listen to patient-provider conversations and write medical visit notes.[6] Now, Epic is integrating this into its EHR to help physicians with their workflows.[7]

These speech recognition systems can potentially automate the creation of accurate clinical documentation in acute care, ambulatory care, and post-acute settings across both physical and virtual encounters. By freeing physicians up from documenting while they speak with patients, they improve the experience of the encounter, lead to improved patient and financial outcomes, and result in higher quality risk-adjusted quality ratings.

The American Academy of Family Physicians has established an Innovation Lab to explore promising technologies that can help in the practice of medicine.[8] They evaluated Suki, an AI assistant that uses voice and commands to help physicians to complete their documentation. Their assessment of Suki showed a 60% adoption rate, and those adopters saw a 72% reduction in their median documentation time per note. This resulted in calculated time savings of 3.3 h per week per clinician. In addition, participants reported improved satisfaction both with their workload and overall with their practice. They reported that physicians described it as a "breakthrough."[8]

They also evaluated Navina, which has an AI assistant that can summarize a patient's chart into a problem-oriented summary. This helps physicians with chart reviews and visit preparations. They saw significant reductions in chart preparation time and more accurate risk-coding. They also observed the identification of missed diagnoses buried in consultant and diagnostic reports.[8]

Rad AI uses AI to turn radiologist dictations into properly formatted reports. Google has also been exploring voice in healthcare applications. It offers two speech recognition models that are trained to understand medical terminology, including diagnoses, medications, and symptoms. The first model is tailored to doctor-to-patient conversations, and the second enables a single medical professional to dictate notes for easy reporting

Virtual assistants and natural language processing (NLP) can integrate real-time, AI-powered clinical intelligence within physicians' workflows and can help to reduce care gaps with contextual diagnostic and treatment guidance at the point of care. For example, NLP-based clinical language understanding generates structured data from an unstructured narrative in radiology reports in real time to document compliance with clinical standards and improve the closure of follow-up exam recommendations related to incidental findings. As I've emphasized before, NLP/NLU (natural language understanding) use cases for AI in clinical notes are work-in-progress, but the fact that they're not ready for prime time shouldn't be a showstopper. These technologies learn over time and putting them out there means that they'll improve with use and feedback.

One of the emerging concepts in this area is that of ambient intelligence. Ambient intelligence occurs when sensors such as microphones and cameras provide data to an AI system that can analyze what's going on in the clinical situation and generate notes for encounters, place the orders, order prescriptions, make referrals, and carry out other actions that come out of an encounter. This could be very powerful when it reaches maturity, since clinicians can forget key aspects of encounters, and it could eventually be better than a human follow-up to a visit. Speech recognition software can transcribe encounters three times faster than a human typing into a clinical system, potentially freeing up a couple of hours a day for a typical caregiver who sees 20–30 patients a day.

One of the benefits of AI technologies is that they're capable of learning and adapting with each interaction. This helps improve the outputs they generate over time and allows for a degree of personalization for each user. The more feedback that AI products receive from users through regular interactions, the better they can become at serving the unique needs of a particular practice, system, or provider.[9]

OrthoIndy, an orthopedic practice in Indianapolis, used Saykara to improve clinical workflows and make documentation easier and better. Saykara is a medical assistant that listens to encounters, creates notes, and places them in the right place in EHRs. It can also make referrals, prescribe meds, and assist with coding. It produces a fully structured note which goes directly into an Allscripts EHR. Physicians only need to review and sign off on the notes in the EHRs.[10] The reason OrthoIndy was so attracted to Saykara was that it promised to remove physicians from hands-on documentation.

At a broad level, ambient intelligence technology's true potential lies in going beyond documentation and becoming an intelligent assistant through effective listening for key issues and to-dos to document. The level of integration between emerging technology tools and core clinical platforms such as EHRs is a significant factor in increasing adoption rates. Today's fundamental challenge for voice recognition in ambient computing is the same for AI applications in general in the healthcare context.[11] Microsoft acquired Nuance as part of its effort to build robust ambient intelligence capabilities in healthcare (Figure 9.3).

Epic has worked with AI-powered voice solutions company Suki to integrate its generative AI assistant into its EHR software through its ambient API. Suki Assistant helps clinicians to complete time-consuming administrative tasks. The company uses generative AI and large language models to listen to the patient-doctor conversation, identify the clinically relevant portions and then summarize that information as suggestions for the note, without human intervention. Clinicians can then review and accept, reject or edit content suggestions to ensure the accuracy of final notes. Once notes are complete, they sync back to Epic.

While acquiring new tools to support clinicians

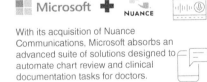

With its acquisition of Nuance Communications, Microsoft absorbs an advanced suite of solutions designed to automate chart review and clinical documentation tasks for doctors.

Nuance solutions are currently used by more than 55% of physicians and 75% of radiologists in the US and are used in 77% of U.S. hospitals.

Ambient device and mobile application
Clinicians engage in conversation with their patients while a dedicated mobile app or purpose-built ambient device with highly optimized microphone array, large interactive display, integrated biometrics, and multi-sensory capabilities securely captures a multi-party conversation.

Ambient skills
Simply say "Hey Dragon" to get information in and out of the EHR. Integrated virtual assistant capabilities enable care teams to complete a growing list of tasks in real time within their EHR and other third-party applications.

Ambient documentation
Deep-learning-based AI securely converts encounter conversations into standardized, structured notes tailored for each specialty that adhere to established documentation standards. AI-generated notes go through a brief quality review process to check for accuracy, omissions, and appropriateness before being delivered to the clinician for signature in the EHR–creating an AI learning loop for continuous improvement.

FIGURE 9.3 **Microsoft Aims to Launch Clinical Ambient Intelligence**
(source: Adapted from CB Insights)

Suki has reported that its ambient note-generation tech is capable of reducing documentation time per note by as much as 72% for family medicine physicians. The company's voice-enabled digital assistant has been integrated into other EHR platforms including Athenahealth, Cerner, and Elation Health.[12]

Here are some salient examples of how this is already making an impact in clinical care from the Health Evolution Summit about the applications of AI in healthcare in 2020[13]:

- Valleywise Health in Arizona added COVID-19-specific documentation templates via the cloud to its existing voice-powered and mobile-enabled documentation solution to eliminate repetitive data entry for stressed care teams. The enhancements enabled physicians to quickly and accurately capture COVID-19 patient acuity, the complexity of symptoms and the risk of mortality.

- Vanderbilt University Medical Center (VUMC) developed a clinical virtual assistant integrated with its Epic EHR to help physicians increase their effectiveness and time with patients while reducing burnout. Doctors can navigate the system, enter orders and talk to the system using natural language commands and questions. The system understands the user's intent and responds in context with visual and spoken summaries.

- Radiologists at Massachusetts General Hospital are expanding the use of speech recognition and real-time NLP for generating structured report data that aids in the early detection and treatment of disease with automated follow-up tracking and compliance. AI also helps ensure the accuracy and completeness of reports, maximizing appropriate value-based reimbursements and reducing duplicate imaging.

- Einstein Healthcare Network in Philadelphia uses AI-driven workflow automation and structured data extraction to reduce radiologist burnout, boost productivity, and improve care quality. Diagnostic AI models augment image interpretation and automate reporting. NLP adds real-time decision support and report quality checks within the normal daily workflow.

- Physicians at the Colorado Center for Reproductive Medicine in New York use mobile speech recognition and speech-enabled clinical documentation to help them engage with patients and their families. Clinicians estimate that they save at least 90 min per day while creating better quality consult notes, op notes, emails, and letters.

- Rush University Medical Center (RUMC) alleviates physician burnout and improves efficiency using a comprehensive, voice-powered EHR optimization initiative. It transformed perceptions of the EHR from a burden to a powerful source of real-time information for improving patient care. Automated documentation templates, clinical scoring, and other process improvements cut documentation time by 45% and raised RUMC's KLAS physician satisfaction score to the highest ever recorded for EHR experience at an academic health system.

- The University of Nebraska Medical Center is continuing to expand its use of ambient clinical intelligence to enable physicians to focus on patient interaction while the documentation essentially writes itself. The system distinguishes between different speakers during the exam, understands the conversation in context, adds clinical intelligence, and responds to clinician queries. After the exam is completed, the AI system creates a clinical note in the EHR and updates the patient's record with other critical data. Physicians report that time spent on documentation has been at least halved, giving them more time for patient care, other professional activities and to be with their families.

- EmergeOrtho in North Carolina uses an ambient clinical intelligence tele-health solution to transform how its orthopedic practices across the state can engage with patients and document care. The technology enables them to focus on patient interaction wherever they're located without having to learn and adjust to new systems and technologies. The system saves physicians significant time that's usually spent on administrative work after-hours and dramatically improves documentation quality during the virtual visit, allowing physicians to review notes that are then submitted directly into the EHR.

- Concord Hospital in New Hampshire extended the voice-powered and mobile documentation solution integrated with its Cerner EHR for physicians to its nurses fielding triage calls. In addition to improving documentation detail and accuracy, it reduced the time needed to complete documentation from 17 min per call to 6 min in just two weeks. That enabled physicians to respond more quickly, resulting in faster callbacks to patients and higher provider and patient satisfaction.

Figure 9.4 shows the documented results of such systems in action.[1] We can see that the use of AI led to saved hours and efforts for physicians.

There are a number of challenges presenting barriers to adoption which need to be continuously improved to make this more universal. One is the challenge of clear voice communication in a noisy and busy clinical setting, particularly when complex medical vocabulary is required. In some situations, it may be necessary to add visual support (such as the screen offering of an Amazon Show device or integrating the voice assistant with screenshots on the computer). Clinical guidelines and graphical displays of data are enhanced when we both "show" and "tell." There are also obvious logistical factors: Wi-Fi access and the need for a secure place to keep the device can be challenging in some units within a hospital.

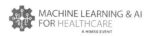

PSJH current work: virtual physician assistants

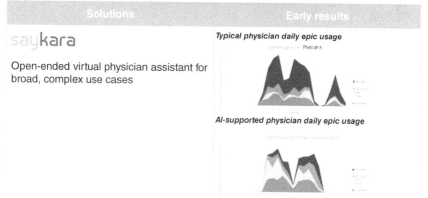

FIGURE 9.4   AI Results in Lessening of the Physician Documentation Work (*source: Adapted from[1]*)

9.2   Quality Measurement

US physicians spend an average of 2.6 h per week reporting quality measures.[14] While most of this time is spent entering information into medical records, physicians are also tasked with tracking quality measure specifications and developing and implementing data collection processes. AI could be used to automatically review clinical documents and either extract information for quality reporting or populate missing data fields. This is especially promising with generative AI, where models trained using large language models are very good at searching through notes and summarizing information or extracting appropriate metrics on command. Today, similar AI-enabled tools are being used for diagnosis coding and risk adjustment. In radiology, Real Time Medical has commercialized an AI-based application to help physicians meet peer review requirements in a way that requires less physician effort yet is more relevant for quality improvement.[4]

9.3   Nursing and Clinical Assistants

AI could be about to improve the way nurses do their jobs. Recent exciting developments include bottles which automatically issue reminders to drink, diapers that sound an alert when wet and sensor-equipped stoma pouches.

AI will change the focus of nursing care, improving nursing documentation, automating data collection, and performing some of the tasks that are currently done by nurses. Professional nursing care will change from being reactive to being predictive, preventive nursing care.

The same types of voice-based technologies that we've previously discussed could also help with nursing activities. In healthcare settings, where sterile operating fields and infection control are priorities, hands-free, immediate access to information has big advantages in terms of safety and efficiency. At Boston Children's ICU, AI-voice assistants allow nurses to ask for key administrative information, such as, "Who is the charge nurse on 7 South? How many beds are available on 8 East?" Clinicians are finding voice most useful for getting information that would otherwise involve picking up the phone, searching through documents, or walking down the hall.[15]

Voice can quickly access guidelines and protocols and save critical minutes in environments where wasted seconds can have a dramatic impact on outcomes. In the future, these AI-based solutions will become learning systems that anticipate information needs and provide just-in-time guidance. AI can save 20% of RN time through avoiding unnecessary visits. As virtual nursing assistants become accustomed to patient diagnoses and conditions, their abilities will grow beyond effective triage into expertise and recommendations around patient treatment.

CareIT Pro provides nursing software that uses AI and supports automation in nursing by reducing the need for information to be entered and linking to content so that further workflows and tasks can be automatically initiated at the right time. The software automatically recognizes patterns, evaluates the planned nursing goals, and recommends necessary adaptations. Combining it with sensors, wearables, and smart devices can further increase automation. Intelligent tools automatically deliver data on the patient to the nursing software and thus allow for automated documentation. Alarms, nursing tasks, and digital processes can be generated and started independently. Nursing staff can receive digital to-do lists and see the current status and quality of nursing processes at all times so that they can react to them at an early stage.[16]

Other such systems include an intelligent drinking cup that can automatically fill based on patient-specific drinking protocols and remind the patient to drink regularly, as well as a stoma pouch sensor that generates an automatic care task for changing the bag when it's almost full. There's also an intelligent nursing mattress that can detect not only the patient's movement, breathing, position, pressure, and sleep but also incontinence.[16]

Gauss Surgical is a Menlo Park-based startup that provides computer vision systems to monitor blood loss in operating and labor rooms to detect potential hemorrhages.[5] This is an area where surgeons, nurses, and technicians often need to collaborate to ensure that correct estimates are made and that the patient is adequately supported. Gauss Surgical's AI solution allows clinical workflows in operating rooms to be improved and for some of the burden to be removed from the busy staff.

9.4   Virtual Assistants

One of the key issues that has always plagued the healthcare system has been the disparity of information between providers and patients. A provider knows where to send a patient if they have a cough with a mild fever (as well as where not to send them), but the patient doesn't know if they should go to the ER at 2 a.m., call their doctor the next day, or just wait it out. The answer depends on factors like their history, general health, and comorbidities. Similarly, many questions and issues that come up in the course of people's daily lives could be answered easily if they had a physician nearby that they could consult.

This seems simple enough, but the reality is that few people have access to an on-demand physician. As such, we have people making decisions about how to use the healthcare system without knowledge or guidance. This leads to over- or under-use of the system, depending on the situation. Also, when patients interact with the healthcare system, it's often a manual and inefficient process. It involves waiting, being rerouted, not being able to reach anyone, being asked to fill out forms, and more.

It's been a dream of many of us to have systems that can guide patients remotely and automatically on the basics of how serious their issues are and where they can seek care. This dream is now closer to reality thanks to AI-based virtual assistants. We discussed these in the chapter on decision support, but they can be considered both a patient decision support system and a clinical workflow tool because with good guidance and by removing a lot of contacts for mundane and basic issues; we can improve the workflow of providers and free them up to focus on their patients. Also, by ensuring that only patients who need to show up to medical facilities are directed there, we can cut down on unnecessary visits and lighten the load of burned-out providers (Figures 9.5 and 9.6).[1, 17]

Soon, medical bots trained using large language models and clinical data can start to impress everyone with their patient triage and support capabilities, just as ChatGPT is impressing everyone now. Given that these systems

How it works

Enter your symptoms

Simply search for the symptoms you're experiencing, select the best fit, and the Symptom Checker will ask you a few more questions to gather details.

Decide on next steps

Based on your symptoms, the Symptom Checker can provide you with information about possible conditions, recommend next steps, and connect you with a doctor if you want to see one.

Start feeling better

The information you get from our Symptom Checker can help you use your time more efficiently and stay focused on your unique health needs.

FIGURE 9.5   An Example of the Workflow of a Virtual Assistant from Babylon Health (*source: CB Insights*)[17]

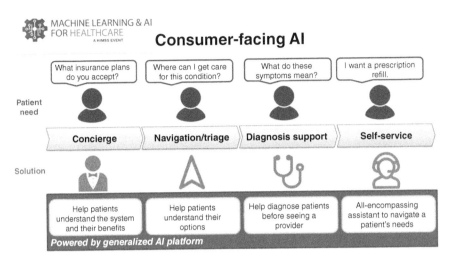

FIGURE 9.6   *(source: Adapted from[1])*

can be trained on large amounts of historical medical literature, they'll be much better than current chatbots at handling patient questions or issues. If they have access to patient data, they can even personalize their interactions with patients and provide responses that are more appropriate given the patients' conditions and medications. Regardless of what system you use, including generative AI systems, the most effective virtual assistants need access to patient data to provide personalized advice.

Many of the solutions here use AI to create voice- and text-based virtual assistants that can talk to patients, analyze the responses they provide, and then offer up guidance. Before it went out of business, Babylon Health offered bots to triage patients to the right setting based on their issues. It then allowed patients to talk to doctors within a couple of minutes and to receive medical advice from phone calls, text messages, and video consultations. Babylon Health's chatbot used NLP to understand symptoms and to check that against the data stored in the patient's medical history. Working within the UK's NHS, Babylon Health trained its chatbot to act as an on-demand symptom checker to evaluate patient symptoms (Figure 9.5).[17] A validation study of the technology found that the bot could safely triage 94% of test patients and that it could match expert decisions for 85% of them. New York-based K Health uses AI to navigate a large dataset of medical conditions and respond to patient inquiries about their medical conditions.[5]

Self-triage chatbots were adopted more rapidly during the COVID-19 pandemic, when they were trained to evaluate COVID symptoms and connect high-risk users with details for telehealth providers or local testing centers.[17] Buoy Health, GYANT, and Conversa Health all launched COVID-19 symptom screeners to support health systems during the pandemic. Providence Health has a bot called Grace that helps with a variety of patient issues and directs them to the appropriate venue (Figure 9.7). The quoted accuracy rates are impressive.[1] These virtual assistants are also helping with the management of chronic conditions, and there are a number of them for conditions like diabetes, hypertension, and weight loss. There are also solutions for helping seniors to manage their health and daily lives.

LLM-powered chatbots could also help care teams to more quickly and easily access training and education resources. Frontline care team members frequently reference these materials as protocols and have to review them to find answers to their questions. LLM-trained chatbot-style search could offer a far more efficient method for users to quickly find the specific information they need to best navigate the technology and shift focus back to their patients.[18]

The Mayo Clinic is exploring the use of search powered by generative AI to make finding information easier for team members. Traditional enterprise search, with queries producing a list of links based on pattern matching and significant manual investigation required to find the more relevant answers, can potentially be improved using generative AI. With generative AI, there's an opportunity to leverage enterprise data from EHRs, practice management software, and other systems to more effectively find answers to questions. This could include applying generative AI to conversational apps that can answer complex questions, produce accurate summaries that synthesize many sources, and help people get the information they need.[19]

Virtual assistants can also be used to respond to patient messages to their providers. Using large language models, responses can be drafted, and after the provider reviews and approves them, those messages can be sent to

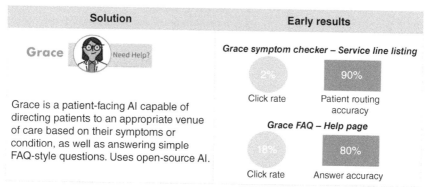

FIGURE 9.7   Consumer – Facing Chatbots in Healthcare Show Promise
(*source: Adapted from*[1])

patients. This would save time for the clinicians but give them full oversight over the responses that are eventually sent to the patients.[12]

Another option is for patients to use a voice-based system to populate medical questionnaires before they visit their healthcare practitioner, saving them time and frustration and cutting down on wasted resources. Voice assistants could therefore be a useful way to educate patients and to engage them at the clinic and continue that engagement at home.

References

1. Using AI and NLP to alleviate physician burnout. Aaron Martin. Machine Learning and AI for Healthcare. A HIMSS Event. 2019
2. Lin, S. Y., Shanafelt, T. D., & Asch, S. M. (2018, May). Reimagining clinical documentation with artificial intelligence. Mayo Clinic Proceedings, 93(5), 563–565. https://doi.org/10.1016/j.mayocp.2018.02.016
3. Arndt, B. G., Beasley, J. W., Watkinson, M. D., Temte, J. L., Tuan, W., Sinsky, C. A., & Gilchrist, V. J. (2016). Tethered to the EHR: primary care physician workload assessment using EHR event log data and time-motion observations. The Annals of Family Medicine, 15(5), 419–426. https://www.annfammed.org/content/15/5/419.full
4. Nundy, S., & Hodgkins, M. L. (2018). The application of AI to augment physicians and reduce burnout. Health Affairs Blog.
5. CB Insights. (2021, January 5). Healthcare AI Trends To Watch. CB Insights Research. https://www.cbinsights.com/research/report/ai-trends-healthcare/
6. Trang, B., & Ross, C. (2023, April 27). 'We're getting much more aggressive': Microsoft's Nuance adds GPT-4 AI to its medical note-taking tool. STAT. https://www.statnews.com/2023/03/20/microsoft-nuance-gpt4-dax-chatgpt/
7. Eddy, N. (2023, April 19). Epic, Microsoft partner to use generative AI for better EHRs. Healthcare IT News. https://www.healthcareitnews.com/news/epic-microsoft-partner-use-generative-ai-better-ehrs
8. Siwicki, B (2022 January 12). Evaluating AI digital assistants for primary care physicians, Healthcare IT News
9. Siwicki, B. (2021, April 28). How to help C-suite leaders and clinicians trust artificial intelligence. Healthcare IT News. https://www.healthcareitnews.com/news/how-help-c-suite-leaders-and-clinicians-trust-artificial-intelligence
10. Siwicki, B. (2021, January 4). AI-powered mobile assistant eliminates after-hours charting for orthoindy docs. Healthcare IT News. https://www.healthcareitnews.com/news/ai-powered-mobile-assistant-eliminates-after-hours-charting-orthoindy-docs
11. Padmanabhan, P. (2022, January 20). Why voice recognition is the new competitive battleground in healthcare's digital transformation. Healthcare IT News. Retrieved September 25, 2022, from https://www.healthcareitnews.com/blog/why-voice-recognition-new-competitive-battleground-healthcares-digital-transformation

12. Landi, H. (2023, May 25). Epic is going all in on generative AI in healthcare. Here's why a handful of health systems is eager to test-drive it. Fierce Healthcare. https://www.fiercehealthcare.com/health-tech/epic-moves-forward-bring-generative-ai-healthcare-heres-why-handful-health-systems-are

13. Health Evolution. (2020, May 18). CEO Guide. Health Evolution. Retrieved September 25, 2022, from https://www.healthevolution.com/ceo-guide/

14. Casalino, L. P., Gans, D., Weber, R., Cea, M., Tuchovsky, A., Bishop, T. F., Miranda, Y., Frankel, B. A., Ziehler, K. B., Wong, M. M., & Evenson, T. B. (2016). US physician practices spend more than $15.4 billion annually to report quality measures. Health Affairs, 35(3). https://www.healthaffairs.org/doi/10.1377/hlthaff.2015.1258

15. Small, C. E., Nigrin, D., Churchwell, K., & Brownstein, J. (2020, March 7). What will health care look like once smart speakers are everywhere?Harvard Business Review. https://hbr.org/2018/03/what-will-health-care-look-like-once-smart-speakers-are-everywhere

16. Matheson, R. (2019, January 4). Startups building integrated nursing ecosystems with AI. Healthcare IT News. Retrieved September 25, 2022, from https://www.healthcareitnews.com/news/emea/startups-building-integrated-nursing-ecosystems-ai

17. CB Insights (2021, March 11). How Conversational AI Can Save Time And Money For Patients And Providers. CB Insights. https://app.cbinsights.com/research/conversational-ai-health-it-tech-stack/

18. Siwicki, B. (2023, June 5). UNC Health's CIO talks generative AI work with Epic and Microsoft. Healthcare IT News. https://www.healthcareitnews.com/news/unc-healths-cio-talks-generative-ai-work-epic-and-microsoft

19. Google Cloud. (2023, June 8). Mayo Clinic working on new generative AI use cases. Healthcare IT News. https://www.healthcareitnews.com/news/google-cloud-mayo-clinic-working-new-generative-ai-use-cases

CHAPTER 10

Administration and Operations

T HE US HEALTHCARE ECONOMY is valued at over $4 trillion. If it was a country, it would have the fifth largest economy in the world, and it equates to nearly half of what the entire world spends on healthcare. We can argue about whether that's a good thing or not and what percentage of it is actually necessary, but we can all agree that it's an inefficient system. It's convoluted and the overall setup creates redundancies and needs lots of approvals and what we used to call paperwork. In fact, it's estimated that about 25% of this $4 trillion is due to administration, which means that we spend $1 trillion a year on paperwork. It's no wonder that healthcare is now the number one employer, passing retail as of 2017 with 17 million jobs.[1]

Administrative money needs to be spent to support activities outside of direct patient care. Given that most economies in the world are smaller than $1 trillion, you could say that the administrative part of the US healthcare system is also one of the largest economies in the world. Part of that is because we have more than 1000 insurance companies, each with its own policies and forms, requiring a major revenue cycle function in each hospital system, and even in small doctors' medical clinics. A typical medical clinic or health system has to deal with so many different payers that many of its employees are occupied with filling out forms and making calls to ensure that they're meeting each payer's requirements, because that's what pays the bills and keeps the lights on. When we think of care delivery institutions, this isn't what typically comes to mind. Unfortunately, it's a reality because of the disjointed payment system in our country and the lack of regulation to solve the problem.

Another contributing factor is the lack of an efficient source of longitudinal patient medical records which would simplify data sharing and access of information for providers, commonly referred to as a health information

AI Doctor: The Rise of Artificial Intelligence in Healthcare: A Guide for Users, Buyers, Builders, and Investors, First Edition. Ronald M. Razmi.

exchange. A single national healthcare database could be achieved through either a commercial or government program that would ensure that all healthcare providers had access to the same data for patients instead of having to waste resources searching for and retrieving data from other institutions.

All of this means that both payers and providers have to expend tremendous resources on administrative tasks. The good news is that we can expect to see future workflow improvements through robotic process automation (RPA), artificial intelligence (AI), and other promising technologies. These technologies are a natural fit to improve efficiency through automating repetitive tasks with minor or moderate complexity. Most of these administrative functions are done electronically, making AI the perfect tool to "figure out" what to do and to perform activities like completing forms, sending information, and scheduling follow-ups. This would bring three economic improvements to the process: first, it would mean fewer healthcare resources, including the time of doctors and nurses, spent on administration; second, it would enable more timely completion of these steps and reduce the time to achieve revenues; and third, for the same budget, it would enable the allocation of more money for actual patient care. As Rock Health put it in their report about AI in healthcare: "*Media has largely centered on the ability of AI/ML to transform how clinical care is delivered through better diagnostics and treatments. But AI/ML is even more quickly transforming the business of healthcare through the automation and enhancement of non-clinical, operational functions—such as claims adjudication, patient engagement, scheduling optimization, risk analytics and documentation.*"[2]

These AI systems could also help us to reduce burnout among physicians that's brought on by the ever-increasing need for doctors to carry out administrative tasks like coding, claims, pharmacy refills, and pre-authorization. Carrying out these manual, repetitive tasks for billing and insurance is frustrating for physicians and costly for healthcare providers. That's why the ability of AI to reduce these tedious and time-consuming workflows in the backend could be one of its biggest impacts on the healthcare industry. It's estimated that AI could lead to time savings of 17% for doctors and over 50% for nurses.

Let's take a closer look at how AI can help.

10.1   Providers

10.1.1   Documentation, Coding, and Billing

The administrative staff of medical institutions deal with a range of revenue-generating activities in support of medical care, like verifying patients' insurance eligibility, identifying the right medical codes based on the services provided, submitting claims to insurers, and following up with patients about outstanding bills. With advances in AI technologies such as computer vision and machine learning-enabled bots, many of these activities can be intelligently automated. RPA, an umbrella term for automating repetitive back-office tasks like onboarding and document digitization, has especially benefited from advances in computer vision and natural language processing. This is very relevant to the major issue of excessive administrative costs. Given that the technology finally seems ready for its moment, more hospitals are weighing the benefits of using AI for coding and billing automation.[3]

Managing billing, revenue collection, insurance filings, and other related activities are at the frontier of AI's entry into healthcare. That's because it's a low-risk area with an immediate financial impact on the health system. It doesn't carry the liability risks of clinical AI applications, where small errors could have large consequences on patient outcomes. Furthermore, medical providers don't need to worry about securing reimbursement, and the business case is much more compelling in the short-to-medium term than clinical AI applications.

More than 40% of submitted claims aren't paid electronically or automatically upon their first submission. The AI applications in this area include more accurate coding from processing provider documentation and identifying the relevant billable medical codes. There are now algorithms that can tap into historical data and use it to predict whether a claim will be approved or denied. The medical insurance industry is increasingly recognizing the potential of AI for improving billing and insurance tasks. There are three main ways that AI is being used to revolutionize healthcare billing and insurance: natural language processing (NLP) for automated, computer-assisted provider documentation (CAPD) and computer-assisted coding; AI for the prioritization of clinical documentation improvement (CDI) and electronic prior authorization; and AI-powered RPA to help with claims management. Generative AI is showing great promise in this area and the large language models (LLMs) at the basis of generative AI will undoubtedly become the basis of AI solutions that will anticipate the words and thoughts of clinicians so that they can further speed access to information and reduce administrative tasks.

Today's AI-powered RPA startups are on a mission to automate the repetitive, manual tasks like claims submission and denial that occur during the end-to-end revenue cycle. In medical coding, players such as Google-backed Nym use NLP to automate the labor-intensive process of translating EHR notes into billable code.[4] Infinitus Systems is developing a "voice RPA" chatbot that asks questions about payment authorization and other procedures and records answers in the relevant fields.

LLMs from Google (Bard) and OpenAI (ChatGPT) have already made impressive progress when it comes to interpreting medical documentation. Healthcare-based NLP tools have also been released on open-source licenses by the National Library of Medicine (part of the National Institutes of Health),

Amazon Comprehend Medical, and Google via its Healthcare Natural Language API. Healthcare AI tools for administrative automation will mostly depend on EHR data. There are tools like NYM that tap into EHR notes to translate health services into billable codes, while RPA platforms are using AI to extract data from EHRs to populate insurance claims forms. This is also known as "charge capture," the process by which doctors translate patient visits and diagnoses into medical codes that can be billed to an insurer. Historically, this has been done by hiring people who read the doctor's notes and update the coding for that visit.

Companies such as Apixio and 3M have developed AI-powered risk adjustment and hierarchical condition category auditors to help practices optimize their coding for quality payment programs.[5] We already know that AI does a better job of spotting patterns than human beings. Traditionally, rules-based engines needed to be constantly updated to reflect changes and to stay accurate over time, but AIs can automatically become better at what they do, especially when it comes to pattern recognition.

One of the companies working with CAPD technology is HITEKS, which provides embedded EHR workflows within Epic to provide timely advice on documentation to support ICD-10 claims coding. Their CEO, Dr. Petratos, is a medical informatics-trained physician who talked to me about some of the issues that medical centers are facing and how their NLP technology is solving some of these issues. According to Dr. Petratos, the sophisticated hospital systems in the United States are now seeking to notify their providers of CDI opportunities in near real-time before they sign their notes, and within the workflows of the EHR. Legacy processes, which include a nurse, physician, or coder manually reviewing each chart after provider notes are written (reactive CDI) and sending a note to the provider's inbox, are inefficient.

"Reactive" CDI takes three times as long and can leave an organization vulnerable to denials due to changed documentation flags by insurance. CAPD software that includes advances in accuracy and timeliness can reduce what's commonly known as "query fatigue," when providers see too many alerts in the EHR and start to tune out. HITEKS developed an approach where they combined certain rules, which are known to be clinically relevant and are required for compliance reasons, with machine learning to suppress inappropriate alerts. "Proactive" CDI is the result of these AI advancements and has been measured to improve the bottom line with a 3% increase in revenues from inpatient accounts, 17% reduction in provider administrative time, and 25% reduction in CDI resources to oversee the CAPD processes.

AI's ability to process and understand natural language (e.g. ambient AI) is also being harnessed to help clinicians create documentation by listening to their interactions with patients to create clinical notes reflective of patients' complaints and providers' assessments and plans. Done well, this could allow us to ease the timeliness and provider burden to simplify the creation of more complete and comprehensive documentation, showing the thought processes of providers much more clearly than our existing approach. It can also help to show the decision-making process that the provider followed, helping with coding and minimizing the risk of denials. As we discussed in Chapter 9, AI could also help to reduce the administrative burden that comes from documentation, allowing us to better highlight the full complexity of each patient's case, leading to better coding and fewer rejected claims. Currently, ambient AI has had limited penetration into US healthcare, but LLMs are showing great promise in this area.

One of the key areas on the administrative side of healthcare is prior authorization. This is when clinicians need to get an approval from the insurance company to perform a service like an MRI for the patient. Insurance companies use prior authorization to control costs by preventing unnecessary procedures. This is always a point of contention since doctors think they should be the ones to make decisions about what's appropriate for their patients. However, insurance companies argue that testing and procedures are often ordered by doctors when medical guidelines don't support them. Most recently, doctors have used ChatGPT to generate these letters to the insurance companies. Although a great time-saver, ChatGPT has shown an ability to provide false scientific references in these letters or fabricate patient data. This underlines the fact that although we're heading for exciting days, the road to get there is not fully paved yet. However, one of the early use cases for generative AI is that of generating prior authorization letters that summarize key information from the EHR and explain why procedures are necessary.

Let's use the example of someone who's presenting with back pain for the first time. The overwhelming majority of patients with back pain improve spontaneously without the use of expensive medical procedures like MRIs. However, some clinicians go straight to ordering an MRI as their preferred diagnostic tool. I can see both sides of the argument, but being a physician, I tend to agree that clinicians know best. There are often circumstances that mean the clinician will deviate from the guidelines for good reason. But they need to do a better job of documentation so that insurance companies agree to pay for it. AI can help with the documentation, ensuring that these extenuating circumstances are included on the forms that will be filed with the insurance company. It would also take care of a lot of annoying and time-consuming tasks for the medical staff.

AI can be used to harvest the appropriate information for prior authorizations and RPA can populate the insurance forms with that information to allow for automatic submission with a higher likelihood of approval. This is good news for providers and their employees because it means they don't have to manually complete forms or set up rules for prior authorization. For example, companies like Epic, HealthFortis, and UIPATH use RPA and workflow software to automate important administrative processes such as eligibility checks, insurance claims, prior authorizations, appointment reminders, billing, data reporting, and analytics.[6]

10.1.2 Practice Management and Operations

AI can help providers and their practices improve operations like scheduling and patient check-ins and check-outs. AI-powered scheduling software could make life easier for patients and their medical providers. It will be able to analyze previous scheduling patterns for each patient and provide suggestions for the best date, time, provider, and location for the patient. It can even automatically schedule appointments to further streamline the process.

If a patient needs to receive multiple treatments or to see several providers on the same day, these tools could develop an optimized schedule for them to follow. This reduces the amount of time spent by both the patient and the scheduling staff to create the next appointment or series of appointments.[7] AI tools can also better understand the complexities that come with every patient and every treatment plan, and these scheduling tools can figure out the optimum visit length for each appointment. A visit for a patient with multiple diagnoses should take longer than a visit for a patient who's normally healthy.

This approach allows us to optimize providers' schedules by customizing the amount of time that each patient receives based on their individual needs. Healthcare providers can provide only the amount of time that's necessary without falling behind in their schedule or rushing from one patient to another. Figuring out these estimates and implementing them into a schedule is prohibitively time-consuming for human beings, but AI can handle it in just a couple of seconds. As we discussed, that can include automatic documentation, better coding, completing forms, and more.

This also ties into the concept of risk-adjusted paneling and resourcing. Risk-adjusted paneling can ensure that primary care physicians have adequate time to address the needs of each patient by increasing or decreasing panel sizes based on patient complexity, which can boost patient satisfaction and lead to better work–life balance for physicians.[8] At UCSF, EHR data on healthcare usage has been used to train algorithms to weigh panel sizes in primary care.[9] The hope is that in the future, we'll be able to use models like these to better determine staffing levels for medical practices based on the amount of care that's required.

AI can also be used to automate certain aspects of pre-visit planning to make physician-care encounters more efficient and rewarding for patients and physicians.[6] This would improve the overall workflow at the physician's office as patients can be checked in faster, physicians can view prioritized information to make visits more efficient and follow-ups can be scheduled automatically.

Another way that AI can improve practice management is through the use of chatbots that are more intelligent due to the fact that instead of being programmed, they're trained with AI and machine learning. This helps to ensure that patients' expectations are met and so they'll start using those technologies more often. Chatbots can save the medical staff from having to spend a lot of time answering the same questions over the phone, and this has been used recently for the management of COVID patient calls. Web-based bots were used to answer questions, address vaccine issues, keep people out of ERs and hospitals, and manage them remotely if they were healthy enough.

Patient-facing chatbots trained on medical literature with LLMs and patient data can build a holistic view of a patient's condition using multiple modalities, ranging from unstructured descriptions of symptoms to continuous glucose monitor readings and patient-provided medication logs. After interpreting this heterogeneous data, the models could interact with the patient, providing detailed advice and explanations. Importantly, these models can facilitate accessible communication, providing clear, readable, or audible information on the patient's schedule.

AI-based chatbots perform a number of functions that could improve operations at medical practices. These solutions can centralize resources, offering location-based information on the programs that are available and providing dynamic answers to specific questions about insurance. An obvious advantage of these chatbots is that they're available 24/7. We just need to make sure that they can integrate with the scheduling tools and EHRs that are currently in use.

Botco.ai's chatbot is deployed on medical practice websites to carry out conversations with visitors, decreasing the amount of time that human employees need to spend on the phone. Implemented at Aspire Indiana Health, Botco's tool operates as an extension of many departments, answering questions about topics like insurance coverage, appointment scheduling, telehealth, behavioral health, addiction, employment and housing, recovery services, and residential and outpatient treatment services.[10] It also integrates with their practice management software and EHR and can schedule and modify appointments to save the staff from having to perform those tasks.

Another important area for medical practices and health systems is ensuring compliance with accepted guidelines and requirements from the government and insurance companies. This is especially critical in coding and billing. There's a long history of providers and institutions engaging in the practice of upcoding, using codes that aren't justified by the level of service provided to achieve a higher level of reimbursement. This is an area where criminal investigations and/or civil lawsuits can create headaches for organizations. As such, detecting and addressing it before the government or insurance companies discover it is important for medical organizations.

AI can help with this, both for payers and providers. As well as spotting fraud faster than human beings, it can stop it from happening in the first place. It does this by processing huge amounts of data and identifying upcoding patterns, looking for appropriate documentation, and flagging anything that seems out of place. As with other areas of healthcare, it's not designed as a replacement for existing fraud detection efforts, but rather as an enhancement that can alert human operators whenever they spot something that's cause for concern.

New AI and machine learning techniques can identify code words that are used in fraudulent situations or patterns of medical coding that could indicate fraud. They do this by understanding both the contents of a document and the context around it, which includes the people involved and the relationships between them. It can spot words that aren't normally used or that are repeatedly used only among a small group of participants. By using AI to automate the process, enterprises can save both time and money, while understanding their data and avoiding issues like potential fraud.[11]

10.1.3   Hospital Operations

AI can be instrumental in helping hospitals improve operational decision-making by using quantifiable metrics to assess the quality of healthcare. As with medical practices, RPA plays a key role in streamlining hospital operations. We mentioned earlier companies that are using AI to improve billing and coding for medical practices. Their use of RPA, computer vision, and machine learning to automate healthcare administrative workflows like checking claim statuses and managing accounts receivable adds significant value to hospital operations.[12]

AI optimization can be critical for managing healthcare assets like hospital rooms, operating rooms (ORs), and radiology scans, as well as vaccine administration, bed allocation, and sequencing activities (room cleaning, discharges, etc.). Companies like LeanTaas are using AI to help hospitals to create capacity. To make this a reality, we need electronic data sources and optimal access to different hospital databases, as well as the ability to aggregate and analyze. This may mean redesigning data systems and processes and introducing technology for optimization and forecasting.[13]

There are a million hospital beds in the United States. Room turnover in hospitals is far less predictable than it is in hotels, so it's harder to manage capacity and operations. Prior to being discharged from a hospital, a patient might need to wait for labs, post-surgery observations, and even a discharging physician who's dealing with an emergency. Using sophisticated AI models that are far better than traditional forecasting tools, you can better forecast and redesign processes to unlock significant capacity.[14]

Given that AI solutions can make sense of data in an ongoing manner and feed those insights to a medical facility, they can improve both clinical and operational decisions, which are very much intertwined. If sepsis is a big issue in a hospital, patients stay longer and that affects the availability of beds, along with other hospital economics. If hospital capacity is better managed using AI's predictive capabilities, more beds will be available, which means patients will get admitted and receive treatment much faster, leading to better outcomes. As such, many of the AI solutions that improve hospital operations are also addressing ongoing clinical issues. Examples of those include:

- Optimizing scheduling and staffing tasks
- Improving clinical workflows by scanning documents and providing recommendations
- Automating tasks like reading scans or interpreting results to expedite decision-making
- Using algorithms to reduce scanning time and radiation to the patients
- Using algorithms to expedite image reconstruction
- Using segmentation to improve radiation therapy
- Predicting hospital-acquired infections such as sepsis and *C. diff*
- Using infrared, computer vision, and sensors to reduce nosocomial infections and track handwashing
- Tapping into reinforcement learning to wean patients off ventilators
- Providing decision support for the use of IVF, pressors, and ventilations
- Powering ICU surveillance of patient vitals and other metrics, as well as ICU discharge
- Monitoring conditions in the OR
- Preventing patient falls
- Using remote monitoring and algorithms to pick up on brewing issues such as sepsis or heart failure

Much of this revolves around better outcome prediction, which in turn leads to better resource allocation. The information required for this type of predictive modeling comes from EHR data and hospital bed data, using metrics like hospitalization length, the number of procedures, and the number of patients with sepsis and other nosocomial infections.

There are various examples of algorithms predicting mortality using structured data from EHRs. One such algorithm by Google had a high success rate when predicting mortality, hospital stay duration, readmission rates, final diagnoses, bleeding complications, kidney failure, and more. Algorithms are showing promise in silico for predicting diseases such as hypertension, kidney failure, diabetes, and arrhythmia by using EHR data, including lab results, trends over time, and more.[15]

Thirty percent of hospital patients who fall experience injury (such as fractures and head trauma), and this boosts the length of their stay by an average of 6.3 days. Each fall that results in an injury costs around $14,000. Qventus analyzes call lights, bed alarms, EMRs, meds, vitals, and ages to assess the risk of falls in hospital. Their deployment at El Camino Hospital resulted in a 29% reduction in falls by identifying when the falls usually happen and the sequence of events that lead to them.[16]

CommonSpirit Health, a combination of Dignity Health and Catholic Health Initiatives, is a nationwide health system of more than 350 hospitals, and it's currently using an AI tool from Lean TaaS that helps to optimize the use of OR suites. The tool, iQueue, uses AI to analyze the use of ORs in an institution, identifies unused OR time, prompts surgeons to release unused OR time, and then allows the hospital to make that time available to other surgeons. Since using the tool, CommonSpirit Health has seen a 21% release fill rate, which means that 21% of the identified available time is being used by other surgeons. This translates to an ROI of 14.5× for the health system.[17]

Another key issue in hospitals (and medical practices) is the security of data and the need to easily transfer it to facilitate better medical care for patients while ensuring privacy and security. Companies are already developing AI-driven privacy tools for healthcare administrators to help them to securely transfer patient data. For example, Baltimore's Protenus has developed healthcare offerings that offer auditing, security, and compliance tools that are powered by AI and which can be used for patient and clinical trial data. San Francisco's Datavant allows users to de-identify patient data so that they can exchange it with other healthcare organizations without compromising patient privacy.[3, 12]

Figure 10.1 shows some of the use cases of AI for hospitals and medical practices. In addition to the ones we discussed, AI can also improve marketing, optimize pricing, and provide competitive intelligence to boost the top line for clinics and hospitals.

AI in Healthcare: Healthcare Management

- **Brand management and marketing:** Create an optimal marketing strategy for the brand based on market perception and target segment
- **Pricing and risk:** Determine the optimal price for treatment and other service according to competition and other market conditions
- **Market research:** Prepare hospital competitive intelligence
- **Operations:** Process automation technologies such as intelligent automation and RPA help hospitals automate routine front office and back office operations such as reporting
- **Customer service chatbots:** Customer service chatbots allow patients to ask questions regarding bill payment, appointments, or medication refills
- **Fraud detection:** Patients may make false claims. Leveraging AI-powered fraud detection tools can help hospital managers to identify fraudsters

FIGURE 10.1 *(source: Original Research)*

10.2   Payers

Like providers, payers can reap enormous benefits from using AI to manage their businesses. That's because insurance companies rely heavily on statistics and numeric analysis. They need to accurately estimate what it will cost to cover the medical care of a population; design benefits based on that; charge the right premiums and monitor as the claims keep coming. If they're not on track, they'll be out of business by the end of the year.

If there's one thing that AI does well, it's to take lots of data, figure out patterns and relationships, and help predict what will happen next. As a matter of fact, payers are already seeing huge benefits from incorporating AI into their business models, especially for combatting fraud and allocating resources.

It's important to step back and reiterate some of what we discussed at the start of this chapter. The United States spends a huge amount on healthcare, more than any other country both in total and per capita (Figure 10.2). However, all of that money doesn't buy better outcomes than other developed nations (Figure 10.3). So where does the money go? You won't be surprised to know that there's been a lot of research into exactly that.

In a seminal paper in *JAMA* in 2018, Papanicolas et al. examined the differences between the United States and other advanced economies in terms of their overall healthcare expenditures and the associated outcomes.[18] They found that back in 2016, the United States spent almost twice as much on medical care as ten high-income countries, despite a poorer performance when it came to population health. Social spending and healthcare usage didn't differ substantially between the United States and other high-income nations. The main drivers of the spending differences appeared to be the prices of labor and goods (including pharmaceuticals and devices) and administrative costs (Figure 10.4).

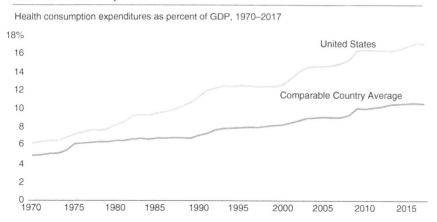

Healthcare in the United States is more expensive than other developed countries

Health consumption expenditures as percent of GDP, 1970–2017

FIGURE 10.2   *(source: KFF Analysis of OECO and National Health Expenditure)*

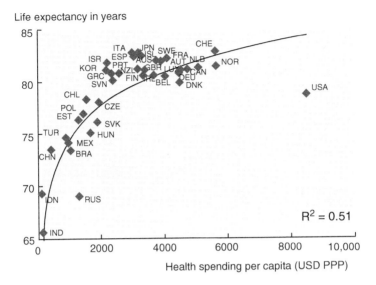

FIGURE 10.3   *(source: OECD Health Statistics 2013)*

For most procedures, the United States pays the highest prices in the world

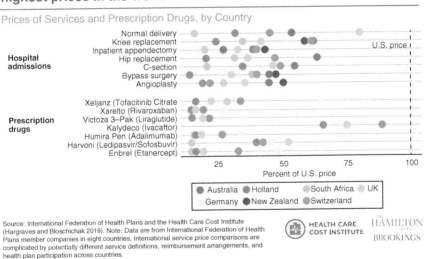

FIGURE 10.4   *(source: Health Care Cost Institute)*

10.2.1   Payer Administrative Functions

The administrative costs of healthcare (which are due to planning, regulating, and managing health systems) is higher in the United States than other advanced nations by a magnitude of 3–8, and a big reason for the United

States having much higher overall costs of care. We've already talked about some of the reasons for this, but the main one is the large number of insurance companies with their own benefit plan requirements (more than 1000 of them!), forms, and filing requirements.

It doesn't look like the number of insurance companies in the United States will shrink any time soon, and our public–private healthcare system is unlikely to become a single-payer system. So how can we lower administrative costs?

One option is to automate as much of it as we can. We've already talked about NLP, computer vision, and RPA, as well as how they're starting to make inroads into taking over administrative functions. The same is true for payers.

Attacking this problem from both sides makes the most sense. Jonathan Bush, the former CEO of AthenaHealth, wrote in 2018 that the greatest near-term opportunity for AI in healthcare isn't for headline-grabbing moonshots but for putting computers and algorithms to work on the most mundane drudgery possible.[19] Using AI to take care of back office and mundane activities that are also resource hungry and that lead to fatigue and burnout instead of better patient care would add a huge amount of value to the healthcare system.

Faxes are still a common method of communication between doctors' offices, payers, and providers, and processing these faxes uses a lot of manpower. Faxes don't use structured text, which is why it takes an average of two and a half minutes to review each document and translate it into inputs for EHRs. Machine learning and business process outsourcing have helped Athena Health to automate faxes and reduced processing time to 1 min and 11 s. This resulted in the elimination of over three million hours of work for one healthcare system. Athena has used AI to further reduce import time to just 30 s, and they've created software that can scan lab results and flag anything urgent that needs human attention. They're also working on an algorithm that could schedule routine follow-ups for high-risk patients. All of this can reduce administrative work for both payers and providers.

The idea of using EHRs to make doctors' jobs easier is yet to become a reality because of the need for manual data entry and how the design of EHRs makes information lookup and retrieval difficult. The next generation of technologies will help doctors. By making it easier to document using voice inputs, increasing coding accuracy, and filling out forms, the potential of intelligent automation could finally reach fruition. This will lessen the workload on the sides of both payers and providers because it's the back and forth between these two sides that generates so much administrative work.

According to a study by Accenture, AI could significantly improve operations and boost the bottom line.[20] One way to accomplish this is by automating processes across billing, customer service, claims, enrollment, and quality and compliance. The report concludes that automating functions could generate $1.5 million in operating income for every hundred employees at payers. According to a different Accenture survey, 72% of executives at payers believe that AI will be among the top three strategic priorities for their company within the year. In the near term, they hope that AI will be used to anticipate and resolve questions from customers, accelerate the prior authorization and clinical review of claims, and improve the process of benefits loading and design.

The biggest potential savings could come from using AI to anticipate and respond to customer demands. AI could unlock $2.1 billion for health insurers in this one area alone, as well as a further $1.4 billion from managing membership and billing, $1.1 billion from managing and supporting reimbursement, $1 billion from managing networks and providers, $900 million from performing health management and $500 million from managing quality improvement and compliance.[20]

Managing customer interactions is the biggest slice of the pie, and AI could allow us to predict what customers will ask based on earlier calls and other data. It could then help a cell center rep to satisfy the customer's needs through a more targeted interaction.

Virtual agents could take care of the simpler interactions and answer questions without human intervention. We could use AI to anticipate needs and to provide just-in-time information based on whatever the customer is asking for. Accenture's analysis also showcases two other areas that insurers should focus on in the short term, which are accelerating prior authorization and the clinical review of claims and improving the process of benefits loading and design. If this sounds like what we discussed for providers, that's because it is. The administrative work in healthcare occurs between payers and providers, so technologies like NLP, computer vision, and AI-enabled RPA will help both sides with coding reviews, prior authorization, and form completion.

Accenture also provided proposals for AI and machine learning that could demonstrate an impact on operating income in the near term. For example, RPA could automatically approve prior authorization requests. In fact, Express Scripts is already doing this, helped along by their acquisition of eviCore for $3.6 billion in 2017.[20, 21] AI could help employees focus on decision-making and those more creative processes that need human intervention and oversight. This could unlock capacity within the institution because payers won't need to scale future jobs if their roles can be automated by AI. As is the case in every part of the healthcare value chain, the key barriers include poorly defined governance, mismatched or poor quality vendors, and unsuitable existing infrastructure.

10.2.2   Fraud

AI could have a significant impact when detecting fraud in health plans. We've already discussed the idea of upcoding and how it's a common method of fraud in healthcare. There are well-documented cases of unusual coding patterns that emerge in health systems or in regions where certain diagnostics or treatments are being prescribed at a rate that doesn't fit the national pattern. In many cases, this turns out to be due to a scheme of kickbacks or upcoding by certain providers. Historically, health plans have detected these abnormal patterns months or years after they've taken place. This usually sets off investigations and attempts to recover those funds, costing health plans significant financial and human resources.

More recently, health plans have started using AI to monitor for fraud and detect abnormal activities before they release payments to providers. As such, they can avoid paying for fraudulent activities, along with the associated costs of investigation and recovery. Insurance company Highmark used AI to save over $260 million by cutting down on fraud, waste, and abuse in 2019 alone. They were able to save more than $850 million between 2015 and 2020.[22, 23]

Insurance organizations are already using AI to detect fraudulent activity. Highmark is tapping into the tech to limit the financial exposure that their customers are at risk of, since payments for fraudulent activities ultimately involve out-of-pocket costs for patients. The AI software used in fraud detection can quickly adapt to changing behavior and pick up on abnormalities much faster than traditional tools, which usually tap into a set of established rules to spot suspicious behavior. The superior performance of Highmark's fraud detection systems was confirmed by Change Healthcare when they reviewed Highmark's Payment Integrity programs. This review found that Highmark's program outperformed the industry standard, saving 10% of medical claims for group customers and nearly 33% more than other national payers.[23]

This is also beneficial to other parts of a health plan's business as they can communicate with their customers about their ability to detect and prevent fraud while simultaneously saving them money through lower premiums and better service.

In an Optum survey of health plan leaders, 43% said they believe that AI will help detect fraud, waste, and abuse in reimbursement.[24] CMS has also adopted AI and other advanced technologies in an effort to reduce Medicare fraud, waste, and abuse.[25] Figure 10.5 shows an example of an algorithm for fraud detection from a McKinsey report about using AI in healthcare.[26]

10.2.3   Personalized Communications

AI can help health plan providers to improve the frequency and personalization of communications between providers and their members. An overabundance of communication touchpoints leads to fatigue on the part of members, and they end up ignoring them. Some members have received more than 200 messages from their health plan in just the space of a year. Even with the best intentions, this excessive communication has led to a problem called "member abrasion," which damages engagement rates and can even cause people to distrust health plans.[27]

AI can help us to develop better health engagement strategies that can reestablish trust. The retail industry has shown that AI can be used to expand traditional data sets for personalized communication, and that this can lead to higher engagement rates. Several health engagement technologies have emerged that can capture data about contexts, channel preferences, behaviors, and values. This data can help us to further personalize communications

Case example: decision model for FWA detection

Using ML techniques, we designed an algorithm to identify claim recovery cases for unbundling of services – *the snapshot below describes an ML algorithm that can be converted into rules to implement in a payer claims editing system*[1]

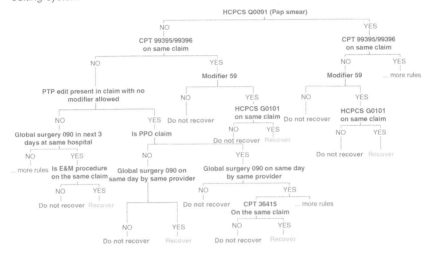

1 Selected portion of algorithm presented (from perspective of Payer claims editing system)
CPT: Current Procedural Terminology (published by the American Medical Association); PTP: Procedure to Procedure; HCPCS: Healthcare Common Procedure Coding System; E&M: Evaluation and Management

FIGURE 10.5   *(source: McKinsey & Company)*[26]

and lead to better health outcomes over time. These systems use AI and machine learning to track responses to campaigns, replicate the ones that are doing well and removing the ones that are failing. They can often do this in real time.

When done well, AI can humanize engagement, empowering healthcare consumers to participate in their own healthcare based on their responses to personalized touchpoints that are sent out in appropriate amounts and via the best channels for the consumer.

References

1. Topol, E. (2019). Deep Medicine: How Artificial Intelligence Can Make Healthcare Human Again (Illustrated). Basic Books
2. Zweig, M., & Tran, D. (2021, July 31). The AI/ML use cases investors are betting on in healthcare | Rock Health. https://rockhealth.com/insights/the-ai-ml-use-cases-investors-are-betting-on-in-healthcare/

3. CB Insights. (2021, January 5). Healthcare AI trends to watch. CB Insights Research. https://www.cbinsights.com/research/report/ai-trends-healthcare/

4. CB Insights. (2021, February 11). How artificial intelligence is reshaping medical billing & insurance. CB Insights Research. Retrieved September 26, 2022, from https://www.cbinsights.com/research/artificial-intelligence-healthcare-providers-medical-billing-insurance/

5. Apixio Launches HCC Auditor, the First AI-Powered Risk Adjustment Auditing Solution. (2018, July 25). GlobeNewswire News Room. Retrieved September 26, 2022, from https://www.globenewswire.com/news-release/2018/07/25/1541847/0/en/Apixio-Launches-HCC-Auditor-the-First-AI-Powered-Risk-Adjustment-Auditing-Solution.html

6. Sinsky, C. A., Sinsky, T. A., & Rajcevich, E. (2015). Putting pre-visit planning into practice. Family Practice Management, 22(6), 34–38

7. Siwicki, B. (2021, June 22). AI deployments accelerating across an array of complex use cases. Healthcare IT News. Retrieved September 26, 2022, from https://www.healthcareitnews.com/news/ai-deployments-accelerating-across-array-complex-use-cases

8. Shanafelt, T., Goh, J., & Sinsky, C. (2017). The business case for investing in physician well-being. JAMA Internal Medicine, 177(12), 1826–1832

9. Rajkomar, A., Yim, J. W. L., Grumbach, K., & Parekh, A. (2016). Weighting primary care patient panel size: a novel electronic health record-derived measure using machine learning. JMIR Medical Informatics, 4(4), e29. https://doi.org/10.2196/medinform.6530

10. Siwicki, B. (2021, August 31). Digital front door chatbot improves the patient experience at Aspire. Healthcare IT News. Retrieved September 26, 2022, from https://www.healthcareitnews.com/news/digital-front-door-chatbot-improves-patient-experience-aspire-indiana-health

11. Siwicki, B. (2021, May 5). Top 5 nightmares hiding in a healthcare organization's unstructured. Healthcare IT News. Retrieved September 26, 2022, from https://www.healthcareitnews.com/news/top-five-nightmares-hiding-healthcare-organizations-unstructured-data

12. CB Insights (2019). From drug R&D to diagnostics: 90+ artificial intelligence startups in healthcare

13. Hess, S., & Giridharadas, M. Using AI to fix broken math and optimize capacity of expensive healthcare assets: The CIO's role in facilitating the transformation. Healthcare Innovation. Webcast. https://www.hcinnovationgroup.com/webinars/webinar/21242825/using-ai-to-fix-broken-math-and-optimize-capacity-of-expensive-healthcare-assets-the-cios-role-in-facilitating-the-transformation

14. State of AI in Hospitals. (2021, February 25). [Video]. Ai4Healthcare

15. Rajkomar, A. et al. (2018, May 8). Scalable and accurate deep learning with electronic health records. NPJ Digital Medicine, 1, 18.

16. Ockerman, E. (2018). AI hospital software knows who's going to fall. Bloomberg. https://www.bloomberg.com/news/articles/2018-06-21/ai-programs-fight-medical-alarm-fatigue-with-patient-fall-alerts

17. Siwicki, B. (2022, July 18). CommonSpirit Health gains huge efficiencies with AI-infused OR. Healthcare IT News. Retrieved September 26, 2022, from https://www.healthcareitnews.com/news/commonspirit-health-gains-huge-efficiencies-ai-infused-or-scheduling-tool

18. Papanicolas, I., Woskie, L. R., & Jha, A. K. (2018). Health care spending in the united states and other high-income countries. JAMA, 319(10), 1024–1039

19. Bush, J. (2018, July 24). How AI is taking the scut work out of health care. Harvard Business Review. Retrieved September 26, 2022, from https://hbr.org/2018/03/how-ai-is-taking-the-scut-work-out-of-health-care

20. Pifer, R., & Byers, J. (2018, August 9). AI can save US insurers $7B in admin costs, Accenture says. Healthcare Dive. Retrieved September 26, 2022, from https://www.healthcaredive.com/news/ai-can-save-us-insurers-7b-in-admin-costs-accenture-says/529578/

21. Bell, J., Bryant, M., & Byers, J. (2018, July 26). Payers, doctors weigh AI's disruptive prescribing potential. Healthcare Dive. Retrieved September 26, 2022, from https://www.healthcaredive.com/news/spotlight-AI-payers-doctors-artifical-intelligence/528424/

22. Highmark Inc.'s Anti-Fraud Department using Artificial Intelligence to reduce fraud, waste and abuse impact. (2020). Cision PR Web. https://www.prweb.com/releases/highmark_inc_s_anti_fraud_department_using_artificial_intelligence_to_reduce_fraud_waste_and_abuse_impact/prweb16874765.htm

23. Kent, J. (2020). Artificial Intelligence Saved Over $260M in Fraud, Waste in 2019 – HealthITAnalytics.com – Cloud Hosting. (n.d.). Retrieved September 26, 2022.

24. Kent, J. (2019). 62% of Execs have implemented an artificial intelligence strategy. Health IT Analytics. https://healthitanalytics.com/news/62-of-execs-have-implemented-an-artificial-intelligence-strategy. https://healthitanalytics.com/news/62-of-execs-have-implemented-an-artificial-intelligence-strategy

25. AI, technology key to reducing medicare fraud and waste, CMS Says. (2019, October 24). DistilINFO POPHealth. Retrieved September 26, 2022, from https://www.distilnfo.com/pophealth/2019/10/24/ai-technology-key-to-reducing-medicare-fraud-and-waste-cms-says/

26. Garg, M., Rayasam, M., Reddy, P., & Tran, J. (2022, September 12). Using machine learning to unlock value across the healthcare value chain. McKinsey & Company. Retrieved September 26, 2022, from https://www.mckinsey.com.br/industries/healthcare-systems-and-services/our-insights/using-machine-learning

27. Beaton, T. (2017, October 5). 80% of Payers Investing in Member Engagement, Satisfaction. Health Payer Intelligence. https://healthpayerintelligence.com/news/80-of-payers-investing-in-member-engagement-satisfaction

CHAPTER 11

AI Applications in Life Sciences

THE CALIFORNIA BIOMEDICAL RESEARCH ASSOCIATION says that it currently takes an average of 12 years for a drug in the United States to go from the research lab to the patient (Figures 11.1 and 11.2). Only one in every thousand drugs that begins preclinical testing ever makes it to human testing, and that has to happen five times before one gets approved. It costs companies an average of $359 million to take a new drug from the research lab to the patient.

It's widely accepted that artificial intelligence (AI) will be a game changer for life sciences. Discovering and creating new diagnostics and treatments will increasingly require dealing with huge amounts of data such as genomics, proteomics, and transcriptomics. This data is large in volume and has many dimensions, and so only AI can analyze it to identify patterns and make predictions. It's impossible for the human mind to understand how billions of genetic codes interact with the various mutations, as well as the relative contribution of each mutation.

AI allows us to look forward to an era of faster drug discovery, better clinical trials, better diagnostics, and faster vaccine discovery (as with COVID-19) (Figure 11.3). To realize this potential, we need to tackle many of the issues we've already discussed, and it all comes back to data.

The data that we need to facilitate this change is in a chaotic format right now. The historic data collected while developing new molecules or looking for new targets isn't in a usable format. The vast libraries of previous experiments by pharma companies contain data that wasn't collected with AI applications in mind. Much of this data is on paper or collected in a narrative format, and so there'll need to be a concerted effort to convert it into a more usable format.

AI Doctor: The Rise of Artificial Intelligence in Healthcare: A Guide for Users, Buyers, Builders, and Investors, First Edition. Ronald M. Razmi.
© 2024 Ronald M. Razmi. Published 2024 by John Wiley & Sons, Inc.

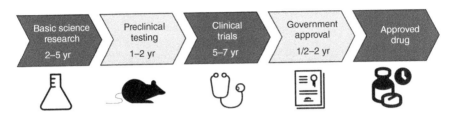

FIGURE 11.1 *(source: Adapted from[1])*

The same issues apply to the use of data to facilitate clinical trials. Many of the key issues that currently plague clinical trials (such as patient recruitment) can be improved using AI, but a lot of the data is unstructured. Until natural language processing (NLP) techniques improve, the benefits will be incremental. The companies that have successfully created valuable databases for drug development, such as Flatiron for Oncology, have done so by manually abstracting key concepts from clinical notes and populating a structured database so that it can be used for drug discovery or development.

Let's take a look at what will be possible and how we'll get there.

11.1   Drug Discovery

AI could identify new targets or molecules that could cure or treat diseases that have been challenging to make progress with so far. Big pharma is struggling with profitability due to the high costs of research and development, as well as the low success rate for new drugs, how hard it is to enroll patients in clinical trials and pressure from various governments to reduce the price of pharmaceuticals. Because of that, pharmaceutical companies are constantly looking for ways to cut the cost of drug development and thus to become more profitable. For AI to help us to understand the causes of diseases, it will need access to huge amounts of data that are currently either inaccessible or don't exist yet.

Creating and analyzing data that can identify promising compounds or targets takes a lot of time. Drug discovery can sift through a lot of data and find patterns. This can shorten the time it takes to discover the right targets and could also add precision to the process. Validating targets and optimizing leads alone can cost over $600 million and take more than four years.[3] AI platforms are cutting down on discovery time by mining medical data—including omics data, scientific literature, and clinical trials data—to identify new drug targets and predict optimal drug designs. They can lower pre-discovery costs by up to 90% and help us to better understand drug mechanisms and the structures of diseases.

Pharma efficiency: challenges

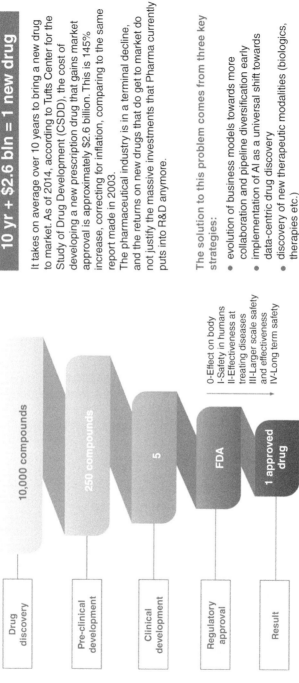

10 yr + \$2.6 bln = 1 new drug

It takes on average over 10 years to bring a new drug to market. As of 2014, according to Tufts Center for the Study of Drug Development (CSDD), the cost of developing a new prescription drug that gains market approval is approximately \$2.6 billion. This is 145% increase, correcting for inflation, comparing to the same report made in 2003.

The pharmaceutical industry is in a terminal decline, and the returns on new drugs that do get to market do not justify the massive investments that Pharma currently puts into R&D anymore.

The solution to this problem comes from three key strategies:

- evolution of business models towards more collaboration and pipeline diversification early
- implementation of AI as a universal shift towards data-centric drug discovery
- discovery of new therapeutic modalities (biologics, therapies etc.)

10,000 compounds

250 compounds

5

FDA

1 approved drug

0-Effect on body
I-Safety in humans
II-Effectiveness at treating diseases
III-Larger scale safety and effectiveness
IV-Long term safety

Drug discovery

Pre-clinical development

Clinical development

Regulatory approval

Result

FIGURE 11.2   (*source: Adapted from*[2])

Application of AI for advanced R&D to address pharma efficiency challenges

Target discovery and early drug discovery	Design and processing of preclinical experiments
• Analyze data sets, form hypotheses and generate novel insights • Identify novel drug candidates • Analyze data from patient samples in both healthy and diseased states to generate novel biomarkers and therapeutic targets • Predict binding affinity and other pharmacological properties of molecules • Allow filtering for drug-like properties of molecules • Reduce complexity in protein design	• Reduce time, money, and uncertainty in planning experiments • Decode open- and closed-access data on reagents and get actionable insights • Automate selection, manipulation, and analysis of cells • Expedite development of cell lines and automate manufacturing of cellular therapeutics • Automate sample analysis with a robotic cloud laboratory

Clinical trials	Repurposing of existing drugs
• Optimize clinical trial study design • Transform diverse streams of biomedical and healthcare data into computer models representative of individual patients • Deliver personalized medicine at scale by revealing optimal health interventions for individual patients • Analyze medical records to find patients for clinical trials • Automate matching cancer patients to clinical trials through personal medical history and genetic analysis • Improve pathology analysis • Identify patients that would benefit from novel therapies	• Rapidly identify new indications for many known drugs • Match existing drugs with rare diseases • Conduct experimental biology at scale by testing 1000+ of compounds on 100+ cellular disease models in parallel • Generate novel biomarkers and therapeutic targets

	Aggregation and synthesis of information
	• Extract knowledge from literature • Generate insights from thousands of unrelated data sources • Improve decision-making • Eliminate blind spots in research • Identify competitive whitespace

FIGURE 11.3   *(source: Adapted from[2])*

Built on language models, AI-powered generators such as ChatGPT can be made to read the codes that make up the building blocks of the human body. Research has found that it's possible to develop a generalizable program—a "genomic language model"—that could be applied to a variety of different tasks, instead of requiring scientists to build fit-for-purpose AIs to chase answers for each major biological question. For example, Nvidia has been working with the synthetic biology company Evozyne to build a large language model focused on constructing never-before-seen proteins.[4]

AI drug discovery platforms drive the following outcomes[3]:

• Lowered drug discovery costs by up to 90%

• Reduced discovery and lead optimization times

• Faster time-to-trial for drugs

• Larger datasets (through medical literature, omics datasets, clinical trials data, and more)

• Better optimized drug designs

• Ability to repurpose existing medications or target diseases that were previously "undruggable"

It can achieve this through several mechanisms[3]:

• Simulating drug interactions, including protein-protein, ligand structure, antibody therapies, and more

• Analyzing omics databases for identifying optimal gene targets

- Using NLP for extracting data from scientific literature
- Using computer vision for cellular image analysis
- Powering molecular databases for predicting optimal small molecule designs

Putting genomics front and center could help us to better understand the biology of diseases, which would drive efficiencies and cut research and development costs while allowing us to bring targeted drugs to patients in record time. Used in combination with genomics, AI could help pharma companies to develop new drugs for rare diseases. The rarer a disease is, the smaller the market is and so the less likely it is to have been addressed. Big pharma is hesitant to take on the high development costs for new drugs if there's no sign of a return on investment.

Biological processes are complex, and that means that they lead to multidimensional data that human beings struggle to wrap their heads around. The good news is that AI is the perfect tool to spot patterns in this kind of data, and startups are increasingly using it to improve drug discovery from start to finish, from identifying biological targets to preclinical testing.

What AI can do in drug discovery[5]:

- Data mining millions of molecular structures
- Designing new molecules
- Predicting toxicity and off-target effects
- Predicting dosages of experimental drugs
- Mining molecular structures in silico
- Analyzing cellular assays on massive scale
- Faster development of more potent molecules
- AI chemical screening of the molecules
- Predicting chemical reactions via machine learning
- Sifting through chemical databases to find the right compounds
- Analyzing genomes and finding disease-causing variants
- Understanding the functions of nonprotein coding sections
- Analyzing interactions between genes
- Determining the patterns of genome methylation
- Planning genome editing and CRISPR targets
- Assessing tumors and sequencing data from tumors
- Analyzing compounds to find a good fit for the targets
- Assessing compounds for the right dose
- In silico labeling of cells and their structures for microscopic analysis

- Ghost cytometry: sorting cells through machine learning
- Assisting in image reconstruction for out-of-focus images or under-sampled data to amplify the data for interpretation

The AI drug discovery market is expected to be worth $40 billion by 2027.[6] Discovery is the largest expenditure for drug development, so if we're able to increase the quality of drug candidates, we'll be able to improve the success rates of clinical trials. A number of well-funded companies have been making noise in this space.

Companies like Atomwise, Exscientia, InSilico Medicine, Insitro, HealX, and Cyclica have been pursuing partnerships with big pharma along with the development of their own compounds. There are two main business models that we're starting to see here. First, there're the biotech startups that are using AI in internal research and development to discover new drugs. Second, there're the SaaS startups that are selling analytics software to pharma companies.

In spite of all this, the progress so far has been underwhelming and partnerships between big pharma and these companies haven't produced any breakthrough drugs (Figure 11.4). That's not unexpected as these partnerships are still in their early stages. However, given the large amounts of capital invested so far and the expectations of investors to see results, further large investments could be in jeopardy.

Neither of these two business models are in the driver's seat yet, as neither have produced key drugs that are being used to treat patients. We've already talked about the quality and format of the data that exists in pharmaceutical databases. The repository of biomedical research data is enormous and, for the most part, digital. Investing resources in making this data ready for AI analysis could be a critical step to unlock the potential value of AI in drug discovery. This can represent a great business opportunity for companies focused on data, rather than drug discovery or AI itself.[7]

There's already a lot of activity in the industry, as well as a number of AI-designed drugs in the works. Startups that partner with big pharma vendors could find themselves on a shortcut to success, and these partnerships could help them to run proofs of concept into potential milestone payments for new drug candidates. These could exceed $1 billion, as we've seen with the InSitro-Gilead partnership, the Exscientia-Celgene partnership, and the Atomwise-Hansoh Pharma partnership. Ultimately, they all aim to find specialized drugs focused on smaller diseases, super-responders to existing drugs and new indications.

As we've already discussed, AI is great at spotting patterns that are hidden in large volumes of data and calculating the effect of small molecular iterations to predict efficacy and specificity. Within this field, the applications are often interrelated and include using AI to analyze clinical, scientific, patient, and genomic data to get a better understanding of disease mechanisms, and

AI for drug discovery market timeline

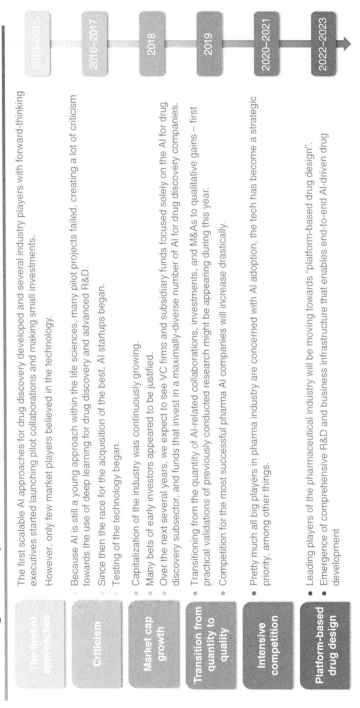

The first AI approaches | 2012–2015
- The first scalable AI approaches for drug discovery developed and several industry players with forward-thinking executives started launching pilot collaborations and making small investments.
- However, only few market players believed in the technology.

Criticism | 2016–2017
- Because AI is still a young approach within the life sciences, many pilot projects failed, creating a lot of criticism towards the use of deep learning for drug discovery and advanced R&D.
- Since then the race for the acquisition of the best, AI startups began.
- Testing of the technology began.

Market cap growth | 2018
- Capitalization of the industry was continuously growing.
- Many bets of early investors appeared to be justified.
- Over the next several years, we expect to see VC firms and subsidiary funds focused solely on the AI for drug discovery subsector, and funds that invest in a maximally-diverse number of AI for drug discovery companies.

Transition from quantity to quality | 2019
- Transitioning from the quantity of AI-related collaborations, investments, and M&As to qualitative gains – first practical validations of previously conducted research might be appearing during this year.
- Competition for the most successful pharma AI companies will increase drastically.

Intensive competition | 2020–2021
- Pretty much all big players in pharma industry are concerned with AI adoption, the tech has become a strategic priority, among other things.

Platform-based drug design | 2022–2023
- Leading players of the pharmaceutical industry will be moving towards "platform-based drug design".
- Emergence of comprehensive R&D and business infrastructure that enables end-to-end AI-driven drug development

FIGURE 11.4 *(source: Adapted from)*[2]

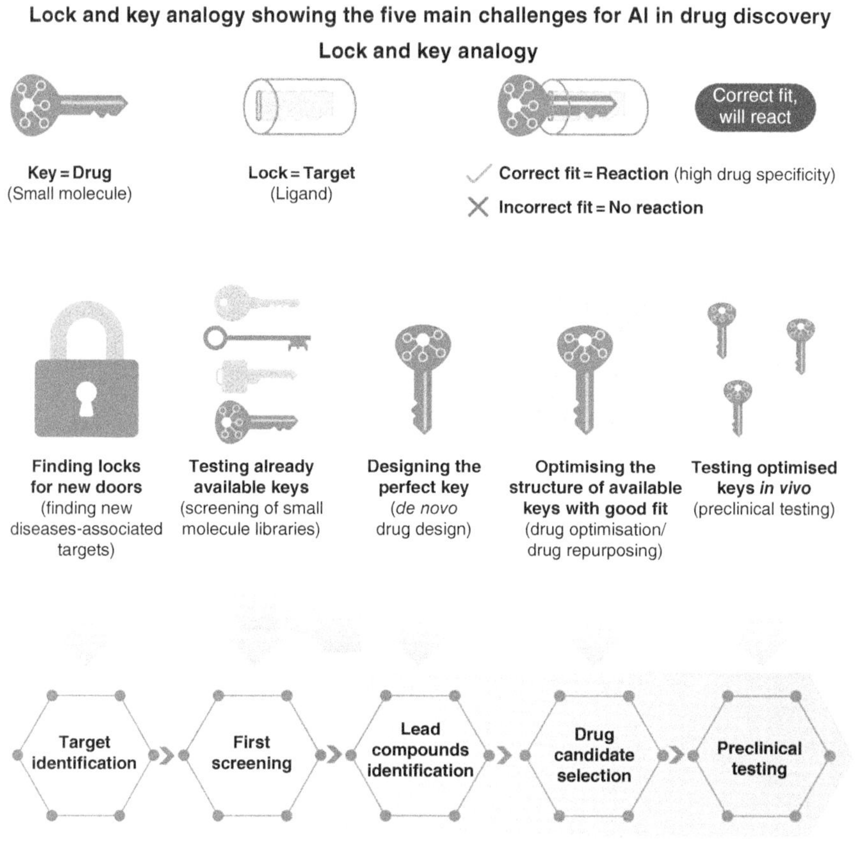

Lock and key analogy showing the five main challenges for AI in drug discovery

Lock and key analogy

| Key = Drug (Small molecule) | Lock = Target (Ligand) | ✓ Correct fit = Reaction (high drug specificity) |
| | | ✗ Incorrect fit = No reaction |

| Finding locks for new doors (finding new diseases-associated targets) | Testing already available keys (screening of small molecule libraries) | Designing the perfect key (*de novo* drug design) | Optimising the structure of available keys with good fit (drug optimisation/ drug repurposing) | Testing optimised keys *in vivo* (preclinical testing) |

Target identification ≫ First screening ≫ Lead compounds identification ≫ Drug candidate selection ≫ Preclinical testing

FIGURE 11.5   *(source: Adapted from Deloitte)*

using this to generate either novel drug candidates or to repurpose existing drugs for new diseases and therapeutic uses (Figure 11.5).[8]

Once potential targets have been identified, AI is also being used to accelerate the drug design process by performing in silico experimentation and conformational analysis on drug molecules to gain insights into the behavior and physical properties of the molecule prior to in vitro and in vivo testing.[8]

AI can also be used for drug screening, the process that happens once a biological target has been identified. Typically carried out in vitro, this is a costly and time-consuming step that's needed to identify the lead candidates for testing. Companies have already started using AI for primary and secondary assays that use computer simulations in silico. For example, Deep Genomics' Project Saturn has created a library of 1000 experimentally verified compounds by testing 69 billion molecules against a million targets.[6]

The companies focused on using AI in drug discovery fall into two categories:

- **Information engines and disease models** inform general drug discovery and can be used by the wider scientific community at the earliest stages of development.
- **Drug design and optimization vendors** produce algorithms design to improve the drug design process and develop candidates from inception through to preclinical testing.

Every biologist understands the concept that proteins are the building blocks of life. Manipulating a protein's function is often the basis of treatment. Understanding a protein's structure and how it influences the cell makes up an important part of the drug development pathway. But a quick method of accurately deducing a protein's structure has proved elusive for scientists, who currently spend years in the lab trying to narrow down potential formations. The CASP (Critical Assessment of Structural Prediction) competition, a worldwide community experiment that aims to solve this problem, was conceived in 1994. This biennial challenge for computational biologists is used to help benchmark methods to predict the structure of proteins from just an amino acid sequence.[9]

The competition made headlines in 2018, when Google's Deepmind joined with its AlphaFold program and significantly outstripped previous attempts. Two years later, the results of AlphaFold 2 were even more exciting: the program managed to determine the shape of around two-thirds of proteins with an accuracy comparable to laboratory experiments. Some experts are now postulating that the team may be able to solve problems that previously took years in a matter of days, leading to a transformative effect in the way that diseases are treated (Figure 11.6).[9]

We spoke earlier about how much of the data from previous experiments with targets or molecules has been collected in a way that makes it hard to analyze. We also discussed how recent breakthroughs with large language models show that these models could effectively digest medical literature and help researchers to find information and results from previous research, identifying hidden insights and helping to design new experiments (Figure 11.7). One of the most promising applications for the new models is to generate protein amino acid sequences and three-dimensional structure from text prompts. Such a model could condition its generation on desired functional properties.[10]

There are emerging machine learning techniques that can help us to prepare data for drug discovery. Machine learning models can be trained to support companies in the life sciences industry and to normalize, index, and structure data. AstraZeneca has been using machine learning for R&D, as well as in pathology to review tissue samples more quickly. Labeling data is always time-consuming, but it's even more of a challenge in this case because it can

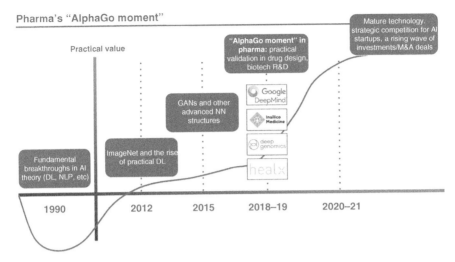

FIGURE 11.6   Advances in AI will Shape the Future of Drug Discovery
(source: Adapted from[2])

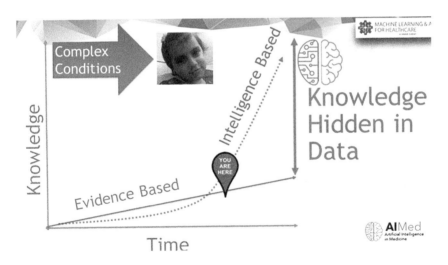

FIGURE 11.7   AI will Uncover Key Insights Hidden in Current Body of Medical Literature *(source: Healthcare Information and Management Systems Society, Inc. (HIMSS), 2019)[5]*

take thousands of tissue sample images to train a model. AstraZeneca uses a machine learning-powered, human-in-the-loop data-labeling, and annotation service to automate some of the most tedious portions of this work, resulting in at least 50% less time spent cataloging samples.[11]

Discovery-stage pharmaceutical company Numerate uses machine learning to quickly and cheaply identify the molecules that have the best odds of progressing through the research pipeline to become candidates for new drugs. The company used its cloud-based platform to rapidly discover and optimize ryanodine receptor 2 (RYR2) modulators, which are being advanced as new drugs to treat life-threatening cardiovascular diseases.[11]

The protein ryanodine 2 is hard to target, but cloud computing has made it much easier. Traditional approaches would make it hard to attack the protein, because the biology is so complex that testing is inherently slow and laborious, and the industry also has a 0.1% screening hit rate for simpler biology. Numerate essentially decided to uncouple the trial-and-error process from the laboratory and found a way to discover candidate drugs at a speed that was five times quicker than the industry average. Data transformation tools can also help to simplify and accelerate data profiling, preparation, and feature engineering, as well as to enable reusable algorithms both for new model discovery and inference.[11]

AI-powered drug miner Exscientia has been able to discover a candidate that targets an enzyme that was previously hard to target because of selectivity and potency. The molecule was found within 11 months of beginning drug design.[12]

In November 2021, a company called Insilico Medicine announced that it had begun its first human trials of ISM001-055, its AI-designed drug candidate that it hoped would treat pulmonary fibrosis. This is one of the most significant milestones in the history of AI-powered drug discovery because this is the first time that a human being has been dosed with an AI-discovered novel molecule based on an AI-discovered novel target.[13]

The first in-human, intravenous dose of this small molecule inhibitor has already been delivered to a healthy volunteer in Australia. To make this happen, Insilico used its AI-powered drug discovery platform, Pharma.ai, to analyze more than 20 disease targets and to predict the most likely successful candidate. It was able to work through the entirety of the discovery process, from identifying a target to nominating preclinical candidates, within a year and a half and with a budget of just $2.6 million. This is the first AI-discovered compound to enter the clinic and more compounds are expected in the near future (Figure 11.8).[13]

11.2   Clinical Trials

Once you find a promising drug or device, you need to take it through trials. This is another long and complicated process. We need to make sure that these products are safe and effective before they're prescribed to large numbers of people. So many things about this process are difficult: deciding which patient population would be appropriate, finding those patients, designing a good study protocol, recruiting the patients, ensuring that they stay with the study, collecting the right data, analyzing the data, and filing it with the

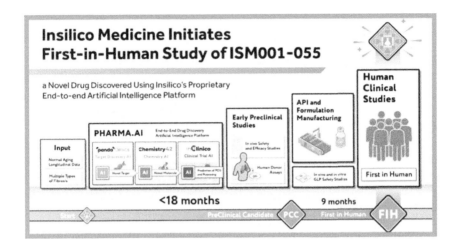

FIGURE 11.8   *(source: Colangelo[13]/Margaretta Colangelo)*

regulatory agency. That's a lot, and it usually takes a long time. Life science companies have been looking for a way to improve this process, and it looks like AI could eventually be one of the catalysts to get the right products to the patients safer and faster.

We covered discovery and preclinical in the last section, but as you can see in Figure 11.9, once you get through the extremely difficult and low-odds process of discovery, the long and low-odds process of clinical development awaits you. This is where you determine the product's safety, the right dose, and its impact on clinical outcomes. Clinical trials are carried out across

Bringing a drug to market is a drawn-out process

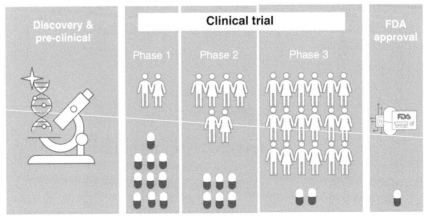

FIGURE 11.9   *(source: Adapted from[14])*

multiple different phases, with their cost and complexity increasing exponentially from Phase I to Phase III. Even though significant amounts of time and money are invested in clinical trials, only 10% of the drugs that enter Phase I will go on to receive FDA approval.

There are a number of reasons why clinical trials fail, ranging from poor study design and insufficient participation from medical centers or physicians to inconsistent data, too few trial participants, and patients dropping out in the middle of the trial. We also need to acknowledge that the huge costs of clinical trials have a subsequent impact on costs for patients, because biopharma companies increase the prices of their approved drugs to write off the costs of failed trials and to stay profitable.

Figure 11.10 shows what it takes for a patient and a clinical trial to get matched with each other. As you can see, it's a highly manual and inefficient

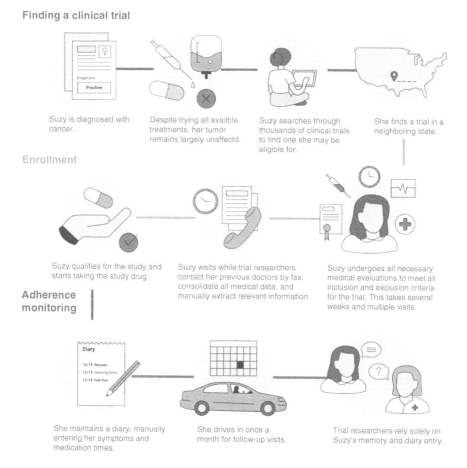

Finding a clinical trial

Suzy is diagnosed with cancer.

Despite trying all availble treatments, her tumor remains largely unaffectd.

Suzy searches through thousands of clinical trials to find one she may be eligible for.

She finds a trial in a neighboring state.

Enrollment

Suzy qualifies for the study and starts taking the study drug.

Suzy waits while trial researchers contact her previous doctors by fax, consolidate all medical data, and manually extract relevant information.

Suzy undergoes all necessary medical evaluations to meet all inclusion and exclusion criteria for the trial. This takes several weeks and multiple visits.

Adherence monitoring

She maintains a diary, manually entering her symptoms and medication times.

She drives in once a month for follow-up visits.

Trial researchers rely solely on Suzy's memory and diary entry.

FIGURE 11.10   Finding and Participating in Clinical Trials is a Challenging Process *(source: Adapted from[14])*

process and luck seems to have as much to do with the outcome as anything else. Patients generally only participate in drug trials when existing treatments have already failed. To make matters more complicated, not all of the patients who are diagnosed are eligible to participate in trials. In fact, determining patient eligibility is a hugely difficult task on its own. Once eligibility has been ascertained, participation is often cost and time intensive. The process in general is inefficient, with drug trials lasting for an average of almost a decade and costing over $1 billion. The overall size of this market is $52 billion annually.[14]

AI can be helpful in various parts of this process. But it's not just AI—it's really data and digital technologies that can transform this long and costly process. AI would be part of the solution. Life science researchers will eventually be able to use machine learning to design optimized trial protocols, identify the best locations for studies, boost patient recruitment, improve adherence to the treatment, and carry out efficient and accurate data analysis.

Machine learning could also be used to speed up the process of regulatory submission, because it could help to capture and analyze the huge amounts of data that are generated during clinical trials. This data will need to be shared to enable collaboration among investigators, sponsor organizations, and contract research organizations (CROs).

For example, Accenture's Intelligent Trial Planner (ITP) uses machine learning to examine forecast recruitment timelines and the overall feasibility of clinical trials. The ITP platform enables study design teams at pharma organizations to run prediction analysis in minutes, not weeks, allowing them to iterate faster and more frequently.[11]

Then there's Teckro, an Irish company, that gives researchers a machine-learning platform for monitoring the progress of clinical trials across teams that are dispersed throughout different geographies. Deep Lens, another startup in this category, uses an AI-based pathology platform called VIPER to identify eligible trial candidates at the point of their diagnosis.[15] Figure 11.11 shows where AI can make an impact in clinical trials.[16]

11.2.1   Information Engines

The goal here is to aggregate and mine data from a number of disparate sources to enhance the efficiency, quality, and success rate of clinical trials. This is done by extracting structured and unstructured data that's relevant to the design and conduct of the trial.

NLP can help us to extract and analyze the information we need from a patient's EHR records, to compare it with the eligibility criteria for all ongoing clinical trials, and to recommend studies that they might be able to participate in. Extracting information from EHRs, labs, images, and other medical

AI in clinical trials

Information engines	Patient stratification	Operations

Information engines

- Enable analysis and decision making from structured and unstructured data.
- Medical records, relevant guidelines, real-world data and other clinical and scientific sources.
- Enhance the quality, efficiency and ultimately success rate of clinical trials.

Patient stratification

- Improved patient stratification to make sure the trial is focusing on the right individuals, and that drug responses are properly and efficiently tracked.
- Biomarkers from speech, behaviour, medical imaging, genomics and other sources.

Operations

- Monitor treatment response and adherence to clinical trial guidelines.
- Reduce patient dropout, developing synthetic control arms, accelerate the recruitment process and making it easier for patients to engage.

FIGURE 11.11   *(source: Adapted from[16])*

records is one of the most highly anticipated use cases of AI in the healthcare industry. The problem is that the solutions that are designed to do this face a range of challenges, such as disparate data sources and unstructured data. Many of the tools that standard NLP algorithms rely on, such as sentiment analysis and word sense disambiguation, struggle with clinical notes because they're often full of acronyms, misspellings, and technical language.

Then there's the fact that structured data can become unstructured due to the way that it's transmitted. For example, if we take a spreadsheet and turn it into a PDF, it loses much of its structure, making it more difficult for researchers to collect the data that they need to determine patient eligibility.

This becomes relevant in many areas of the trials, including the design, site selection, patient recruitment, and more, such as finding super-responders and evidence for new therapeutic approaches. All of these activities will benefit from us being able to analyze clinical information and figure out what and whom to focus on.

Antidote.me has made the information for clinical trials machine-readable and easy to search. It started out by gathering thousands of clinical studies from the World Health Organization and **ClinicalTrials.gov**, and then it hired experts to manually standardize all of that data into structured language that an algorithm could understand. Models were then trained to categorize and identify studies. Antidote has annotated more than 14,000 trials—about 50% of what's listed on **ClinicalTrials.gov**—spanning 726 conditions.[17] This is vital work because poor study design has hugely negative impacts on costs, efficiency, and success rates.

AI tools can help us to select the optimal primary and secondary end-points in clinical studies to define the most relevant protocols for patients, payers, and regulators. The goal is to optimize study design by identifying the best possible country and site strategies, patient recruitment and startup plans and enrollment models. Better designed studies inherently lead to more predictable results, reduced development times, higher recruitment rates, fewer amendments to protocols, and higher efficiency from start to finish. These improvements increase the chances of success and facilitate realistic and accurate planning.[18]

A technique called adaptive design, which relies on a more flexible approach to clinical trials, has become a key trend for researchers tackling COVID-19. Traditional studies are more rigid about endpoints and dosing reg-imens, while adaptive designs allow researchers to make modifications as the trial progresses.

One of the biggest ongoing challenges is that of identifying trial sites with access to enough patients who meet inclusion criteria (Figure 11.12). As studies continue to target more specific populations, recruitment goals become harder and harder for them to meet. This increases costs, lengthens timelines, and adds to the risk of failure. The Tufts Center for the Study of Drug Development (CSDD) says that nearly half of all sites miss their enrollment targets, while only 3% of cancer patients are currently enrolled in clinical trials. As many as 80% of all clinical trials miss their enrollment time-lines, while about a third of Phase III trials are halted due to the challenge of enrollment.[18]

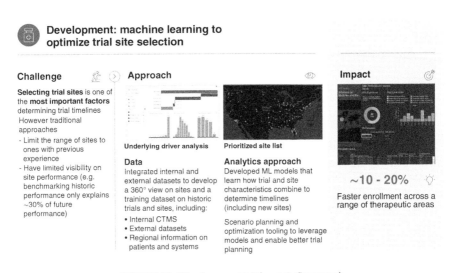

Development: machine learning to optimize trial site selection

Challenge

Selecting trial sites is one of the **most important factors** determining trial timelines However traditional approaches

- Limit the range of sites to ones with previous experience
- Have limited visibility on site performance (e.g. benchmarking historic performance only explains ~30% of future performance)

Approach

Underlying driver analysis

Data
Integrated internal and external datasets to develop a 360° view on sites and a training dataset on historic trials and sites, including:

• Internal CTMS
• External datasets
• Regional information on patients and systems

Prioritized site list

Analytics approach
Developed ML models that learn how trial and site characteristics combine to determine timelines (including new sites)

Scenario planning and optimization tooling to leverage models and enable better trial planning

Impact

~10 - 20%

Faster enrollment across a range of therapeutic areas

FIGURE 11.12   *(source: McKinsey & Company)*

Fortunately, AI and machine learning can help us to cut down on these risks by identifying the best sites and the recruitment strategies that are most likely to work. This requires them to map patient populations and to spot the sites with the highest amount of potential for delivering a large number of patients before any of the sites are ever opened. This would allow sponsors to open fewer sites, to speed up the recruitment process, and to cut down on under-enrollment.

Real-time scenario planning can be powered by machine learning and used to facilitate smarter trials by helping researchers to pick the best sites, countries, and protocols to follow. By cutting down on wastage from poor resources, researchers could reduce costs by 20%. As if that wasn't enough, these more accurate decisions based on data can be used to carry out trials more rapidly, leading to further savings and improving patient outcomes.

Technologies like deep neutral networks, NLP, and optical character recognition (OCR) are already being used to format structured and unstructured data to carry out safety reviews faster and more efficiently. Companies in this category include Aetion, Concerto HealthAI, Owkin, TrinetX, and COTA. Each one of these uses a combination of NLP and ML to introduce intelligent automation to the process. These information engines work with other digital and manual processes within clinical trial design and operations, guiding decisions toward better patient stratification.[16]

11.2.2   Patient Stratification

Here, we're talking about technologies that help with finding, screening, selecting, recruiting, and keeping study patients. A variety of AI technologies can assist in this process. You can use NLP on clinical notes as a first pass to find patients with the right stage of disease once you know their diagnosis from the ICD-10 codes.

For example, if you're recruiting non-small cell lung cancer patients who are in stage III or IV, the staging information isn't coded in ICD-10. You'd need to find those patients by examining the clinical notes. Well, this might be a simple enough ask from the less-than-perfect NLP technologies we have access to today.

This would reveal patients who could then be further screened by study staff, but identifying more patients at the top of the funnel would mean faster recruitment timelines. Solutions are increasingly turning to AI to extract information from medical records to simplify the enrollment process by vetting inclusion and exclusion criteria. Deep 6 AI is using NLP to extract clinical data like diagnoses, symptoms, and treatments from EHRs, and it can even identify patients with conditions that aren't mentioned in EHRs to improve the match rate between clinical trials and patients.

Other opportunities for AI in this category include using it to identify and track digital biomarkers in voice, movement, and other physiological biomarkers. This allows more precise diagnosis and monitoring, although many of these digital biomarkers haven't been fully established for specific diseases or endorsed for this purpose. However, that's clearly the direction we're headed in. Companies in this category include nQ Medial, WinterLight Labs, VIDA, Perspectum, Quibim, IAG, and IXICO. These companies are using AI to track digital biomarkers in voice, patient movements, and imaging (radiology and pathology) to facilitate clinical trials.[16]

Other solutions focus on capturing physiological data. When combined with wearable devices, AI can provide continuous, real-time monitoring for physiological and behavioral changes in patients, reducing the cost, frequency, and difficulty associated with on-site checkups. AliveCor provides a wearable EKG device that uses machine learning to pick up on abnormal heart rhythms like atrial fibrillation. Meanwhile, Biofourmis is using wearable devices to track patients' vital signs and to provide predictive health insights. The startup partnered with the University of Hong Kong to capture the temperature, heart rate, and oxygen levels of patients infected with COVID-19 to detect subtle changes in health and accelerate virus research.[14]

Another group of companies is using AI to better assess patient genetics and to identify biomarkers that better diagnose and subtype patients for more efficient treatment matching and monitoring. Companies here include Tempus and WuXi NextCODE.[16]

11.2.3   Clinical Trial Operations

AI can introduce key intelligent automation to different processes in the actual running of trial operations. Some examples of this include using AI in monitoring medication adherence, creating digital twins and synthetic arms that help reduce the number of patients needed, and identifying optimal patients for recruitment by analyzing clinical information.

Nonadherence often leads to adverse effects on patients' health, and it can also boost costs by forcing researchers to find new patients or compromising the accuracy of their studies. As a general rule, therapeutic efficacy is proven with adherence rates of 80% or above. The problem is that as many as half of the medications prescribed in the United States aren't taken correctly. That's why the sponsors of clinical studies are investing in emerging technologies that could cut down on nonadherence (Figure 11.13). Patients are being asked to note when they're taking the drugs, what other medications they're taking, and any adverse effects that they're experiencing, such as stomach aches, muscle aches, and headaches.

This process is adversely affected by issues such as reliance on patient memory, outdated recording systems, and the risk of dropout.[19]

Medication adherence tracking is prone to human error

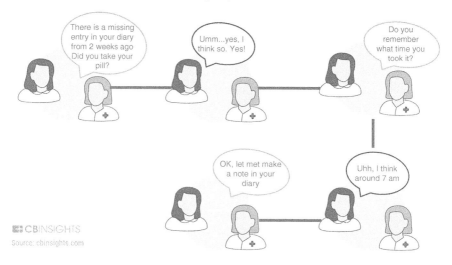

FIGURE 11.13   *(source: Adapted from CB Insights)*

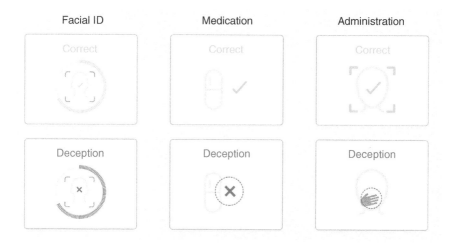

FIGURE 11.14   **AI can Help in Improving Medication Adherence** *(source: AiCure)*

AiCure uses an interactive medical assistant (IMA) that is designed to identify patients who are most at risk of nonadherence. The patients shoot a video of themselves taking the pill, and AiCure confirms that the right person is taking the right pill (Figure 11.14). Then there are other emerging technologies, like speech analytics and digital phenotyping, which are being used to assess adherence to medication. Mental health startup Mindstrong uses digital phenotyping technology to measure mood based on how users interact with their mobile device.[14]

Aural Analytics uses speech detection to pick up on subtle changes to users' brain health, and the company recently partnered with Mass General Hospital to carry out a trial for amyotrophic lateral sclerosis (ALS). As part of this, they're using connected devices to facilitate the real-time study of medication adherence. For example, optimize.health (previously Pillsy) launched a smart medication bottle with a corresponding mobile application that provides reminders, educational content, dose tracking, and patient-reported data for providers.[14]

As can be seen in Figure 11.15, data generated by patients (such as through Project Baseline) could help us to create digital twins to reduce the number of patients who need to be recruited and assist in quicker analysis of the data. Most trials consist of an experimental group of patients who get the drug in the study and a control group that is given a placebo. The goal of the control group is to provide a baseline that we can compare the experimental group to.

Unlearn.ai is being used to reduce the number of subjects that we need for clinical trials through the use of digital twins as a type of synthetic control group (Figure 11.15). This cuts down on patient resistance to the trial because it reduces the chance of them being given the placebo. This also reduces the number of patients who are required for a trial to be carried out.

Synthetic data can also provide us with data that imitates real-world data, offering a potential solution to the problem of not being able to find enough patients. Computer-generated synthetic data can be used instead of manually

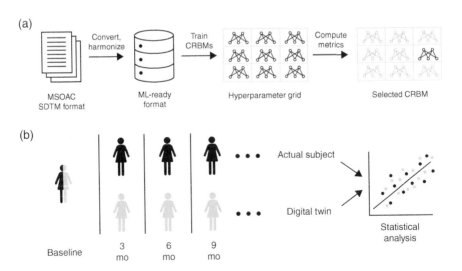

FIGURE 11.15 **Aggregating and Normalizing Diverse Data Allows for Creation of Digital Twins for Improving Population Health** (*source: Reference 14*)

collecting and labeling data from the real world. The goal here is to speed up the training for AI and machine learning models, driving greater cost efficiencies and bypassing the constraints that come from real-world data collection. This type of data comes in different forms, including demographics, labs, imaging, and more. And because the synthetic data is created by a computer, it's not based on real data or health records. Companies like Simerse create synthetic data to train AI and machine learning models.[20]

11.3   Medical Affairs and Commercial

Machine learning can also accelerate the regulatory submission process, as the massive amounts of data generated during clinical trials can be captured and effectively shared to collaborate among investigators, CROs, and sponsor organizations.[11]

In pharmacovigilance, huge amounts of structured and unstructured data need to be reviewed so that we can provide oversight. Machine learning and NLP models are allowing us to address many of the challenges that PV teams face when it comes to harnessing data to provide enhanced quality and oversight. These kinds of tools allow us to automate some of the highly manual processing tasks, and they can also translate and digitize documents on safety cases and adverse drug reactions (ADRs) to make them easier to use. They can also perform data listening tasks to monitor conversations on social media and other platforms, ensuring adverse events are promptly identified.[18]

Also, the commercialization of life science solutions is an area that's ripe for innovation with data, analytics, and AI. Novartis made headlines in 2019 when it armed its sales force with an AI-driven service to tell sales reps which doctors they should visit and what topics they should bring up once they got through the door.[21] The COVID-19 pandemic meant that sales reps couldn't see doctors face-to-face, and so many pharma companies switched their focus to AI in an effort to get their brands noticed by the right doctors at the right time.

Applications for AI in the commercial side of life sciences include weeding out content that regulators would disapprove of and building relationships with patients. Recent innovations like ChatGPT have shown that companies might even use machines to write promotional copy. Experts expect more drug makers to follow in the footsteps of other industries and to use AI to further boost their brands in the coming years as they figure out how to use patient and provider data in a way that allows for better commercial activities without violating privacy.

More pharma marketers are expected to use chatbots in the near future. Novo Nordisk debuted its digital concierge chatbot Sophia back in 2018, and they're becoming more mainstream.[21] As well as appearing more human, these bots will work more closely with other services, scheduling telemedicine appointments or helping patients to find pharmacies and specialist physicians. AI will expand the possibilities for truly engaging with patients.

Other key applications of AI in commercial life sciences include content creation, audience targeting, and compliance automation. Companies are already using AI tools to generate routine promotional material like personalized subject lines for emails. This allows for a truly one-to-one marketing program that's scaled to an entire HCP or patient database.[21]

The increasing amount of online patient data and the rich databases of providers allow AI solutions to know about patients and their provider histories, as well as what their interests or issues might be. As such, life science companies can take a far more intelligent approach to content strategy and content engagement. For example, a patient in the middle of cancer treatment might welcome information about a drug maker's patient support program or tips for managing side effects from an IV infusion, even though that kind of messaging might not appeal to the masses in a broad marketing campaign.[21]

Although there are concerns around privacy and doctor-patient relationships, good controls could allow patients to benefit from the AI-based personalized marketing that we see in other industries. Given the increase in customized digital marketing, there's been a noticeable rise in the amount of promotional content that we see. This shows us another promising use of AI, which is to review content to ensure it's consistent with drug labeling and regulatory guidance. Using AI, errors can be found in marketing content earlier in the process, and as a result, companies can get that content out quicker. Just like other applications of AI in healthcare, it would be augmenting humans and not replacing them.

AI can process large amounts of content and allow personalization at scale for life science campaigns by taking a first pass at screening a marketing message and determining if it's fully compliant.

References

1. Arnold, D., & Wilson, T. (2017). What doctor? Why AI and robotics will define new health PwC. https://www.linkedin.com/pulse/what-doctor-why-ai-robotics-define-new-health-alexandra-schimmelpfeng
2. Iqbal, R., Amimer, D., Kiel, M., Wadhwa, P., Ha, A., & Lerner, I. (2022). Deep Pharma Intelligence webinar. https://www.deep-pharma.tech/conference-ai-in-drug-discovery-2022
3. AI drug discovery platforms. (2021). CB Insights. https://www.cbinsights.com/reports/CB-Insights_ESP-Vendor-Assessment-Matrix-AI-Drug-Discovery-Platforms-Healthcare.pdf

4. Hale, C. (2023, January 12). JPM23: Not just for chat generators, Nvidia turns AI language models toward genomic, protein data. Fierce Biotech. https://www.fiercebiotech.com/medtech/jpm23-not-just-chat-generators-nvidia-turns-ai-language-models-toward-genomic-protein-data

5. Chang, A. (2019, February 11). Artificial intelligence in medicine, synergies between man and machine. [Presentation]. AI in Medicine Symposium, Orlando, Florida.

6. CB Insights. (2020, December 22). Can applying AI to genomics improve healthcare? CB Insights Research. https://www.cbinsights.com/research/ai-genomics-healthcare/

7. HealthEconomics.Com. (2021, May 27). The State of AI in Pharma. https://www.healtheconomics.com/webinars/the-state-of-ai-in-pharma

8. Kristensen, U. (2020, April 2). VC funding for AI in Drug Development & Clinical Trials hits $5.2B. Signify Research. https://www.signifyresearch.net/healthcare-it/vc-funding-ai-drug-development-clinical-trials-hits-5-2b/

9. Fitt, I. (2020, December 18). DeepMind triumph – too much hype for little real-world impact? Signify Research. https://www.signifyresearch.net/healthcare-it/deepmind-triumph-much-hype-little-real-world-impact/

10. Kucera, T., Togninalli, M., & Meng-Papaxanthos, L. (2022). Conditional generative modeling for de novo protein design with hierarchical functions. Bioinformatics, 38(13), 3454–3461. https://doi.org/10.1093/bioinformatics/btac353

11. Siwicki, B. (2021, June 16). AWS leader talks about technologies needed to take precision medicine. Healthcare IT News. https://www.healthcareitnews.com/news/aws-leader-talks-about-technologies-needed-take-precision-medicine-next-level

12. LaHucik, K. (2021). Bristol Myers' $1.2B discovery pact with Exscientia strikes gold as first drug candidate selected. Fierce Biotech. https://www.fiercebiotech.com/biotech/bristol-myers-pays-exscientia-20m-1-2b-deal-for-first-drug-candidate

13. Colangelo, M. (2022, June 28). AI in healthcare highlights & milestones Q1 2022. LinkedIn. https://www.linkedin.com/pulse/ai-healthcare-highlights-milestones-2021-margaretta-colangelo/

14. CB Insights. (2022, August 16). The future of clinical trials: trends to watch in 2022 and beyond. CB Insights Research. https://www.cbinsights.com/research/briefing/clinical-trials-trends/

15. CB Insights. (2021, January 5). Healthcare AI trends to watch. CB Insights Research. https://www.cbinsights.com/research/report/ai-trends-healthcare/

16. Fitt, I. (2021, September 29). AI in Drug Development & Clinical Trials. Signify Research. https://www.signifyresearch.net/reports/ai-drug-development-clinical-trials/

17. Molteni, M. (2018, January 30). Meet the company trying to democratize clinical trials with AI. WIRED. https://www.wired.com/story/meet-the-company-trying-to-democratize-clinical-trials-with-ai/

18. IQVIA. (2019). AI IN CLINICAL DEVELOPMENT: Improving safety and accelerating results. https://www.iqvia.com/-/media/iqvia/pdfs/library/white-papers/ai-in-clinical-development.pdf

19. Glass, L., Shorter, G., & Patil, R. The future of Clinical Trials: how AI & big tech could make drug development cheaper, faster, & more effective. (2018, August 7). CB Insights. https://www.cbinsights.com/reports/CB-Insights_Future-Of-Clinical-Trials.pdf

20. Siwicki, B. (2021, May 26). Synthetic data's growing role in healthcare AI, machine learning and. Healthcare IT News. https://www.healthcareitnews.com/news/synthetic-datas-growing-role-healthcare-ai-machine-learning-and-robotics

21. Missakian, N. (2021). 2022 forecast: From copywriting to compliance, expect pharma marketers to find new ways to tap AI's potential. Fierce Pharma. https://www.fiercepharma.com/marketing/from-copywriting-to-compliance-expect-pharma-marketers-to-eye-new-ways-to-tap-ai-s

PART III

The Business Case for AI in Healthcare

CHAPTER 12

Which Health AI Applications Are Ready for Their Moment?

A **KEY (AND VERY LEGITIMATE)** question about artificial intelligence (AI) in Healthcare is whether it's ready for prime time.

If all of the hospitals, physicians, nurses, patients, and insurance companies lined up and said "give me AI now," could the applications we've discussed deliver consistently and with good form? That's the question we'll tackle in this chapter. Is the use of natural language processing (NLP) on clinical notes for point-of-care decision support ready to deliver consistently if used in the management of cancer patients? Is the use of deep learning to find ischemic stroke on computed tomography (CT) scans of patients in the emergency room (ER) consistently and accurately predictive? Will decision support models developed with large language models be useful to physicians at the point of care?

In the end, the path for the adoption of AI in healthcare will be through the in-demand use cases where AI performs at an acceptable level. That intersection tells us where we'll see the initial wave of application adoption and, as the needs of users evolve and the technology matures, we'll see the next use cases gain traction. Professor Pete Szolovits, Head of the Clinical Decision-Making Group at MIT's Computer Science and Artificial

AI Doctor: The Rise of Artificial Intelligence in Healthcare: A Guide for Users, Buyers, Builders, and Investors, First Edition. Ronald M. Razmi.
© 2024 Ronald M. Razmi. Published 2024 by John Wiley & Sons, Inc.

Intelligence Laboratory, told me that one of the key barriers will be the lack of cross-functional expertise in medicine and computer science under the same roof. This can lead to models that perform well but which don't solve an urgent clinical problem, or models that solve important problems but aren't well-trained.

To some extent, technological maturity could be the driver here: if AI performance reaches a certain level for a use case, such as clinical trial patient recruitment, it would make sense for every life science company to start using it for their trials. That's where recent advances in generative AI are making a splash. Using large language models on historic structured and unstructured healthcare data to train proficient models for different use cases could lead to performance that's better than expected. It certainly holds the promise to upend projected timelines and make applications like documentation, patient identification for clinical trials, and decision support available sooner than we thought.

12.1   Methodology

Let's go back and revisit some of the key concepts from earlier chapters.

Figure 12.1 reminds us that AI should be thought of as an umbrella term for a range of technologies, and this includes NLP and machine learning (ML). Although NLP is mostly ML-based these days, for the purposes of our discussion here, we simplify things by talking about ML for identifying patterns and making predictions on structured data, and NLP/NLU (natural language understanding) as understanding meaning in written or spoken words.

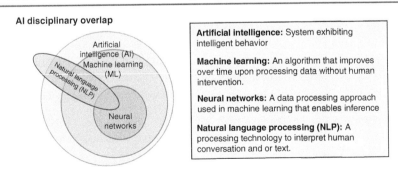

Artificial intelligence encompasses machine learning and neural networks. NLP cuts through the three

AI disciplinary overlap

Artificial intelligence (AI)
Natural language processing (NLP)
Machine learning (ML)
Neural networks

Artificial intelligence: System exhibiting intelligent behavior

Machine learning: An algorithm that improves over time upon processing data without human intervention.

Neural networks: A data processing approach used in machine learning that enables inference

Natural language processing (NLP): A processing technology to interpret human conversation and or text.

FIGURE 12.1   *(source: HIMSS 2019)*[1]

Although we can go several layers deeper and get into what's included under each, given that the focus of this book isn't the technical side of AI, we can keep it high-level and simple here.

Figure 12.2 shows another nice breakdown of AI technologies. Starting with sensing, AI technologies can do things like looking at an image (e.g. magnetic resonance imaging [MRIs]) and finding abnormalities or looking for abnormal signals on a digital audio file (e.g. an Alzheimer's patient's voice). This is ultimately the main methodology used for the analysis of structured data to find patterns.

Then there's the comprehension of meaning and intentions. This is where natural language NLP/NLU comes in. NLP can be applied to text or voice. In both instances, we're not just analyzing a digital file and identifying abnormal patterns; we need to understand the meaning of the sequence of words that have been written or spoken. This is proving to be more challenging in healthcare, and given that, most healthcare data is unstructured and most of the interactions are personal with voice, the fact that this technology has been slower to come to fruition has meant that some of the most promising applications of AI in healthcare remain conceptual.

Much of that may start to change with the emergence of large language models that can consume large amounts of unlabeled and unstructured historic data and be ready to answer questions, extract insights, and support decision-making. As such, we're now at the dawn of a new age of AI in healthcare. I've recently been playing with a system that uses large language models

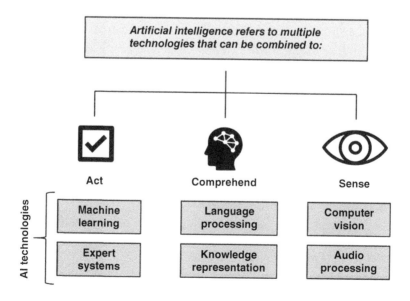

FIGURE 12.2   *(source: Accenture)²*

trained on medical literature. As a cardiologist, I've been asking a lot of questions about complex cardiac topics and feeding it radiology reports and labs and asking it to interpret the data. So far, I've not seen any errors and I've found the responses to be complete and nuanced. This system isn't currently publicly available, but there are other systems that already have beta versions out. However, it can still be tricky to use these models to process clinical notes because sentiment analysis and word sense disambiguation are more difficult when the content is full of acronyms and misspellings.

The performance level of NLP in healthcare is related to the actual use case, but it's historically been nowhere near the performance of deep learning models using structured data. Professor Szolovits has often said to me that NLP isn't yet ready for prime time for clinical notes as a tool in individual decision making because it has too many false negatives and positives, but for use cases where some errors are tolerated, such as cohort selection, clinical trials recruitment, etc it is already a useful tool. The recent release of Chat-GPT hints at the fact that training on large amounts of unstructured data without significant manual annotation is becoming more possible, even given the complexity of this data as compared with what ChatGPT was trained on (the internet). Although clinical information such as clinical notes and clinical trial results may need more preparation work for training generative AI models, there's no doubt that we're at the dawn of a new age for AI with the pace of progress accelerating. Google has released its Healthcare Natural Language application programming interface (API), a cloud-based ML solution that can parse and analyze text-based health data. This is a step forward in the field, but its accuracy and impact remain to be fully defined.

The third area, "Act," is all about combining ML and NLP to come up with the optimal course of action and instructing the system to carry out that action. Examples of this include using computer vision (ML) in the operating room to analyze the patient's anatomy and to direct a robot to perform the next action in surgery based upon its findings. Generative AI is in this category since it creates new content as the result of the on-demand production of output based on a user's instructions. It can answer questions, provide decision support on demand, create new data, generate letters and education materials, and more.

AI can be broken down into four key functions:

- **Perception:** Revolves around collecting and interpreting data that allows it to sense and describe the world around it. This covers audio processing, computer vision, and NLP.
- **Prediction:** Revolves around tapping into AI-based reasoning to make predictions around behavior and results. This is often used for population health management and risk analysis.
- **Prescription:** Revolves around understanding what needs to be done to achieve certain goals. This is used in a variety of ways, including for clinical decision support, drug discovery, and logistics.

- **Combinations:** Resolves around partnering AI with other technologies (e.g. robotics) to provide fully integrated solutions. Examples of this include household robots, self-driving cars, robotic surgeons, and other tools that are able to respond to external stimuli.

Putting it all together, we can conclude that the various forms of AI have made progress but that some have progressed more than others and that some problems are more challenging than others. Sensing is easier than comprehending. Finding abnormal patterns in an image or voice file is easier than understanding the key elements of a physician–patient discussion, deciding which parts of that discussion should end up in the clinical notes and what orders to place as a result of that conversation.

Recent breakthroughs in deep learning have allowed us to create AI systems that are as good as or better than human intelligence at certain key tasks. However, we're still a long way from being able to create "general AI," the term that's used for machines that can carry out all of the cognitive tasks that we humans can do.

To examine these use cases to decide how robust AI methodologies are at delivering on their promise, we can look at clinical care, including population health, administrative and operations, and research and development.

12.2 Clinical Care

In clinical care, we have single-file diagnostic use cases such as reading radiology, pathology, dermatology, and ophthalmology images. The more structured the data is, the better the ML can perform in analyzing it. Signals and images are well structured by time and geometry. Files that might often be stored in a relational DB are structured as tables and by the foreign keys they contains. Text such as discharge summaries may be structured by sections and sub-sections, though this structure is frequently not as "clean" as the others because it's not enforced by software or and contains narratives. A note describing a physical exam is a narrative and less structured than a relational database. Computer vision, a form of deep learning methodology, performs very well on digital images and can potentially surpass human capabilities. We need to remember that this doesn't mean that the algorithm will be sufficient in reading the image. The image may have several other findings that have nothing to do with what the algorithm was trained to do and need a comprehensive human review. Also, for images like skin images or fundoscopic pictures, if the quality is poor due to lighting issues or movement, the accuracy of the AI interpretation can be significantly compromised. Although that's not an issue with the AI methodology, it can still impact adoption since if data acquisition doesn't yield a high-quality image on a regular basis, the users will lose patience and stop using the AI reading.

Most of today's research is focused on diagnostic applications in radiology, ophthalmology, and pathology, according to Dr. Kang Zhang, an ophthalmologist and medicine professor at the Macau University of Science and Technology.

More than 90% of this research focuses on imaging-based diagnostics, as shown in examples of fundoscopic assessment for diabetic retinopathy, reading of CTs, MRIs, and X-rays, and assessment of skin lesions. Why? Because the deep learning models that perform these functions are well-developed and these types of structured data files are compatible with what deep learning models do.

A series of promising studies have looked into the use of deep learning algorithms for detecting abnormalities on images. Qure.ai's chest X-ray tool, qXR, can automatically detect and localize as many as 29 different abnormalities, including those that could suggest the presence of lung cancer. There are a number of indications to look for, such as sharply circumscribed nodules and masses with irregular margins or ill-defined lesions. The qXR algorithm is CE-marked and can detect lung cancer nodules at a high rate of accuracy in less than a minute, as well as revealing the size and position of the nodules. The aim is to help clinicians to pick up on tiny nodules that could be missed even by the experts. One study identified a 17% improvement in sensitivity when AI was used to interpret chest X-rays as opposed to trusting to traditional readings by radiologists. These early detection aids could provide huge long-term benefits in the war against cancer and result in a lower cost per-life-year saved.[3]

Deep learning algorithms can be very valuable for certain types of radiology images that are especially challenging for the radiologists. These relate to diseases that are slow growing and subtle findings that are diffuse and subtle, such as changes in the brain before the diagnosis of Alzheimer's. Historically, radiologists have used positron emission tomography (PET) scans in an attempt to spot Alzheimer's by looking for reduced glucose levels in the brain, especially in the frontal and parietal lobes. The problem is that Alzheimer's is a slow progressive disorder, and so these changes can be subtle and difficult to spot. That's where deep learning comes in, a technology that's particularly good at spotting subtle differences. Human radiologists are great at finding focal findings like those we see in brain tumors, but they struggle at spotting slower, global changes, although if the lesions are too small for human eyes, computer vision algorithms can be more accurate than humans in detecting them.

Applying deep learning algorithms to PET scans shows great promise.[4] In one experiment, the algorithm was able to correctly identify 92% of patients with Alzheimer's in the first test set and 98% in the second. It was also able to do this an average of 75.8 months (or a little more than six years) before the patient was given their final diagnosis.

Deep learning algorithms have also shown great efficacy at identifying abnormal patterns on fundoscopic images to detect eye disease, such as diabetic retinopathy. In the evaluation of retinal fundus photographs from adults with diabetes, an algorithm based on deep ML had high sensitivity and specificity for detecting referable diabetic retinopathy.[5] Moreover, fundus photographs can be used to predict many systemic diseases, such as chronic kidney disease, stroke, cardiovascular disease, hypertension, and type-2 diabetes.

Researchers from Google were able to take a neural network and to train it on retinal images to find risk factors for cardiovascular issues. The research found that as well as identifying risk factors such as age, gender, and smoking patterns through retinal images, it was also "quantifiable to a degree of precision not reported before."[6]

This area is ready for prime time now and promises to provide value beyond what was expected just a few years ago. One example is the area of radiomics, where we find radiographic findings that can distinguish between different subtypes of a disease. For example, findings on CT scans of the brains of different types of Alzheimer's patients may be different, even if to human eyes, they look similar. Different types of tumors may have different radiomics even if they look like a mass to human eyes. This could obviate the need for molecular testing and additional steps to identify subtypes of certain diseases. The ML methodology is mature enough to do this consistently and at a high-level. We just need to apply it now to see how far it can go in accurately finding pathology on images using computer vision.

Similar to the single-file, narrow applications of deep learning for reviewing images in various areas of healthcare, we're now ready to use deep learning for pattern recognition in other areas dealing with a single digital file with structured data. Examples of this include diagnosing arrhythmias like atrial fibrillation from a remotely acquired electrocardiogram (ECG), assessing seizure or other brainwave abnormalities from an EEG file, using a facial image acquired by a cell phone to assess distress, using cell phone cameras to analyze urine strips, using a sound file to diagnose the cause of a cough and combining hardware with an AI algorithm to listen to heart and lung sounds or evaluate images of throats or ears.

In all of these cases, the deep learning algorithm evaluates a structured data file and, based on its previous training, identifies and quantifies abnormalities. The deep learning methodology seems to be advanced enough to do this well and consistently. Now, we need to do the real-world studies to confirm its performance and establish the benefits.

A study from Cardiogram has shown that diabetes-induced changes in heart rate variability can be detected using a combination of off-the-shelf wearable devices and deep learning. One algorithm was able to demonstrate 85% accuracy when it came to detecting diabetes from heart rates.[6] Apple watch was used to collect the data that the algorithm used to make this determination.

Some of the more novel ways to collect data and look for disease fall into this bucket. This includes areas such as the analysis of voice, device interactions, activity levels, and data collected from sonar and radar for passive monitoring. Although this category isn't as straightforward as using computer vision on an image or deep learning on an ECG file, it's similar in that data is collected in a digital, structured format and that the AI is charged with detecting abnormal patterns from the file.

What makes it different is that these are novel data sources that haven't historically been used to diagnose or monitor disease. As such, collecting the data, establishing normal and abnormal patterns, and having enough data to train and validate models will take longer. But the deep learning technology to analyze and yield results is already at an acceptable level of performance and consistency. We put this in the medium-term adoption category.

One emerging application is using blood work to spot cancer. Startups like Grails and Freenome are tapping into AI so that they can spot patterns in cell-free biomarkers in blood that could be associated with cancer. The ability of AI to spot patterns is set to lead to more and more new diagnostic methods and the ability to identify risk factors that were previously unknown.[6]

Another big category is 'omics, by which we mean genomics, proteomics, transcriptomics, epi-genomics, metagenomics, and similar biological molecules. Deep learning is well suited for this as we're dealing with large volumes and high dimensions of data.

The issue here is that we're once again learning what's normal or abnormal with these molecules and building large enough databases to study and use them for training and validating models. Even with the power of AI, there are so many permutations and so many relationships between the different biological entities that it will take time to make this a part of the everyday practice of medicine. However, we're already seeing that AI is an incredibly powerful tool for studying these emerging biological entities and understanding how to better diagnose and treat diseases. These applications will be in the long-term adoption category.

The next wave of applications in the clinical setting involves analysis and interaction with written and spoken speech using AI for patient management. This is where NLP and understanding comes in. The issue here is that spoken and written text can produce structured and unstructured digital files. So, if the data file is unstructured (text), the NLP needs to analyze it for meaning of the sequence of the words. For voice, the file is structured but the analysis of the meaning of the interaction is more difficult than identifying abnormal patterns in the quality of the voice.

Prior to the emergence of large language models, the approach to training NLP models was to annotate the concepts that the NLP model would need to abstract from the unstructured data and train it extensively before using it in production. For the most part, the output of these models has been to extract key concepts and data out of the unstructured file to produce a structured file out of that, which could then be analyzed. There are many ways for people to say or write the same concept. In healthcare, no standard has ever been established for how to write a clinical note or to verbally communicate with patients. As such, preparing NLPs for healthcare has meant training the models for different specialties and specific applications, such as radiology vs pathology. This is not nearly as developed as the more straightforward applications of training algorithms to detect specific patterns or abnormalities in structured data files. Here, the emergence of large language models could lead to a breakthrough as the self-supervised training on historic structured and unstructured data without labeling them first could make the development of these models easier. The applications in healthcare may take longer to show results due to the messiness of the data and the issues with the clinical notes, but significant progress in the short-term seems inevitable.

Applications of this on the clinical side of medicine include the analysis of clinical notes for risk assessment, analyzing social determinants of health, carrying out patient triage, diagnosing complex conditions, assessing the complexity of patients, predicting complications or adverse events, providing point of care decision support and matching the best treatments to patient conditions. Other applications of NLP for clinical settings that don't necessarily involve clinical notes but still require the analysis of written language include triage bots, text-based health coaching, and cognitive behavioral therapy (CBT). These applications are poised for a significant jump in performance given the power of large language models. They can be instrumental to bringing the promise of population health to life.

In all of these cases, especially in real-time applications for decision support, NLP has acted as a barrier because it wasn't fully developed for healthcare applications, and the range of data it needs to process from unstructured text and digital audio files has posed a challenge to its capabilities. As such, the current applications are neither scalable nor reproducible. For example, when it's analyzing clinical notes that include the acronym VA, it could mean either Virginia or veteran administration. Also, there's the issue of drift: language evolves quickly, rendering classifiers ineffective.[7]

The launch of new, state-of-the-art NLP solutions are based on decades of deep learning models and use various types of neural networks. Transformer-based deep learning models use self-attention mechanisms like bidirectional encoder representations from transformers (BERT) and generative pre-trained transformer (GPT) and are the current state-of-the-art solutions. They work by splitting training into pre-training and fine-tuning. In the pre-training stage, the models use unsupervised learning to train based on large unlabeled datasets, such as those provided by Wikipedia, PubMed articles, and clinical notes. In fine-tuning, transformer models fine-tune the pre-trained models for specific downstream tasks using supervised learning.[8]

In an article in Health IT News, Yonghui Wu, the NLP director at the University of Florida Health's Clinical and Translational Science Institute, explained, *"The key step is pre-training, where transformer-based models learn task-independent linguistic knowledge from massive text data, which can be applied to solve many downstream NLP tasks. However, to make the transformer-based models effective, they're usually very huge with billions of parameters which can't fit into a single GPU memory, be trained with a single computer node, and apply traditional training strategies. Training these large models requires massive computing power, efficient memory management and advanced distributed training techniques such as data and/or model parallelisms to reduce training time. Therefore, even though there are big transformer models in the general English domain, there are no comparable transformer models in the medical domain."*[8]

The team at UF Health developed GatorTron, the world's largest transformer-based NLP model—with around nine billion parameters—in the medical domain and trained it using more than 197 million notes with more than three billion sentences and 82 billion words of clinical text from UF Health.[7] GatorTron is currently being tested for downstream tasks like relation extraction, named-entity recognition, semantic similarity of text, and answering questions using EHR data in a research setting. The team is working to apply GatorTron to real-world healthcare applications such as patient cohort identification, text de-identification and information extraction.[8]

The GatorTron model was evaluated by UF Health on four key NLP tasks: medical natural language inference, medical Q&As, clinical relation extraction, and clinical concept extraction. For the first two tasks, it was able to achieve a state-of-the-art performance on both of the benchmark datasets. For clinical relation extraction, it outperformed other BERT models that had been pre-trained in clinical or biomedical domains, while for clinical concept extraction, it achieved state-of-the-art performance levels on all three benchmarks.

Seymour Duncker told me, "The emergence of large language models such as BERT is giving rise to the concept of highly generalized foundation models. These multi-billion parameter models are generated through the unsupervised training of general data at a massive scale. The field has been surprised by the ability of these models to generalize and support a wide range of tasks, such as classification, sequence labeling, span relation classification and generation tasks, which previously all required distinct architectures. The practice is quickly shifting to using foundation models that are adapted to specific downstream tasks. There's already significant research underway to expand the power of foundation models to other AI domains such as vision, robotics, reasoning and search as well as multi-modal models that span multiple domains such as vision and NLP. The multi-modal approach is especially exciting for healthcare as healthcare data is intrinsically multimodal (e.g. imaging, EHRs and clinical records) that combine to tell the whole picture. Practical applications of foundation models are already happening. For example, Google Search already depends on the BERT model."

Researchers at the University of Florida indicated that well-trained, large language models could improve downstream NLP tasks through fine-tuning, such as automated summarization, clinical decision support systems, medical chatbots, and medical Q&As. There's clear progress with NLP in healthcare, but the hardware and software requirements, the vast amount of data needed, and the expertise required to pull it all together make for slower progress than we all want. Many of the mentioned applications of NLP with the large language models (LLMs) has been in the long-term adoption bucket but it may be moving into the medium-term adoption timelines.

AI can be super powerful when it comes to evaluating risk because it can tap into data from a variety of sources, including EHRs, lab work, claims data, pharmaceutical data, social determinants of health, and more. This risk assessment could be done using ML-based models. In the past, health systems and providers have used claims-based risk models like the adjusted clinical group (ACG), Center for Medicare and Medicaid Services-Hierarchical Condition Category (CMS-HCC), and Diagnostic Cost Group (DxCG). It is woth remembering the discussion about bias in chapter 2 and how Obermeyer et al realized that using claims data and cost as a proxy for risk introduces a bias toward those who have insurance. These claims-based risk models were built to forecast population risk at an overall level, rather than looking at individuals. This means that while they can predict population health as a whole, they're no good when it comes to predicting individual risk. The good news is that ML can be used to detect risk at a small scale. Before much of this data can be used for the risk prediction model, key concepts will need to be pulled out of the unstructured notes, and that's where NLP comes in.[9]

The processing and understanding of spoken language (rather than written language) leads into some juicy potential use cases like audio patient support applications, analyzing the physician–patient encounter for note generation, auto-documenting diagnoses and medications, auto-entering orders and referrals, responding to patient issues using smart speakers, performing searches, providing information in response to patients' voice inquiries, powering CBT with voice and companion robots. It could also lead to us carrying out patient engagement using automated calls that ask questions and respond to patient inquiries and supporting nurses and physicians through voice commands.

We need machines to understand spoken words and to respond appropriately. This involves NLP and NLU and requires training on specific use cases and using historic files to train these applications. Even though the accuracy has improved in recent years, the level of performance might not be at a level where we can confidently predict brisk adoption. The historic data to train these models isn't plentiful, but companies like Nurance have large libraries of clinical transcriptions from doctors dictating their patient encounter notes. There is emerging evidence that the language used in a doctor–patient conversation is quite different (and more diverse, thus harder) than that in a dictated note. We continue to see errors and frustration on the part of the users and a significant amount of human involvement and oversight is still required. These applications will take longer to integrate into the practice of medicine and population health management.

We've already reviewed some promising progress in this area. For example, we've discussed Saykara, a voice-based medical assistant that listens to encounters, creates notes, and places them in the right place in EHRs. Saykara can also make referrals and prescribe meds.[10] This is an example of

NLP technology that's trained for a specific application in orthopedics and which already has a good level of performance. The key here may be to focus training in one specialty and to make sure that it can understand the language used by specialists. For this use case to become more ubiquitous, similar applications will need to be developed in other specialties.

We also discussed the use of voice at Boston Children's Hospital to allow nurses to ask for key administrative information such as "Who's the charge nurse on 7 South?" and "How many beds are available on 8 East?" Clinicians are finding voice useful for getting information that would otherwise involve picking up the phone, searching through documents or walking down the hall.[11] However, the use of voice in clinical settings isn't widespread. The reasons for this include patient privacy and logistical factors like the need for Wi-Fi access and a secure place to keep devices. We also need to tackle the complex challenge of understanding the human voice in busy clinical settings, especially when physicians are using complex vocabulary.[11] This would be in the medium-term adoption bucket. In addtion to the issues mentioned, the business case may not get priorty over those that immediately increase revenue or lower costs.

We discussed the use of voice at home and the use case of KidsMD, a widely available tool for Amazon Alexa which allows parents to ask questions about common illnesses. They can learn about the symptoms of ear infections, fever, the common cold, and other common ailments and then receive tailored guidance from Boston Children's Hospital. This includes receiving suggestions about whether they need to visit a doctor and how they can care for their child at home.[11] Amazon recently debuted an Alexa feature with Giant Eagle Pharmacy which allows users to track and refill medications by saying, "Alexa, manage my medications."[12, 13]

Analyzing patterns in voice and text has already shown to have powerful diagnostic promise. A team from Stevens Institute of Technology has developed an AI tool that can diagnose Alzheimer's disease with more than 95% accuracy, eliminating the need for expensive scans or in-person testing.[14]

The Stevens Institute of Technology team was able to create an explainable AI tool which taps into convolutional neural networks and attention mechanisms to identify signs of Alzheimer's. As well as accurately spotting the more well-known symptoms, the tool can also spot subtle linguistic patterns that have previously gone undetected. The algorithm was trained on texts that were written by both healthy people and known Alzheimer's patients and which described an image of children stealing cookies from a jar. Each sentence was converted into a unique sequence of numbers (a vector) which represented a specific point in a 512-dimensional space. By doing this, even the most complex sentences could be given a numerical value, which made it much easier for algorithms to analyze the structural and thematic relationships between different sentences. This is an example of the promise of speech in diagnosing disease and, in time, NLP will most likely do much of the heavy lifting in analyzing the written speech.

The second part of the speech analysis would involve using digital biomarkers in voice such as speech patterns, speed, and voice quality to assess mood and cognition. This is similar to the analysis of a digital, structured file where the deep learning applications look for patterns and deviations from the established baseline. This is readier for prime time than the processing and understanding of written or spoken language and is already showing some promising applications.

The Mayo Clinic partnered with Beyond Verbal, a startup from Israel that analyzes acoustic features in people's voices to spot signs of coronary artery disease (CAD). The study found two voice features that were strongly associated with CAD when subjects were describing an emotional experience.[6] This would be in the medium to long-term adoption category since studies will need to be conducted to validate the utility of these digital biomarkers in the everyday practice of medicine.

Another category here is the use of computer vision for the analysis of food for precision nutrition and the assessment of patient movement for remote therapy and fitness. Although the analysis of food for its caloric and nutritional content is not very accurate at this time, it is a computer vision (deep learning) application. As such, given the intense focus on using AI for weight loss and disease management, better datasets to train more accurate models are a focus of intense efforts. This would be in the medium-term bucket. As for the analysis of patient movements and remote therapy, companies like Hinge and Sword have already launched proficient applications. This is mainly computer vision and combined with large language models, it can deliver acceptable performance in analysis and coaching today. Deep learning can also be applied to applications that monitor for patient falls, home movements, and other applications that require the detection of abnormal patterns from digital structured files that are created by cameras, microphones, sonar, and radar. These applications achieve pattern recognition with deep learning and are already being used successfully in other sectors, as well as being rolled out in healthcare.

12.3   Administrative and Operations

As with the clinical applications of AI, the administrative and operational use cases can be categorized depending upon whether they use ML to recognize patterns in data (like claims, appointments, capacity data, and staffing) and whether they require the comprehension of notes and voice records. There seems to be much more in the comprehend category for administration since the administration of healthcare involves creating codes from clinical notes, completing and submitting forms, carrying out capacity management based on when the patient will be discharged, note generation from physician and patient interactions, and responding to physician or nurse commands.

This is a frontier area for AI applications because it doesn't involve direct clinical care and patient health issues, and so a lower level of performance can be tolerated. It's easier to experiment with such applications because even if they only take you 70% of the way there, they're still saving lots of work and showing a return on investment.

At the core of a lot of these applications is a combination of NLP for the abstraction of data from unstructured notes, analysis of that data with ML-trained algorithms and the ability to complete forms using robotic process automation or communicate with ML-trained bots. This allows them to carry out tasks like clinical code generation, prior authorization workflow, claims management, smart scheduling based on patient complexity, staffing based on patient panel complexity, account receivables management, compliance, and more. You can put chatbots that understand patient issues and provide information or guidance in this category. Here, generative AI is relevant since it can automate key administrative tasks (probably where it's the safest to use initially), but only with enough review and supervision. The initial experience with generative AI, such as ChatGPT, shows that it holds potential but can definitely make serious mistakes and "fake" a perfectly reasonable but incorrect response to a request. As such, generative AI's use cases in healthcare are limited for now and anyone who uses it should do so with great caution and plenty of reviews built-in for the output. This is because it was trained on massive datasets from all over the internet and can have serious biases and false assumptions underpinning its output.

Another category here includes the areas we mentioned under the clinical bucket, such as the use of voice for note generation for physicians and nurses, listening to commands and performing tasks, literature search based on user needs and other applications that require pattern detection in the voice file, and understanding the intent behind it, so that the "act" algorithms can respond appropriately or complete an activity. This is an area where an initial set of narrow applications are making their way into healthcare, but they're not fully automated and still require human involvement and therefore the adoption will be slower. We'll see rapid progress in this area with the use of language models for training new algorithms for specific use cases in generating prior authorization letters, creating education material, deploying patient-facing bots, creating documentation, and more.

We've talked about the emerging capabilities of NLP for text and voice and how ML applications for structured data are readier for immediate performance. In the context of automating documentation from voice, the combination of NLP and ML allows solutions to be personalized to each user. They can identify each user's preferences, from the terminology they use to the way they want their documents to be formatted. This will in turn allow them to create more accurate documentation that reflects the user's thought processes and preferences. All of these benefits will be made available in real time, rather than them coming into play hours later in solutions that rely on human labor. Companies like Suki are showing good performance with this type of ambient intelligence technology for clinical encounter documentation, and this category has become a short-term adoption thanks to the LLMs.

Then there are other semi-administrative and semi-clinical applications, such as the collection of data from patients from sensors in hospital or clinics and using ML-trained models to fill out documentation or to perform other tasks. These are more about sensing and acting, which is in the structured data realm, and as we've discussed, ML algorithms are now very proficient at this. The same goes for the analysis of claims data for fraud patterns, using hospital operational data for improving capacity management or ordering supplies, staffing based on predicted demand, benefits design, and similar uses cases.

12.4   Life Sciences

In life sciences, we can expect the same patterns of adoption based on the level of performance of the underlying AI methodology and the data used in each potential application. Applications that use structured pattern detection in data such as genomics, labs, clinical trial structured data, cellular pattern detection, computational biology for conformational analysis and in-silico experimentation in drug discovery, digital biomarker collection in clinical trials, medication adherence using computer vision, synthetic data generation for clinical trials and for developing AI models, digital phenotyping, and analysis of prescription data are more accessible today because they deal with more structured data. ML is being used with large databases such as National Center for Biotechnology Information (NCBI) and similar experimental datasets, and this is central to what life sciences researchers do when finding new, life-saving treatments. AI is already making an impact in public and private sector research in use cases like learning how proteins fold or learning to recognize enhancer regions in genetic sequences.

However, a large number of AI applications in this area also require the analysis of unstructured data and the abstraction of data and concepts or for the analysis and search of existing medical literature and trial data. Across discovery, development, medical affairs, and commercial areas, there's a significant need to analyze unstructured data in medical literature and clinical data.

This has proven to be quite challenging and requires a lot of human input. Based on the historical capabilities of NLP models, the traditional thinking has been that processing the vast amount of medical literature for insights requires humans to pick keywords and findings, differentiate the quality of literature, identify the right insights, and annotate the literature for the AI to extract and aggregate. Here again, that thinking is starting to change as large language models showcase their capabilities. Training the emerging foundation models on large amounts of historic medical literature without having to label them means that these applications may be much closer to real-world use and these massive datasets can now be searched for insights and be better used as part of ongoing research. These models can be fine-tuned for specific applications such as clinical trial patient recruitment, adverse reaction analysis, and commercial activities. This means that many of the applications of AI in life sciences may be on the precipice of delivering much better results than they have to date.

Other applications that can benefit from new foundation models include the analysis of historic discovery experimental data, trial design, site selection, patient recruitment, clinical trial data analysis and submission, safety case analysis and submission, data listening on social media, marketing content analysis and generation, personalization of content based on patient and provider profile, compliance activities, and more.

Ideally, AI software could extract the relevant information from EHRs, compare it with the trials that are currently in progress and then suggest any matching studies. The use of AI to extract information from EHRs and lab images is one of its most widely touted applications in healthcare, but to do this, it will need to take on challenges like disparate data sources and unstructured healthcare data.

Despite the federal government spending more than $28 billion to digitize electronic health records in the last decade, there's no centralized repository or standard format for patient medical data to be stored in. It's difficult for patients to even access their *own* records, especially when they've visited a number of healthcare institutions. The challenge is made more difficult by the fact that different providers use different EHR software to enter their data. When it comes to clinical trials, researchers are still relying on fax requests for patient records. They'll contact each hospital individually, and the facilities will then fax or email the information, often as images (including images of handwritten notes or PDF files). It doesn't take a genius to know that this system is archaic and labor intensive, and it makes it even harder for researchers to collect the data that's needed to determine whether a patient is eligible for a clinical trial.

Another emerging category which can use ML but which still needs significant human input is that of data preparation and annotation. Obviously, this is needed to train the ML algorithms, and labeling data for training purposes has historically been done by humans. It's now hoped that we can use AI models to automate significant amounts of data preparation and annotation. This can save a significant amount of human hours and lead to faster development of the AI models that will assist in life sciences research.

Given the hard work of the bench research to discover new treatments and take them through clinical trials, the impact of AI models that can automate and shorten key parts of this process can't be overstated. As such, with the one-two punch of ML models for structured data and large language models for unstructured data, life science companies can choose where they feel that they can get the highest return on investment in the short and medium-term and start working with some of these AI models. From a methodological standpoint, many of the discussed AI models seem ready for their initial intended use cases.

References

1. Martin, A. (2019). Using AI and NLP to alleviate physician burnout. Machine Learning and AI for Healthcare. A HIMSS Event.
2. Artificial Intelligence is the Future of Growth | Accenture Canada. (2016). Accenture.
3. Mageit, S. (2020, December 8). AstraZeneca partners with Qure.ai for early stage diagnoses of lung. MobiHealthNews. https://www.mobihealthnews.com/news/emea/astrazeneca-partners-qureai-early-stage-diagnoses-lung-cancer
4. University of California San Francisco. (2019, January 3). Artificial Intelligence Can Detect Alzheimer's Disease in Brain Scans Six Years Before a Diagnosis | UC San Francisco. Artificial Intelligence Can Detect Alzheimerâ™s Disease in Brain Scans Six Years Before a Diagnosis | UC San Francisco. https://www.ucsf.edu/news/2019/01/412946/artificial-intelligence-can-detect-alzheimers-disease-brain-scans-six-years
5. Gulshan, V., Peng, L., Coram, M., Stumpe, M. C., Wu, D., Narayanaswamy, A., Venugopalan, S., Widner, K., Madams, T., Cuadros, J., Kim, R., Raman, R., Nelson, P. C., Mega, J. L., & Webster, D. R. (2016). Development and validation of a deep learning algorithm for detection of diabetic retinopathy in retinal fundus photographs. JAMA, 316(22), 2402. https://doi.org/10.1001/jama.2016.17216
6. CB Insights. (2020, June 29). Artificial intelligence trends to watch in 2018. CB Insights Research. https://www.cbinsights.com/research/report/artificial-intelligence-trends-2018/
7. HIMSS. (2019). Building a real-time community insights: engine for a healthcare system: challenges and opportunities. https://365.himss.org/sites/himss365/files/365/handouts/552672016/handout-MLAI13.pdf
8. Siwicki, B. (2021, October 14). NLP powers clinical concept extraction, medical Q&A and more at UF. Healthcare IT News. https://www.healthcareitnews.com/news/nlp-powers-clinical-concept-extraction-medical-qa-and-more-uf-health
9. Advisory Board, Population Health Advisor. (2018). Addressing the needs of your rising-risk patients.
10. Siwicki, B. (2021, January 4). AI-powered mobile assistant eliminates after-hours charting for. Healthcare IT News. https://www.healthcareitnews.com/news/ai-powered-mobile-assistant-eliminates-after-hours-charting-orthoindy-docs
11. Small, C. E., Nigrin, D., Churchwell, K., & Brownstein, J. (2020, October 24). What will health care look like once smart speakers are everywhere?. Harvard Business Review. https://hbr.org/2018/03/what-will-health-care-look-like-once-smart-speakers-are-everywhere

12. Jiang, R. (2019, November 26). Alexa can remind you to take your medication. US About Amazon. https://www.aboutamazon.com/news/devices/new-ways-to-manage-your-medications-at-home-using-alexa

13. Bulik, B. S. (2019). Can you hear me, pharma? Voice-enabled apps are on the rise—and please don't freak out about privacy. Fierce Pharma. https://www.fiercepharma.com/marketing/can-you-hear-me-pharma-voice-enabled-apps-rise-and-please-don-t-freak-out-about-privacy

14. A.I. tool promises faster, more Accurate Alzheimer's Diagnosis. 2020, November 19). Stevens Institute of Technology. https://www.stevens.edu/news/ai-tool-promises-faster-more-accurate-alzheimers-diagnosis

CHAPTER 13

The Business Model for Buyers of Health AI Solutions

WHICH OF THE USE CASES we've mentioned will actually be relevant and of high value to the intended users? The reality is that some of the artificial intelligence (AI) applications we've discussed are nice to have while others are urgently needed. Here, we'll try to examine which of the many use cases will solve problems that need solving right now and will provide immediate boost to the business models of the buyers. Will the quantification of ejection fraction (EF) on echocardiograms using computer vision be something that cardiologists want and that medical centers will spend money on? Will physicians use ambient intelligence to lessen the burden of note-taking, placing orders, and making referrals? Ultimately, AI, as with any other technology, is worth buying if it creates meaningful return on investment (ROI). This can be in the form of saved dollars, better patient outcomes, improved workflow for the staff, and more. As such, the business case analysis for any health AI application is its own bottoms-up analysis. Here, we will examine what use cases may provide strong ROI now and in the medium and long terms. And, we will discuss how to approach this analysis for each use case.

If AI applications can perform to an acceptable level and the various barriers such as data issues, disparate systems, bias, and local training can be solved, what use cases are compelling enough today for immediate adoption? We've reviewed many clinical, administrative, and life science applications, and many are aspirational. But some are ready to solve the myriad of problems

AI Doctor: The Rise of Artificial Intelligence in Healthcare: A Guide for Users, Buyers, Builders, and Investors, First Edition. Ronald M. Razmi.
© 2024 Ronald M. Razmi. Published 2024 by John Wiley & Sons, Inc.

that lead to poor outcomes and high costs. We can assume that like any other technology, there will be short-, medium-, and long-term adoption of the various use cases. Assuming that methodology isn't an issue and the barriers are addressed, which use cases will be in high demand to begin with?

In the healthcare industry, we owe it to our patients to focus on use cases. Even if an algorithm works well for a use case, if its value to clinicians (the user) or health systems and payers (the buyer) isn't compelling, it probably won't see much adoption. An algorithm that expedites care to a stroke patient in a chaotic emergency room (ER) has a good chance of adoption. An algorithm that reads a routine scan and provides some quantification of what the physicians can already estimate won't be in as much demand. There are good reasons for algorithms to parse patient records to look for signs of rare diseases, but there are fewer good reasons for using them to evaluate clinical symptoms. It's cool that AI tools can make diagnoses from scratch, but for most clinical encounters doctors are already pretty good at it.

In a KPMG survey of healthcare executives, 89% of respondents said that AI is already creating efficiencies in their systems, while 91% say that AI is increasing patient access to care.[1] However, many noted that so far it's increased cost rather than lowering it, so the business case for their use is still emerging. However, in a Chartis Group survey of 226 health system executives, there was a strong indication that their investments in AI will significantly increase.[2] The executives were asked about a range of artificial intelligence use cases, including cybersecurity, insurance, surgical robots, clinical trials, triage and a dozen, or so other areas. Chartis encountered widespread agreement that AI could help with all of them.

In the Third Annual Optum Survey on AI in Healthcare, the top three applications that healthcare executives plan to tap AI for include monitoring data from Internet of Things devices (such as wearable technologies), accelerating research for new therapeutic or clinical discoveries, and assigning codes for accurate diagnosis and reimbursement. A majority indicated that their plans to implement AI have accelerated since the pandemic (Figure 13.1).[3]

However, as AI has been rolled out in clinical practice, there have been concerning developments in certain cases and that could have an impact on the pace of adoption. Recent examples that highlight the growing concern over inappropriate and disappointing AI solutions include racial bias in algorithms supporting healthcare decision-making, unexpected poor performance in cancer diagnostic support, and inferior performance when deploying AI solutions in real-world environments.[4]

For AI in healthcare to continue development, we'll require practicality and intelligence from innovators. They'll need to identify gaps in the market instead of just finding new ways to do something that we can already do to a high standard. Doctors can plan tumor therapies and read the latest studies themselves. They could choose the best possible patients for the recently

Top 3 priorities for AI deployment, by sector

	Hospitals	Health plans	Life sciences	Employers
Priority 1	Improve reimbursement coding 45%	Improve reimbursement coding 40%	Accelerate research 47%	Monitor IoT data 47%
Priority 2	Monitor IoT data 38%	Automate administrative processes 40%	Identify patients for trials 44%	Accelerate research 45%
Priority 3	Accelerate research 36%	Detect fraud, waste and abuse 39%	Enable personalized communications 39%	Enable personalized communications/ automate administrative processes 35% each

FIGURE 13.1   Administrative Use Cases are High Priority for Buyers of Health AI Solutions *(source: Adapted from[3])*

approved expensive immunotherapy.[5] But, helping them document patient encounters, better coding for submitting charges, better patient triage that improves the mix of patients in their offices are all use cases that they need now (Figure 13.2).

Professor Szolovits of MIT indicated that many of the applications in early use focus on diagnostics because that data is easier to get, cleaner to prepare for analysis and the outputs are easier to integrate into existing workflows. Others indicated that the most important long-term benefits will be the

Where AI is already delivering value in hospitals?

AI/ML use cases being pilot tested or in production

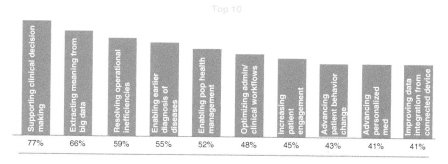

FIGURE 13.2   *(source: Adapted from[6])*

discovery of new therapies and matching those therapies with individuals. This has a lot of us excited, but progress has been slow and the underlying AI methodologies are still works in progress.

When we discussed the barriers to the adoption of AI, we discussed physician and health system economics. This will have a lot to do with the demand for such technologies. All things being equal, the applications that improve physician and health system economics will see greater demand. The applications that have a detrimental impact on economics, even if they're ready for immediate use, will be de-prioritized. As such, if the income of radiologists is threatened by some of the deep learning applications in that area, their adoption will be slower than expected (if not never!) However, if an application of AI, such as improving the accuracy and speed of performing colonoscopies, will result in more procedures, it will see faster adoption.

The issue of reimbursement by payers is an important factor that should be discussed. Is it possible that if radiologists use AI to read scans, they'll receive less reimbursement? Or to approach this from the other angle, if payers are reimbursing for the use of AI, will they pay radiologists less as a result?

My discussions with insurance executives have shown that they don't think this is likely. If the use of these technologies will improve patient outcomes and lead to fewer errors, there are benefits to them that will motivate executives to pay for them in addition to radiologists' reading fees. It may become part of the technical fee, which is separate from the reading fee. An analogy here is that cab drivers don't get paid less if their car has better technologies like navigation or cruise control that help them to drive better and safer.

It's important to mention that not all innovations that improve care are reimbursed. If certain AI technologies result in improved efficiency and productivity, these benefits will accrue to the medical centers and payers won't pay for those technologies. Payers usually require prospective trials with outcomes as endpoints before reimbursing. An example of this is a pill that's inserted with a chip to help with adherence, which is yet to receive reimbursement. Likewise, inhalers with sensor technologies haven't shown outcome improvement and have therefore not been considered for reimbursement. Value is measured in patient outcomes, not proxy endpoints such as the number of pills taken or the frequency of usage for inhalers.

In this section, we'll examine those use cases that have the highest demand and which will see the fastest uptake (Figure 13.3).

13.1   Clinical Care

There are immediate use cases for deep learning algorithms for the initial examination of radiology images for acute conditions that require immediate intervention for optimal medical outcomes such as pulmonary embolus or

Key stakeholders are indicating that they see immediate benefits for AI technologies and they will buy or pay for these benefits

Clinicians

- Improve accuracy in reading radiology scans
- Speed up current clinical workflows
- Novel care pathways

Medical centers

- Improve productivity and efficiency,
- Reducing medical errors
- Cost reduction and improved margins

Health plans

- Improving quality of care and patient outcomes
- Reduction of erroneous diagnoses
- Accelerating patient management

FIGURE 13.3   *(source: Original Research)*

pneumothorax. These algorithms can read scans before a radiologist does, flag those that show abnormalities and prioritize them for the radiologist to expedite care. This is an example of a clear-cut use case that improves outcomes, streamlines clinical workflows, improves operations, and saves money.

The use case here is very strong as the technology will serve as an immediate screener for these issues and can alert the medical team to immediately check the images to confirm the presence of abnormalities and intervene in a timely manner.[7] In specialties such as oncology, where radiology findings can be subtle and slow growing, AI can be a game changer in detecting disease earlier, monitoring its change over time and identifying characteristics that point toward a diagnosis or subtype of cancer. One important caveat here is that the workflows need to be such that the radiologists don't do anything extra and can benefit from the AI pre-read by having their scans prioritized automatically with a mark next to the ones that have already been reviewed by the AI algorithm.

These are examples of the compelling use cases that will be able to gain traction in the clinical setting and provide value in the short term. In fact, the acute setting application of the viz.ai system that reviews head computed tomography (CTs) for strokes and alerts the medical team is one of the first ones to receive a code and reimbursement. This means that the regulatory and reimbursement authorities see immediate value in this type of application. Not all use cases are as compelling or have an immediate return on investment. For the buyers here, the improved patient outcomes that result in reimbursement, better workflows that result in clinical team satisfaction, and improved operations in their hospitals make for a very strong business case.

Radiologists are under increasing pressure to read more scans, and AI could make them faster and more efficient. In my discussions with health system executives, they indicated that radiology is one of the most lucrative business lines in the health system and that any tool that improves clinical quality will be a differentiator against local competitors. This means more patients and more dollars for the health system: strong business case indeed! Also, if radiologists come to view these tools as necessary to their job, health system executives won't wait for reimbursement as they view radiologists' satisfaction and efficiency as very important to overall radiology business lines. Historically, for most add-on software that's used for clinical quality improvement, the business case hinges on an increased volume of cases and differentiation against local competitors.

Overall, there's a strong business case in radiology. Given the increasing number of scans and the shortage of radiologists in many countries, coupled with the maturity of deep learning and single, digital structured data files in radiology, it's poised to be the initial frontier for AI in clinical care.[8] The business case to acquire such technologies in radiology doesn't hinge on reimbursement by insurance companies, and improving the workflow of the radiologists and worklist triage of cases will have immediate benefits for everyone involved.

There are other applications, such as facial recognition technology to use in the ER for patient triage, that are similar to the radiology applications that can help prioritize patients with critical issues. These are on the radar but their deployment involves significantly more risk and is still in the experimental stage. The intersection of AI and human decision-making (datasets that capture human decision-making and skill sets) will be a long-term application due to the technical issues mentioned before and still unclear ROI for users and buyers. One example of this is decision support systems that help clinicians to risk stratify patients in the ER and to avoid over- or under-ordering tests.

We've already discussed the use of AI as an autonomous technology for the widespread screening of diabetic retinopathy. Well, diabetes is a major issue that's exploded over the last few decades. Screening for diabetic retinopathy usually isn't done by primary care physicians and there aren't enough ophthalmologists to do it on a routine basis. Given that the FDA approved this application as an autonomous technology with no physician supervision, it's a great initial clinical application of AI. Interestingly, with more screening and identification of cases that will need to be seen by ophthalmologists for management, we actually increase the number of patients that they'll see. So much for "replacing" them!

In the acute care setting, we talked about the application of AI for better managing sepsis in the hospital. Sepsis is a major issue affecting patient outcomes, hospital quality metrics, and their bottom lines. It leads to longer hospital stays and higher costs that can turn a profitable hospital visit into a nonprofitable one. That means that all of the incentives are aligned to use AI to better manage sepsis. This is a great example of improved patient outcomes, decision support for clinicians and economic benefits for institutions. This trifecta leads to a strong business case.[9]

The demonstrated benefits of AI for the management of sepsis highlight one of the most promising short-term clinical use cases for AI: the management of critical patients. First, diagnostics and treatment for these patients are overly challenging and need vast expertise. If AI can take over some of these challenging steps, they'll be standardized and improved. Second, a humongous amount of data is gathered when treating critically ill patients. Third, outcome measures in critical medicine are truly black and white. In many AI projects, the study group can't even agree on the study feature, such as whether a spot on a lung x-ray scan is a tumor, infection, or an artifact. Teaching AI with debatable data measures and features will rarely, if ever, lead to success. In critical medicine, death or bleeding in the brain on a computed tomography scan is rather unambiguous.[9] Fourth, imaging studies of critically ill patients are often associated with outcome. Therefore, these imaging studies consist of highly meaningful and important pixel data, which is the best petrol for AI engines.

In these types of patients, creating and running real-time risk algorithms that are constantly updated based on clinical data will be important as they monitor and identify those that are about to experience complications and allow the medical team to take proactive actions to address the drivers of those risks before those patients experience a deterioration in their condition. At Oschner, AI was able to predict patient deterioration before it happened, with 85–90% accuracy when predicting critical codes. This led to a reduction of 40–45% of codes by intervening before they happened. They were also able to reduce the incidence of C. Diff infections by 50% by changing the drug regimen after AI predicted its likely occurrence.[5] The inpatient decision support business cases are quite strong. Given the Diagnosis-related Group (DRG) reimbursement for inpatient visits, shorter length of stay and use of less resources to resolve the issue means dollars flowing to the bottom line of the hospital.

Some of the applications that are gaining traction in clinical settings such as the Mayo Clinic are the diagnosis of intermittent A Fib from remote-acquired electrocardiogram (ECG) and determining genetic components of tumors without using biopsies by looking at radiology features (radiomics).[10] The same applies to using remote monitoring data and algorithms to manage hypertension, diabetes, and other chronic diseases. One theme here is that algorithms developed on machine-generated data like ECG machines are better than those developed on human-generated data since they're more standardized and structured. This goes back to our earlier discussion about the fact that deep learning models using structured data are readier for primetime than the use of natural language processing (NLP) on non-standardized and nonstructured data, and thus the initial demand by the buyers will be for the use cases that are at an acceptable level of performance.

The issue here is that receiving data from outside the clinical setting, combining it with electronic health record (EHR) data, figuring out what it means, and then formulating a plan of action is currently aspirational. These use cases are in the medium- to long-term adoption bucket because our current healthcare system doesn't have the pipelines to make this work. It's not just the data issues. Clinicians and care teams are already burned out and overwhelmed, and adding to their to-do list just makes things even more difficult for them. Of course, AI solutions can do some of the heavy lifting, such as analyzing the data and figuring out what needs to be done. That will become the new reality when the unified patient record issue has been addressed and we've built strong data pipelines to combine clinical data with remotely collected data. Also, reimbursement for these types of activities is not well-established yet. True, value-based care is a focus for payers but providers have yet to find their footing in this area. As such, although they may represent the future of healthcare, the business case for their adoption is not so strong today.

These use cases can be the catalyst for health systems and providers to finally manage high-risk patients outside of the clinical setting. If the world moves toward value-based care, the economic value of using algorithms to facilitate this move could be clearer to providers. At Oschner, they used patient data to identify issues with members, and when those members called in for a service call, those issues were automatically flagged and the rep transferred them to nurses to help them while they were on the phone.[5] At Cambia Health, a salient use case for AI is for care managers to become more efficient. The AI algorithm analyzes claims history plus additional data such as social determinants of health and evaluates risk, identifies the drivers of risk, matches the patient to a care manager with the right skillset, predicts clinical deterioration, and allows nurses to intervene before the process starts.[11]

Patient communication material can be created using generative AI, and it can be personalized if there's access to enough patient data. We've already discussed applications for automated interactions with patients outside of the clinical setting, such as the one from MyndYou which calls patients and asks about their clinical and social issues, and then alerts the care team if any problems are identified. This type of intelligent and automated patient engagement can help care teams to scale up and increase the number of patients they manage, as well as allowing them to manage them more effectively. Also, the more personalized plans that can be created using generative AI will improve the chance of patient adherence. This use case is here and now and is already adding value in patient management. The business case for this is strong if used with certain types of patients to avoid readmission or to generate revenues with the new chronic care management codes. Also, if this type of technology is used in engaging patients about their preventive or follow-up procedures, it can generate revenue for the health system in fee-for-service contracts.

As reimbursement to providers becomes more value based, AI can be their secret weapon to perform well on those contracts. AI's ability to incorporate

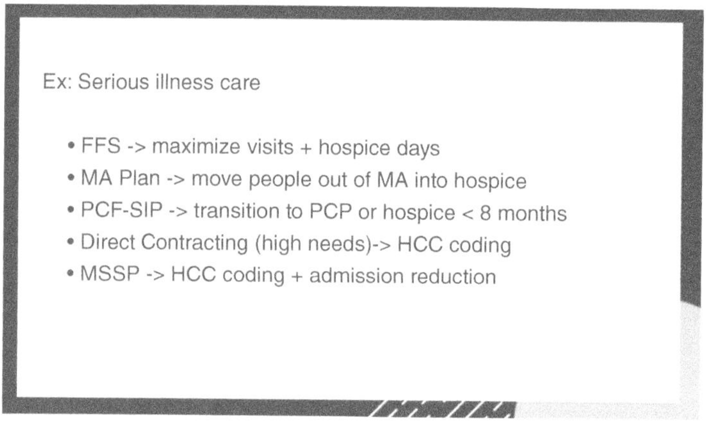

Ex: Serious illness care

- FFS -> maximize visits + hospice days
- MA Plan -> move people out of MA into hospice
- PCF-SIP -> transition to PCP or hospice < 8 months
- Direct Contracting (high needs)-> HCC coding
- MSSP -> HCC coding + admission reduction

FIGURE 13.4   AI can Assist with Choosing the Best Next Step Based on the Patient's Insurance Type *(source: Adapted from[12])*

different data to create better risk models, personalize recommendations for high-risk patients, communicate with patients, generate educational content, and learn from its performance over time makes it an ideal tool for value-based contracts. For example, for serious illness care, you can develop models that help you maximize your financial performance (Figure 13.4) As you can see, depending on whether the patient is in a Fee-for-Service plan, a Medicare Advantage plan, or a Shared Saving plan, your AI models can help you choose the right course of action to optimize your financial performance.

Chatbots represent a here and now use case for AI in healthcare. The initial wave of these applications with Babylon, Ada, and Buoy has shown promise at introducing intelligence into the patient's decision on where to get care and handling basic follow-up issues that don't need human intervention. This technology isn't without its critics. Babylon faced a huge backlash after the company announced that its triage chatbot could outperform new doctors in a simulation of the MRCGP exam. Martin Marshall, the vice chair of the Royal College of General Practitioners, released a statement to say, "The potential of technology to support doctors to deliver the best possible patient care is fantastic, but at the end of the day, computers are computers, and GPs are highly trained medical professionals. The two can't be compared and the former may support but will never replace the latter. Much of what GPs do is based on a trusting relationship between a patient and a doctor, and research has shown GPs have a 'gut feeling' when they just know something is wrong with a patient."[9] The fact Babylon became one of the most high-profile failures in digital health should serve as a cautionary tale for any technology company that assumes early traction will necessarily translate into eventual success.

At the moment, most triage chatbots are directing people to medical professionals, rather than totally replacing them. Without chatbots, patients without any medical expertise are making those decisions on their own. Most current chatbots aren't AI-based and use a conditional logic that's pre-programmed. However, with the emergence of large language models, training new chatbots on clinical literature could mean that AI-powered chatbots will be in use sooner than we thought. This will be especially true if the chatbots or AI voice interactions are offered by the health systems that have the patient data. The quality of the interactions and recommendations by AI systems will be far higher if they're based on patients' conditions and current treatments. The business case here would be to offer support to patients in their decision-making process in their care journey. This will most likely result in patients choosing the center offering this as their destination for care, hence higher volumes and revenues.

The fact that these technologies aren't perfect and can't handle every case shouldn't keep us from using them in the large number of cases where they can actually add significant value. We discussed their use cases with COVID and how Providence Health successfully used them to triage patients to the right care setting at a time when healthcare resources were stretched and keeping healthier patients out of ERs was critical.[11]

According to an Accenture survey, more than 75% of US consumers were willing to use AI-based tools to better manage their health.[13] This includes a willingness to share their data from wearables, mobile apps, and other sources. This shows that as the healthcare system tries to incorporate AI in the provision of care and population health management, and an increasing number of tools become available for consumers to manage their own health, the public is mostly open to using them.

Other use cases that are seeing some initial traction and demand from buyers include the use of AI in the genetic analysis of tumors and treatment matching, the diagnosis of rare diseases, passive monitoring of patients in in-patient settings with alerts for nurses, virtual assistants for nurses, the use of AI with robotics in the surgical suite, chatbots for mental health issues, assistance with pathology workflows, and AI-enabled therapy for musculo-skeletal issues. Each of these use cases can have immediate benefits to the users, and while they may or may not get reimbursement in the short term, their implementation doesn't face huge barriers in terms of data or workflows. However, the economic benefits of the use case and the implementation issues aren't as clear cut as the use cases in radiology or critical patient risk analysis. I put these in the medium-term adoption category. This is because it is not clear yet if the dollars required to purchase and implement them will immediately translate into new revenues, cost savings, or significant improvement of workflows. They very well might, but the evidence for the magnitude of their impact is still emerging.

There are, of course, many aspirational cases that are in development, and we're anxiously waiting to see them validated in trials and launched into the practice of medicine. These include use cases like the collection of novel digital biomarkers for diseases like multiple sclerosis and Alzheimer's, real-time decision support for chronic diseases based on device data, the use of novel biomarkers in radiology or genetics for sub-typing psychiatric illnesses, the recognition and management of chronic pain using mobile devices and immersive technologies, remote examination of patients with AI-powered devices, diagnosis of the causes of respiratory issues from the characteristics of coughs, analyzing passive monitoring data from home and providing digital coaching, and optimizing staffing levels and patient scheduling based on risk levels and disease severity. Here, the technological issues need more work, use cases and the required evidence need to be further developed and economic impact needs to be better quantified.

13.2   Administrative and Operations

Health systems are already experimenting with low-risk applications of AI in areas like hospital operations management, scheduling, claims processing, prior authorization, accounts receivable management, coding, cybersecurity, fraud detection, and other back office use cases. Certain productivity applications such as voice recognition to help with physician note generation and workflow are seeing adoption across the care delivery spectrum.

In the Chartis Group survey of health executives' attitudes toward AI that we mentioned earlier, there was a notable difference between use cases that received the highest scores—operational use cases such as insurance and cybersecurity—and clinical interventions like care planning, care triage, and diagnosis, which came in much lower.[2] This indicates that the administrative and workflow use cases will be at the frontier of AI's adoption in healthcare (Figure 13.5). There's great optimism about the ability of AI-based tools and systems to improve the overall business model for health systems. This is now truer than ever due to the promise of generative AI, which is particularly well-suited for many administrative use cases such as generating prior authorization letters, creating codes based on physician notes, generating referrals to specialists, creating patient communication material, and more. As such, many are now doing live installations of AI-based tools that predict insurance denials for claims that will allow them to prevent denials and ensure reimbursement. The business case here is quite strong: automation of manual activities for the care team or the administrative staff and higher chance of speedy payment by payers.

At the Health Evolution Summit in 2020, it was revealed that the top two applications of AI at the Mayo Clinic are voice recognition for transcribing physician notes and computer-assisted coding.[10] This is interesting given the fact that the Mayo Clinic is one of the most respected medical

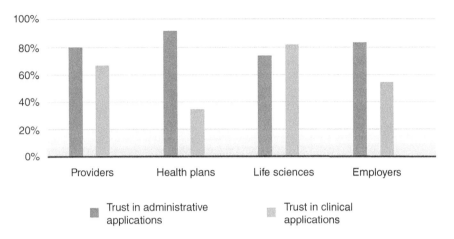

FIGURE 13.5   Which AI Applications the Healthcare Stakeholders Trust Most
(source: Adapted from[14])

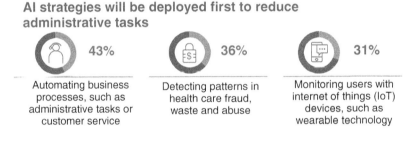

FIGURE 13.6   *(source: Adapted from[14])*

institutions in the world. The assumption would be that some of the clinical use cases would be their initial foray. But, as we discussed before, some of these administrative and workflow applications can generate immediate ROI and present less risk to patients and physicians. Also, the issues of overworked physicians and burnout are real, so these use cases are relevant to keeping physicians sane and sharp. Figure 13.6 shows that amongst providers and payers, there's currently more trust in the administrative applications of AI.

There are many possible explanations for the trust gap that we see between using AI for administration and using it within the clinic. We've long known that administrative functions are the ideal place for AI to launch given the less complex nature of the data and the lower risk. As trust in AI increases, more investments will be made and we'll start to see the clinical validation that we need to convince clinical stakeholders of AI's future role. In the meantime, we can expect to see a short-term boost in clinical operations and the better use of staff and resources through better billing, scheduling, and revenue cycle management.

Some of the lower risk use cases that will see earlier adoption by health systems and payers include customer service and patient navigation. This is in line with the premise of lower risk applications being where these entities will dip their toes into AI. For example, self-service platforms for patient flow and navigation can improve the revenue mix for health systems, along with their margins.

As the number of AI use cases increases and they improve in quality and lower in cost, some of these benefits will also accrue to the health plans and they'll be more willing to reimburse for their adoption. Companies like Qventus and LeanTaas are tapping into predictive algorithms so that health systems can better optimize labor, supplies, and throughput at hospitals. These applications will be at the frontier of AI adoption by health systems and providers as they promise to deliver an immediate ROI and improve workflows (rather than create more work).

As is shown by the surveys, helping provider workflows by minimizing data entry and automating their documentation, order entry, referral generation, and coding will be amongst the initial use cases that will see the most rapid adoption. These are lower risk applications with significant benefits to providers so the business case is easy to make. AI-enabled speech recognition alleviates physician burnout by automating the creation of accurate clinical documentation in acute care, ambulatory care, and post-acute settings across both physical and virtual encounters. The business case here is quite strong given the improvement in staff satisfaction and potential for better coding and charge capture (Figure 13.7).

Current AI opportunities in health care

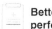 **Better performance**

- Clinical documentation
- Coding
- Payment integrity
- Prior authorization

 Better outcomes

- Early diagnosis and treatment
- Prescription benefit management
- Risk adjustment
- Simplified population analysis

 Better experience

- Call centers
- Care coordination
- Employee benefits

FIGURE 13.7   *(source: Adapted from[9])*

It is important to keep in mind that the adoption rate will be different for larger health systems, smaller hospitals, and independent provider groups. Health systems or larger hospitals might invest in AI solutions to see benefits to clinician workflows, operational efficiencies, and patient outcomes, but the cost will be a factor for physician offices, independent outpatient surgical centers, and smaller hospitals.

One of the most promising business cases for AI for health insurance companies is population health management, and payers are pushing health systems to use the best technologies to successfully approach population health. This could help payers given the expected lower cost of care when it is done proactively and preventively. Value-based payment is continuing to be rolled out, and AI could be one of the enablers of value-based care. Also, AI is perfectly suited for the task of reviewing and processing the millions of claims that are filed each day, and so we shouldn't be surprised that health plans report being the furthest along when it comes to AI adoption. Payers will carry out health economics assessments to assess the impact on quality and overall cost of care and will start reimbursing for those that can show results in one or both of these areas.

To carry out population health management, we need to be able to gather large amounts of data about patients' day-to-day behavior. The good news is that healthcare consumers are getting better at using wearable devices, virtual assistants, and smartphone apps to monitor and report their health information. Human activity is one of the largest sources of healthcare data, and AI can be used to extract and segment it before carrying out data analysis to help us create community-based health strategies. We could also use this data analysis to research the impact that social determinants of health have on overall population health.

Maintaining the security of patients' personal health information will be an even more pressing consideration for healthcare organizations as the quantity of data increases. Healthcare breaches are already estimated to cost organizations $429 per patient record, according to an IBM report.[15] This same study projects that AI could save $2 billion each year by reducing health record breaches through its ability to detect abnormal interactions with patient data. As regulators increase scrutiny of AI security, it's possible that innovations in data management could safeguard proprietary information. That's another lower risk application of AI that could gain traction with providers and payers in the short term.

Insurance companies seem poised to reap significant benefits in various areas, such as benefits design, customer service, care management, and fraud detection. This mix of applications relies on machine learning and NLP to deliver results, and most are already showing acceptable performance. Of course, applications that rely on NLP as opposed to machine-generated structured data might not be showing the level of performance that some would like to see before using them. However, large language models promise a significant jump in performance for these applications and could expedite their adoption. These applications mean immediate benefits to the payer's bottom line and don't represent high-risk use cases. As such, they're examples of strong business cases for buyers to immediately proceed with initial projects.

13.3 Life Sciences

Using AI in discovery in medical science is currently a key focus area, and there's been robust demand from life science companies. It looks like the promise of more drugs and faster timelines is too good to resist for these companies. However, given the level of expertise required, most are partnering with AI discovery companies. This usually means that the AI company gets access to the historical experiment data of the biopharma company and uses that to find promising molecules or targets. We already discussed how much of that data isn't really usable, and from a methodological point of view, there are a number of barriers to overcome in the short term. However, there's enough usable data involved in the process that these companies are pushing ahead to find the next wave of drugs using AI.

A key area for drug discovery is the analysis of the medical literature and data from previous experiments. In both of these cases, we need to analyze unstructured and specialized data. Extracting insights from medical literature is an area where large language models have led to significant progress. Using normal language, researchers can ask questions about previous learnings about a topic in clinical literature. This can accelerate the process of synthesizing medical literature to help researchers in every therapeutic area. Similarly, much of the data from previous experiments could be made more accessible for research by using large language models to train on that data. That means the insights from previous experiments could soon become far more available to researchers.

We've already discussed how machine learning could power human-in-the-loop data annotation and labeling services. These are some of the most time-consuming and tedious aspects of carrying out research at life sciences companies. This has resulted in less than half the time being required to catalogue samples. There's already evidence of demand from life science companies in this area. The business case for all of this is fairly strong but the benefits are not immediate. Although these use cases will improve R&D and will lead to better pipelines and faster development, it will still be years before the ROI will be realized. As such, everyone is not diving in head first. Many life science companies are monitoring the space and waiting for the right time to invest.

Those biopharma companies that don't want to be left behind and are taking tangible steps to invest in these capabilities. aren't necessarily developing in-house capabilities to do this on their own. Most are choosing partnership as their path into AI, but are not yet betting the house on it. Most will wait until we see a few compounds successfully come out of the billions of dollars that have been invested so far.

Most biopharma companies see the future of their industry in personalized diagnostics or treatments. As such, they're increasingly engaging in R&D efforts that involve large and multidimensional data, such as genomics, proteomics, clinical data, and behavioral data. This is where AI is no longer a luxury and you either need to build, buy, or partner for these capabilities. Most are partnering at the moment, but it's entirely possible that they'll start bringing some of these capabilities in-house since it will become core to their businesses. Roche's acquisition of Flatiron Health is an example of that. Flatiron possessed a large set of oncology data and had the capabilities to mine and analyze that data.

The various applications of AI in clinical development, such as protocol design, site selection, patient recruitment, and trial management, are now gaining traction. It's clear that most life science companies are taking tangible steps to incorporate some of these capabilities into their upcoming trials or even developing groups in-house that function as experts for the various business units who'd like to take advantage of these emerging technologies. I've advised many of these companies over the years and have seen their desire to use AI in their clinical development programs, but many of them don't know where to start or they're not sold that AI is fully ready.

In many ways, it isn't. They can be useful when there's complete and mostly structured data that can be used by AI models to facilitate some of these steps. However, the real barriers to most of these applications are the fragmented state of data, unstructured and messy data in EHR and clinical trial systems that they can't access, and the limitations of NLP technology. Fortunately, this last issue is becoming less of a barrier with the promise of large language models and their ability to synthesize insights from historic unstructured data. This means that the next generation of models trained by life science companies could be more effective at identifying patients for clinical trials if they have access to EHRs and other clinical data. Faster design of clinical trials or patient recruitment for them means getting drugs to the market faster and reaping billions of dollars in rewards. Given the capabilities of large language models, the business case for using them is becoming stronger.

Also, the use of machine learning techniques for computational biology (e.g. in silico experimentation and conformational analysis) allows us to develop new insights into the behaviors and physical properties of molecules before we carry out in vitro and in vivo testing. The same is true of cellular analysis using computer vision for the preclinical analysis of promising compounds. These applications are here and now and the only steps that need to be taken are to prepare the data (for example, digitizing the cellular slides) and re-designing research workflows around their capabilities. Given the rapid progress in this space, initial investments in these capabilities present a strong business case for R&D groups in pharma, but the ROI will take time to realize.

In life sciences research and development, we also see biopharma companies pursuing novel disease biomarkers, such as those that can be spotted with computer vision on scans. This seems to be an area where tangible steps are being taken by companies developing solutions for multiple sclerosis and dementia, where subtle radiological findings are often present years before the disease is diagnosed. The evidence of disease progression or regression on radiological scans can be very subtle and not obviously visible to the human eye, which makes it perfect for computer vision. For life science companies, this is an excellent way to show the benefits of their treatments or to identify patients that are advancing in their disease in subtle ways and need more intensive therapy. This can expedite drug approval or improve reimbursement and makes for a strong business case to engage in them.

The use of digital biomarkers such as activity levels, interaction with devices, facial analysis, sleep parameters, and voice features make for excellent use cases and are already being pursued by life science companies. They add another layer of data to substantiate the case for their products with regulators and payers. However, these digital biomarkers aren't fully established in most diseases, and their association with a disease and their value has to be validated before they're fully accepted by the medical community. As such, I'd put this category in the medium-term adoption bucket with still unclear ROI.

Treatment adherence is in the short-term adoption bucket. This is where AI technology such as computer vision can verify that patients are adhering to their treatments in a trial. Companies like cure.ai are already working with pharma companies to improve drug adherence in clinical trials. The business case for monitoring adherence in clinical trials is quite strong and represents a "here and now" investment for life science companies. Also, the use of chatbots to support patients during trials is a prime use case that may gain momentum with the emergence of large language models that allow for better and faster training of these bots on historic medical literature and clinical data. The use of synthetic data for conducting experiments and doing trials is another application that shows promise. Synthetic data can help to develop AI models for research use cases and lead to faster clinical trials. The business case here will be strong once the regulatory bodies like the FDA begin to accept synthetic data for approvals.

Many of the use cases in medical affairs and commercial areas involve NLP and AI-enabled RPA. This involves collecting data and organizing it for submissions, completing forms, social media listening, content analysis, content generation, compliance automation, content personalization, audience targeting, and more. Many of these use cases will see faster progress and adoption with the use of generative AI. LLMs can allow medical affairs and commercial teams to glean insights from that data and generate outputs for patients and providers. There are use cases where AI can introduce intelligent automation, and with human review of generative AI's output, they're prime for immediate investment by life science buyers.

13.4   Guide for Buyer Assessment of Health AI Solutions

Now that we've covered many applications around clinical, administrative, and life science use cases and discussed whether their business case for buyers is strong or not, we need to lay out a simple but practical approach for decision-making. There are many shiny objects out there and it can be daunting to decide which ones make the cut for your technology budget in the near future. That's why I recommend using a scorecard-based approach, where the use cases with the highest impact become the top ones to go shopping for solutions. You can also use a score-card approach for choosing the right companies.

Assessing the use case:

- How large is the impact of the targeted problem on patient outcomes, staff workflows, or corporate profits?
- How urgent is the need to address this problem?
- Will the purchase of this type of AI solution have an impact on the intended results within 12–18 months?
- How strong is the evidence for the readiness of this type of AI solution for the intended use case?
- Does this type of AI solution require regulatory approval? If so, has it been obtained?
- Is there insurance reimbursement for this type of AI solution? If not, how will its economic benefits be assessed?
- What's the total dollar cost of acquisition of this type of AI technology? This includes licensing, implementation, training, maintenance, and any other costs.
- Does the organization have the necessary staffing to fully implement and support the solution?
- Does the organization have the necessary governance in place to provide ongoing monitoring of the performance of this type of AI solution?

- How will the ongoing benefits be assessed and quantified?
- Are the potential users aware of any changes to their workflows and have they definitely confirmed that they'll embrace those changes?

Assessing the companies:

- How long has the company been providing its AI solution?
- How many customers are currently using it?
- What's the customer feedback to date?
- What makes their particular solution unique and differentiated from other companies providing similar solutions?
- How does the company provide ongoing monitoring and improvement of the performance of their AI solution?
- What adjacent needs does the company address now or plan to address in the future? Choosing companies with a product roadmap that matches the organizations' other unmet needs will avoid having to find new vendors for each need.

References

1. Kent, J. (2020). 53% of Execs Say Healthcare Leads Artificial Intelligence Adoption. Health IT Analytics. https://healthitanalytics.com/news/53-of-execs-say-healthcare-leads-artificial-intelligence-adoption?fbclid=IwAR2k00duF6UldzXfSJMSoKjbBtCyqYbIdHy37Hhp0M7zMh1KoJSe3WWy0cU
2. Miliard, M. (2021, July 23). 68% of health system execs plan deeper AI investments to meet. Healthcare IT News. https://www.healthcareitnews.com/news/68-health-system-execs-plan-deeper-ai-investments-meet-strategic-goals
3. Third Annual Optum Survey - AI in Health Care. (2020). Optum. https://www.optum.com/business/insights/page.hub.2020-ai-survey.html
4. Siwicki, B. (2021, September 1). Can healthcare avoid another AI winter? Healthcare IT News. https://www.healthcareitnews.com/news/can-healthcare-avoid-another-ai-winter
5. CEO insights: realities of leading an AI-enabled organization. (2020, October 25). [Presentation]. Health Evolution Summit, Digital.
6. Sullivan, T. (2019, February 10). 3 charts show where artificial intelligence is making an impact in healthcare right now. Healthcare IT News. https://www.healthcareitnews.com/news/3-charts-show-where-artificial-intelligence-making-impact-healthcare-right-now
7. Ventech Solutions and MedCity News. (2019, May 16). Aidoc gets FDA nod for AI pulmonary embolism screening tool. MedCity News. https://medcitynews.com/2019/05/aidoc-gets-fda-nod-for-ai-pulmonary-embolism-screening-tool/

8. Monegain, B. (2018, November 1). Where hospitals plan big AI deployments: diagnostic imaging. Healthcare IT News. https://www.healthcareitnews.com/news/where-hospitals-plan-big-ai-deployments-diagnostic-imaging

9. von Grätz, P. G., Lovett, L., Postelnicu, L., Rouger, M. (2018). Clinical Artificial Intelligence. [E-book]. HIMSS. https://pages.himss.org/HIMSSInsights2.html

10. AI insights: from new business models to patient care. (2020, October 25). [Presentation]. Health Evolution Summit, Digital.

11. Business use cases: progressive AI/ML initiatives to drive efficiencies. (2020, October 25). [Presentation]. Health Evolution Summit, Digital.

12. Perez, S. (2021, December 13). Machine Learning & AI for Healthcare. HIMSS. https://www.himss.org/event-machine-learning-ai-healthcare

13. Wilson, J., & Daugherty, P. (2018, March 27). AI will change health care jobs for the better. Harvard Business Review. https://hbr.org/2018/03/ai-will-change-health-care-jobs-for-the-better

14. UnitedHealth Group. (2020, February 24). OptumIQ survey on artificial intelligence reveals confidence and growth opportunities. https://www.unitedhealthgroup.com/newsroom/posts/2019-10-08-optumiq-survey.html

15. IBM. (2020). Cost of a Data Breach Report 2020. IBM. https://www.ibm.com/account/reg/us-en/signup?formid=urx-46542

CHAPTER 14

How to Build and Invest in the Best Health AI Companies

IF THE METHODOLOGY WORKS and the customers have a need for an artificial intelligence (AI) technology, then all systems should go for AI in healthcare, right? Well, not quite! Those two requirements are a great place to start and mean that someone will eventually figure out the right business model. I spent a few years doing just that for various healthcare companies at McKinsey & Company—figuring out the best business model in light of market dynamics, technological innovations, and the competitive environment. I also built a company that sold care management software to providers, which isn't an easy set of customers to sell to. AI-based solutions will face skepticism and have a tough road ahead before they gain adoption, even if they're solving clear, unmet needs. That's just how it is in healthcare. Changing the practice of medicine isn't easy, but changing the business of healthcare is a little easier. So, what are the right business models for companies that are innovating in healthcare AI? How can the investors separate the winning companies from the pack.

First, there are several business models that could work. Successfully commercializing these technologies to providers, consumers, or life science companies will probably require different business models. Within the healthcare delivery system, business models are notoriously complex and not for the faint of heart. The end users of healthcare products (providers or patients) are usually different from the people who decide if they should be using the AI solution (executives or providers); those who pay for it are different from

AI Doctor: The Rise of Artificial Intelligence in Healthcare: A Guide for Users, Buyers, Builders, and Investors, First Edition. Ronald M. Razmi.
© 2024 Ronald M. Razmi. Published 2024 by John Wiley & Sons, Inc.

those who prescribe it; and those who approve the marketing of the products (e.g. the Food and Drug Administration [FDA]) are different to the ones paying for it. For technologies like radiology AI applications, which could be used by healthcare providers to do their jobs more effectively, the FDA approves it, health system executives decide if they can buy it for providers, and payers decide whether to reimburse for it.

This is why it's worth identifying the right business models for any AI solutions before you spend years building it. Unless innovators figure out how to successfully commercialize AI-based products or services, the sector will struggle to grow. We've seen many of the companies that are developing healthcare AI solutions raise a large amount of capital and show increasing valuations with subsequent rounds of financing or with successful initial public offering (IPOs). However, we've seen less evidence of significant adoption and revenue growth from commercializing those technologies. This may be because the buyers of these technologies—such as providers, payers, and life science companies—are still learning about the use cases and their impact on their business model. As they become convinced of their value and their impact on the bottom line, we can expect them to accelerate their expenditure on AI technologies as a new way to deliver care, develop new diagnostics or treatments, and improve their operations.

Life science companies are dipping their toes into drug discovery and development. For both of these areas, the jury is still out on how much they can improve on traditional approaches. Massive investments have been made in AI for drug discovery, and although some drugs are making their way through initial clinical trials, it remains to be seen how much time and money can be saved—if any can be saved at all. Despite the promise of AI in trial design, site selection, patient recruitment, and patient engagement, the clear return on investment (ROI) for these applications is yet to be established. As such, life science companies are still cautious buyers of AI-enabled solutions, and although attractive use cases are being reported, we still haven't seen a clear ROI.

14.1   Barriers to Entry and Intellectual Property (IP)

One of the keys to the success of any business is the protection of IP. If people could just copy your technology as soon as it was available, how would you protect your long-term profits? In life sciences, the drugs are under strict patents for 20 years and nobody can create the same molecule until your patent expires. That makes it worthwhile for drug companies to invest billions of dollars to develop these drugs. For device companies, their devices are patented and they have a period of protection that ensures they can recover their investments and create the desired ROI.

With digital technologies, there's always been more of a question mark. How can you protect computer code? If you have hardware, like a wearable device, you can create IP protection for the device and the software that runs inside it can be covered by the patent. But what if you only have software? If you only have code, can you protect it? What if you've developed an AI model as the basis for your software? Most of the algorithms used to develop AI models are open source, which means that anyone can use them to develop their own models if they have access to the right data.

If you work for a commercial entity that has a model for reading computed tomography (CT) scans for strokes or tumors, can you protect your model by stopping others with access to good data and open-source algorithms from developing a similar model? What if there's a medical center using its own data? What if another commercial entity develops a model that's more accurate because it uses a richer dataset to develop and validate the model? As an investor, that would give me pause to write a check for such a company.

Academic medical centers are making significant investments in creating long-term datasets and incorporating them into their workflows and patient care. Massachusetts General Hospital (MGH) has launched the Center for Clinical Data Science, a full-sized team that's solely focused on creating, promoting, and translating AI into tools that will enhance clinical outcomes, improve efficiency, and enhance patient-focused care.[1] In 2018, they signed an agreement with Nuance to carry out rapid development, validation and deployment for radiologists at the point of care. We're seeing something similar at the Cleveland Clinic, the Mayo Clinic, and many other academic medical centers.

There's now more than two decades' worth of patents that have been granted for digital products. Many of these are about novel ways of collecting remote data or using data and code to manage patients. A study of these patents shows that they're less about the core technology used—such as remote data collection or the actual code—and more about the method of use. The core technologies used to collect data from wearables or the use of that data to manage health can't be patented, so the specific system design or method of use is patented instead. This provides some protection and keeps others from just copying the system, but it's not nearly as strong as the patents that protect molecules or medical devices. With digital technologies, there's usually a different way to do the same thing without designing the system in the exact same way. As such, most investors discount these patents for the most part.

Since 2021, there have been 321 filings for AI-related patents in the pharma space, according to research firm Pharmaceutical Technology, nearly as much as in the previous six years combined.[2] But while digital health companies can patent their initial algorithms, the US Patent and Trademark Office has ruled that AI can't be the inventor of new patents. This means that once a company's algorithm starts generating novel insights on its own, they can't be patented and protected. The US Eastern District of Virginia ruled in favor of this finding in September of 2022.

"Data isn't patentable," says Anne Li, an IP lawyer at Crowell. This doesn't mean that digital health companies are out of luck, she says, they just need to protect themselves. "When you're entering into joint agreements or doing clinical trials, it's very important to have the correct structures in place to protect patient confidentiality and your dataset."[2]

GE Healthcare was granted a patent in 2018 discussing the use of machine learning to analyze cell types in microscope images.[3] The patent proposes an "intuitive interface enabling medical staff (e.g. pathologists and biologists) to annotate and evaluate different cell phenotypes used in the algorithm and be presented through the interface." This shows how AI patents are less about protecting a concept or an approach and more about a specific system that makes the workflow and user interface more streamlined for developing the algorithm. Although interesting, there are many other approaches being used to evaluate cell phenotypes in pathology and none would violate the patent, which only protects GE's specific system and workflow.

14.1.1   Creating Defensible Products

Given that many entities have access to large datasets and the foundational algorithms are mostly open source, the barriers to entry are rather low. As such, barriers other than IP should be used to build sustainable businesses over time. Prototype AI models can be surprisingly easy to build, but there's little precedent for preparing them for clinical use. We need to be able to integrate them into multiple disparate systems using all sorts of different data types. We also need to be able to commercialize them, which requires us to demonstrate the value of them when it comes to reducing costs and improving outcomes.

One possible approach is to build end-to-end systems that introduce intelligent automation to the entire process and which aren't just an algorithm that sits in the cloud and solves one problem in the value chain. This provides a more defensible model, as solving healthcare workflows end-to-end requires deep expertise and a combination of skills that are hard to come by. You can see that today with many of the companies that have built AI solutions. Most of them were able to get hold of data and to develop models that are point solutions. However, the deep thinking required around the workflow issues that need to be solved to successfully operationalize their algorithm is often missing. As such, most are surprised when they learn that FDA approval isn't their ticket to rapid adoption and successful commercialization.

Another approach to create competitive differentiation and barriers to entry is to develop a brand and to establish a reputation for building great models. One of the key concerns about AI models is that they were built and validated on limited datasets and that their performance in the real world often falls short of what they showed in their FDA trials. There's already evidence of this with some of the models by Epic (electronic health record [EHR] system) and other vendors.[4]

Researchers at Mount Sinai's Icahn School of Medicine found that the same deep learning algorithms diagnosing pneumonia in their own chest X-rays didn't work as well when applied to images from the National Institutes of Health and the Indiana University Network for Patient Care.[5] Also, when clinical algorithms were launched at Mount Sinai hospital, a number of issues were encountered including inconsistent data quality, the difficulty of managing different data sources, and a lack of standardization.[6]

This all points to an opportunity to create a brand in this emerging field as a purveyor of top-notch models that are trained and validated on large and heterogeneous datasets with robust performance in the real world and across different settings. Also, given the potential bias for AI models in healthcare, being known for practicing responsible AI will be a differentiator. The Coalition for AI Health (CHAI) is developing recommendations for dependable health AI technologies that can be used by buyers when vetting these products. The CHAI has previously produced a paper on bias, equity, and fairness which is being used to develop the recommendations. The result will be a framework, the *Guidelines for the Responsible Use of AI in Healthcare*, which will intentionally foster resilient AI assurance, safety, and security. This presents an opportunity for companies that are serious about using a robust approach to building responsible AI models to differentiate themselves and gain a competitive advantage.[7]

One other powerful way to create barriers to entry and to differentiate is to undertake large-scale clinical studies that establish the benefits of your AI solutions and show stakeholders that the algorithms achieve their expected results. These results could include improving patient outcomes, reducing costs, improving institutions' operations, and boosting clinical and administrative staff productivity. This isn't the kind of effort that most companies have the appetite for, know how to do, have the funds for, or can execute well.

It can be surprisingly easy to build AI algorithms, but it's often difficult to understand the associated workflows and challenges. That's why it's so difficult to convert algorithms into sophisticated products that work consistently in general clinical applications. Showing how these AI products reduce costs and improve outcomes will require clinical translation and industrial-grade integration into routine workflows.[8] That would be a powerful barrier to entry, and better than any patents!

14.2   Startups Versus Large Companies

Allow me to introduce Nuance AI Marketplace, an open platform that's designed to help developers, data scientists, and radiologists accelerate the development, deployment, and adoption of AI in medical imaging.

The company has a partnership with the MGH to make its internally developed radiology algorithms available in the Nuance AI Marketplace. Some are FDA-approved. This means that commercial companies with FDA-approved radiology algorithms that perform the same function are competing with MGH on the Nuance marketplace.

Once on the Nuance marketplace, the algorithms can be directly embedded into radiologists' workflows using reporting tools like Nuance PowerScribe One. This shows that larger companies, like Nuance, are carving out key roles for themselves. They don't necessarily need to develop the algorithms, but they can make them available to everyone once they're cleared by the FDA. Since Nuance is helping with the implementation of medical algorithms for health systems and providers, it incentivizes them to buy the Nuance platform so that they can find and activate AI solutions quicker and more easily.

For smaller companies, there are many pitfalls in getting into the AI business. They include having to assemble large, well-annotated datasets, the ability to use huge amounts of computing power, and the technical skills required to build the models and integrate them into the complex web of information systems at health centers. This may be beyond the reach of smaller, more innovative companies which could develop algorithms, but which might struggle to operationalize them. As such, larger companies like Nuance could create the ecosystem that these algorithms will launch in. This means that the established companies with diverse capabilities will be vital for the future of AI in Healthcare.

Philips has developed an AI-based tool called Illumeo, for radiologists, which can display contextual information about patients alongside their images so that physicians don't need to hunt around for that information.[9] Better still, it can anticipate radiologists' needs, such as by automatically suggesting the right tools to use to measure and analyze blood vessels. It can even learn individual user preferences, or what's known in the industry as radiologists' "hanging protocol."[10] Phillips is one of the major hardware and software vendors for radiology, and incorporating new AI solutions into their existing user-base would allow their customers to benefit from these solutions inside their existing workflows. This highlights opportunities for the companies developing these solutions to interface and fit inside legacy systems—or even to develop them specifically *for* those systems. That would improve the odds of a successful exit.

Another key factor giving established companies an edge is that they'll be able to bring a suite of AI applications to their users. Too many small companies will only have one or two solutions, and dealing with multiple companies will be difficult for buyers. They'll prefer to deal with larger companies that consolidate those solutions into multiple modules in a single application. Vendors with practice management software, hospital claims and payment vendors, and analytic providers will all be natural choices. Hardware vendors and PACS vendors will be natural consolidators for radiology solutions. A vertical focus will likely be critical to success when it comes to collecting data for developing and testing models in the real world and then optimizing them for wider rollout.

It's important to note that even larger companies have struggled with AI in their health offerings. Ten years ago, IBM's Watson was able to beat humans at the popular quiz show "Jeopardy!," supposedly marking a huge shift in the way that machines could answer questions. Pundits said that this would open up new revenues for IBM and for major tech companies in general. Healthcare is an obvious target, a trillion-dollar industry that's full of inefficiencies. So far, AI has been unable to live up to that promise. IBM has even sold Watson Health, despite spending billions of dollars to build it up in an effort to help doctors diagnose and cure cancer.

Unfortunately for IBM, Watson Health struggled for market share and was never really profitable.[11] Alphabet Inc.'s Google DeepMind, which famously developed a Go-playing algorithm that vanquished a champion human player in 2016, later launched several healthcare-related initiatives focused on chronic conditions.[12] DeepMind has also lost money in recent years with their healthcare initiatives, as well as being criticized for how health data was being collected.[13, 14]

All of this helps to highlight how hard it can be to apply AI to healthcare, with hurdles including human, financial, and technological barriers. Even the largest technology companies struggle to fully understand how an AI solution that "works" can be incorporated into the practice of medicine. Developers need to understand what clinical workflows look like in the trenches, as well as where they can insert AI without slowing things down in the clinic. When we add that to the reimbursement and business challenges, we can see how monumental the challenge is to create a successful business, whether large or small.

14.3   Sales and Marketing

In my discussions with leaders at cutting-edge companies with FDA-approved products in healthcare AI, I've noticed a common thread. Most were surprised by how difficult it's been to successfully sell FDA-approved solutions in radiology, pathology, ophthalmology, and more. They noted that medical centers aren't sure how to use the solutions and are therefore cautious about pulling the trigger. They explained that the caution stems from uncertainty about how healthcare AI solutions will fit into their existing technology portfolio, how it will interface with their legacy systems, what their ROI will be, and whether they'll be reimbursed. They also asked, "Is it really necessary?"

Here are some of their comments:

- "Medical centers are interested but they're not moving rapidly to buy FDA-approved algorithms to incorporate into their daily operations. Although the data used for FDA approval establishes the safety and efficacy of the algorithms, it doesn't establish improvements to efficiency or patient outcomes."
- "We're finding that medical centers don't yet have the expertise to operationalize algorithms and selling them algorithms doesn't seem conducive to their operating model."
- "Changes to workflow in radiology departments is a barrier to adoption."
- "Medical centers are asking for more evidence than what they've been shown so far when buying these algorithms."
- "The FDA only cares if [the algorithms] are safe or efficacious in performing the required task, but it's not currently asking providers to show endpoints such as time savings or improved patient outcomes."

As you can see from these comments, AI healthcare developers are running into issues with buyers, and a lot of it is centered around two areas—buyers aren't sure how to operationalize AI solutions, and the evidence used to gain FDA approval isn't enough to convince buyers to make a purchase. Often, several committees are involved in making a final decision and each application is reviewed and decided upon in isolation. Key questions include, "What problem does it solve?," "How much better is it than the current solutions?," and "What value does it add?"

The sale of these solutions to buyers like health systems, payers, and life science companies is complicated and bureaucratic. The sellers need internal champions to navigate clinical and administrative minefields to get the software adopted and paid for. The internal champion is someone in the clinical or operational team at the healthcare customers or someone in the R&D or commercial team in the life science companies who will make the case to the organization to buy your solution. They make the case that you solve an important issue for their group and do so in a way that makes its adoption easy. They present to multiple committees and make the clinical and business cases for buying the new technology. The more these people have been equipped with evidence of the benefits of your technology, the more convincingly they can make the case for it and the better the chances are of their company buying it.

You often need to create a pipeline of customers and continue to do product demonstrations and provide evidence of the ROI of your solution to potential customers. In healthcare, the rule of thumb is that your customers are looking for at least a 4 or 5 to 1 ROI. That means that they'll gain $4–5 of new sales or cost savings for every dollar they pay you.

Buoy Health has a free chatbot that helps people figure out the best setting to seek care for their specific issues. Their revenue comes from partnering with medical centers that can benefit from the patients choosing them for their medical problems. This can be described as a business-to-consumer-to-business model. By showing adoption by consumers, you can get the attention of decision-makers at provider institutions that will see it as a way to drive patients to their facilities. This leads to more revenue, and there's no better way to get their attention than to drive more business to them.

If you work for an innovative company with an FDA-approved healthcare AI solution, it can be a shock when you realize that no one is lining up to buy your well-designed and full-of-value product. But there are no shortcuts, and you have to stand in line with everyone else unless you've generated evidence that your product can improve the customers' business model. This can be in the form of a well-designed trial or carefully collecting evidence of the benefits of your solution while doing pilots with initial customers.

When it's time to make the sale, you need to decide how to price it. Will you go with a subscription model, a SaaS model, or a pilot model? How about a percentage of the value created as part of a value-based contract that the provider is participating in?

The answer will vary depending on the type of solution you're selling, but a good rule of thumb is to stay out of any model that pays you based on the adoption of the solution or the demonstrable value provided. Both of those are poison for a young company. It always takes longer than you expect for users to adopt your solution, and showing the value you've added in a value-based contract is difficult to quantify and takes time. This can mean that you'll go out of business before you see any of the money.

You should aim for contracts that pay you at least a minimum annual fee, regardless of usage or value shown. This minimum fee should cover your costs of servicing the contract and include some margin. This will at least keep the lights on for your business until the widespread adoption of AI solutions becomes commonplace. In order to maximize revenues, a transaction or user-based revenue model will ensure that you capture as much value as possible from the solution you're providing. Generally, AI-based platforms are in the cloud and there are variable costs associated with the amount of cloud space you use that are proportional to the amount of data that's processed through the system. As such, figure out the drivers of the variable costs and ensure that your pricing model reflects that.

I've never been a fan of the cost-plus pricing model. When I was a McKinsey consultant, I saw how companies left significant amounts of money on the table because they opted for some arbitrary margin above their costs, when the customer would have paid much more since they got significant value from the solution. As such, figuring out the economic value to the customer and trying to capture a portion of that value ensures that you maximize your pricing power. However, making sure you know what it costs to provide the solution and ensuring that your pricing is at least in line with your competitors is a simple way to make sure you're not significantly underpricing your offering.

Another key issue is that healthcare customers are slow to pay. The cash cycle is even longer than the sales cycles, and the sales cycles are really long! What I refer to as the cash cycle includes sales cycle, contracting time, implementation time, and collection of the first invoice. This can be quite long and perilous to your business. At Acupera, we often had to wait four to five months to get paid when our contracts had payables of 30–60 days. This means calling repeatedly to collect, and since you're not sitting on top of a big cash cushion, you may have to go to your investors to bridge you until you get paid. It's not a good situation to be in, and they'll eventually run out of patience and cut you off. As such, be sure to estimate all of this and to carefully manage your cash. Raise more money to anticipate and be covered for these long cash cycles or keep your burn rate lower since it'll be a while before you get paid, even after you make the sale,

14.4   Initial Customers

While we've examined the issues that are keeping the majority of buyers from immediately adopting healthcare AI solutions, there are still pockets of potential buyers who could become the early adopters. These buyers can see an immediate ROI and don't need to wait for additional evidence or reimbursement.

One such group consists of independent radiology groups and teleradiology businesses, which can differentiate themselves by improving their output in terms of quality and speed. If the AI algorithms can make them more accurate when reading scans and add more quantification, such as the progression of a tumor over time, it will allow them to make their end product of a higher quality than that of their competitors. Also, providers value the speed with which they receive these reports. If providers can get reports faster and offer more expedient care to their patients, they'll most likely direct more business to the radiology group that offers the fastest reports.

The diagnostic imaging provider RadNet, which maintains a US network of 350 outpatient imaging centers, has its own subsidiary that develops AI solutions that can improve the quality and speed of the radiology workflow. They've also secured two software clearances from the FDA to help radiologists spot breast and prostate cancer.[15] This highlights the fact that if you work for a healthcare AI company that's developing radiology algorithms, RadNet could be an ideal customer thanks to its radiology centers around the country. However, if your potential customers are developing and gaining approval for their own algorithms, how can you stay in business? Can you be accurate with your forecasts if you don't know which target customers are developing their own solutions?

For teleradiology businesses, their value proposition is that they can quickly and accurately read scans. If these tools allow them to better triage and contact medical centers for the acute cases that need immediate attention, they can become a more highly valued partner. Teleradiology vendors often provide evening and weekend coverage. This means that there are fewer resources in hospitals to take care of acutely ill patients. The timely mobilization of those resources could save lives and create a less chaotic environment. Because of that, the ability to quickly identify those cases and notify providers will be of high value to those providers.

Academic medical centers (AMCs) could provide another important group of early customers. AMCs usually handle large volumes of patients as they're often the destination for the uninsured and underinsured. They're trauma centers that receive complicated patients sent to them from other centers. If AI technologies are showing promise as assistive devices to improve or hasten diagnosis, to make their clinical staff more productive, and to improve operations, they're more likely to be first movers. If they see an immediate benefit, they'll work with the solution provider to generate the real-world evidence that can accelerate commercialization of that solution (probably for a discount!).

Of course, these medical centers can develop their own models. They have plenty of data and the resources to use that data to develop high-quality models. So, what's stopping them? In a lot of cases, nothing! Some are busy developing models for various clinical and administrative issues and gaining experience. Some are trying to commercialize their models to other providers, although they're in the minority. Most will use models that are developed by outside entities since they don't have the bandwidth to develop their own models. My discussions have shown that most medical centers say that the key benefit of externally developed models is that they save time. Building a model from scratch takes a lot of time and effort, and so finding a relevant model from an outside vendor and then training it on local data is a much faster option.

My interviews with AMC leaders have suggested that they'll continue to invest in AI and to learn from their experiences. At the moment, most of them are using hybrid models which combine self-developed algorithms and commercially available algorithms from industry vendors. This approach allows them to focus on key niches through their own algorithms while simultaneously using the commercial algorithms to tackle broader opportunities. Because of that, they're able to harness their own internal expertise as well as the wider expertise of the industry.

14.5　Direct-to-Consumer (D2C)

One of the major benefits of AI-enabled healthcare solutions is that they provide a higher degree of personalization. As such, they could be a wise choice in the emerging D2C health market.

Companies are selling products that are meant to address basic health and wellness issues by providing personalized nutrition, personalized exercise programs, home screening for diseases like skin or colon cancer, and more. In these situations, rather than selling to providers or payers, companies market and sell directly to consumers. In recent years, we've seen companies like RO, HIMS, and ThirtyMadison engage in the D2C health market. Some of the products are touted to be personalized based on consumers' genetics, skin types, and other factors.

Some of the key benefits to the D2C model include that it allows companies to market to people before they enter the healthcare system, build a brand with the consumers, identify lower acuity needs, and provide a personalized service. There's a notoriously slow sales cycle for enterprise customers in the healthcare industry, so D2C affords a much shorter sales cycle and ramping up revenues faster. Therefore, D2C can offer direct access to consumers, quicker transactions, and fewer barriers.

This all combines to make it an appealing model for startups that are entering the market. However, in spite of all of these benefits, it's proven to be a tough business model for digital health companies. That's because many people believe that since they pay their insurance premiums, any health-related products should be paid for by their insurance company. Also, customer acquisition costs can be quite high in a D2C business model. That's why the recovery of those costs isn't guaranteed, since many people don't continue to use digital health products like wearables or apps long-term

In a report about the subject, Rock Health indicated that D2C business models aren't always conducive to achieving the scale and widespread impact that healthcare innovation can offer due to high customer acquisition costs.[16] One big issue is that the burden of payment often falls at the feet of consumers. This has historically spelled doom for healthcare companies as people want their insurance to pay for health products.

That's why some digital health companies are adopting a dual approach in which they compete in both the D2C and business to business (B2B) markets. This allows them to engage those users directly, to raise awareness, and to bring in some revenue while they take on the slow enterprise sales process.

If the solutions that are offered to people actually work and there's solid evidence for it—especially in the health, wellness, and preventive space—then I'd take that approach every time. In areas such as nutrition and fitness, where the consumer already shoulders the burden of payment, it's likely that they'll be open to solutions that help them make better choices and receive personalized health benefits.

The major advantage is that you can bypass the long and complex enterprise sales process. However, with higher customer acquisition costs and the need for standing out in the crowd, you'll need to be well-funded to bear the costs of sales and marketing. Also, you'll need to roll up your sleeves and generate the evidence that allows you to differentiate and to get endorsement from the medical community.

14.6 Planning Your Entrepreneurial Health AI Journey

Selling to providers and life science companies is always difficult. Health systems, independent hospitals, and medical groups aren't high-margin businesses. They usually operate on single-digit profit margins and have to jump through a lot of hoops to be paid for the services they provide. As such, they're very deliberate with their technology investments, despite being bombarded by different companies trying to get them to try the latest and greatest technologies. They're hearing messages about how each of those technologies will increase their revenues, lower their costs, improve patient outcomes, and boost productivity. As such, they have various processes in place to review new technologies, usually involving committee after committee to prepare the ultimate business case that will be presented to decision-makers.

Given the limited budget for technology at clinical institutions or life science companies, one indisputable question that has to be asked before you develop any AI solutions is if it solves a problem that's mission-critical. If you successfully develop your AI solution and start offering it to your customers, will it provide a major improvement in how they're doing something that's core to their business? If you're helping with reading routine radiology scans and your benefit is that the radiologist can become a little more efficient and a little more accurate, that may not be enough to make the cut for the health system to buy your system. If you do a first-pass screening of patient charts to identify potential clinical trial participants but that needs to be reviewed again by pharma screeners, your value may lack the wow factor.

That doesn't mean these systems aren't an improvement over the current approaches and don't create value. It's just that their value might not be enough when stacked up against other solutions that solve more critical problems and do so in a more complete manner. If the current approach to the issue you're solving is good enough, your customers might not be able to justify spending on a fancy new toy. In order to carry out this analysis in the most methodical way, you need to figure out what the costs of the current approaches are and estimate the impact that you'll have on that cost. If the cost is high and you have a high impact (two highs), you might be on to something. If the answer to either one of those questions is a "low," you might not be able to get much traction for your solution.

The next key question to ask is whether your solution makes life easier for users or whether it creates extra work. The workflow issue is very important. If you solve a mission-critical problem but you're too disruptive to existing workflows, the chances of adoption aren't good. We have a decade of experience with promising digital health solutions that worked outside of the EHR (and good luck asking the clinical team to work in a system outside of the EHR) and resulted in extra work for the team. Extra work for the team doesn't bode well for your chance of adoption, even if you create a lot of value.

Needless to say, those systems didn't see a large amount of adoption. Examples include the many analytic platforms that have tried to bring more of a business analytics approach to the practice and operation of medicine. None gained much traction because they didn't fit with the existing workflows. It's possible to create new workflows using a superior technology, but the new workflow has to make things easier for everyone involved, automate steps, save time, and more. Otherwise, good luck getting people in clinical medicine, life science company R&D or commercial teams to change their workflows.

The next important factor to consider is whether your solution will be paid for out of their own pockets or whether they'll expect it to be reimbursed by insurance companies. If the answer is the latter, you have a much steeper hill to climb. If the benefit of your solution is better patient outcomes, health systems and providers would like to see it reimbursed by payers. Of course, the payer will only reimburse if they see strong evidence. So, we're back to the issue of having to do well-designed trials or generating evidence with initial deployments. You'll need to generate the ROI evidence regardless of the reimbursement issue, but if the payers are involved, the process gets longer and the evidence required is far higher.

For AI solutions that improve health system operations or life science business models, there wouldn't be a reimbursement. In those cases, your ROI is based on the money saved, new revenues, faster development timelines, higher patient adherence to the prescribed therapies, and faster provider adoption of new diagnostics or treatments. If your solution improves the use of an existing pharmaceutical or device (e.g. an adjunct digital therapeutic), you might come back to the reimbursement issue. If the life science company can see a higher use of their product with your AI solution, they may decide that gaining market share is worth the price they'll pay you. However, if most of the benefit accrues to the patient, you might need extra reimbursement beyond what's already paid for the drug or the device.

Another interesting business model is using AI solutions as tools that are used internally to provide services at a lower cost with increased automation. This can translate into higher quality output (e.g. better and faster reads of radiology scans) at a competitive price that makes your offering a better value. Many health systems or life science companies don't have certain skills in enough quantity in-house and would be willing to pay outside vendors to help them if the price isn't too high. Examples of these for health systems include disease management programs, community outreach services, and telehealth programs. For life science companies, these can include drug discovery, clinical trial management, patient engagement, provider content generation, and more. In these situations, you can build a business with a high-quality service that's enabled by your internal use of AI and which potentially has better margins.

14.7   Assessment of Companies by Investors

As an investor in this area, I see many opportunities for the next decade and beyond to invest in AI solutions that will improve population health. This will be one of the most exciting areas for investors. To find the right companies, investors need to be very discerning, as many of the solutions that sound great (discovery AI, anyone?) will take a long time to show results. That means that many of the companies tackling those problems won't make it. There's a long list of companies that have built health AI algorithms that got FDA approval and never gained any clinical traction.

There are many AI companies that developed solutions in drug discovery and created partnerships with big pharma but are now worthless. How do you avoid investing in future zombie health AI companies? Based on my past operating and investing experience and my research in this space for the last few years, I offer the following areas to explore as you're considering a health AI company to invest in. This is for both public and private companies. Some of the supposedly best health AI companies that went public with valuations of billions of dollars didn't hold up to public market scrutiny. Examples of that are Babylon and Benevolent AI.

14.7.1   Key Areas to Explore for a Health AI Company for Investment

- Are they solving a mission-critical unmet need? What's the cost of the current approach? What's their estimated impact on this cost?
- Will they fit into existing workflows or will a new workflow be created for users? If so, does this make things easier and remove work, or will it add extra work?
- How strong is the evidence that this health AI solution will work in the real-world environment? Will the necessary data be available for it to create its output?

- How involved will the implementation be? Will it require multiple data interfaces with existing systems?
- Will the customer need to devote significant resources to launch the system?
- What's the realistic ROI for the customer?
- What's the total cost of ownership for the customer?
- How complex will the sales and marketing be for such a novel technology? What are the length of the sales and cash cycles?
- How difficult will it be for another entity to develop a similar or better solution if they have access to good datasets? What are the real barriers for the competitors?

Although some of these questions are part of any investment analysis, they take on extra importance for health AI solutions since the technologies are novel and unfamiliar to buyers. As such, carefully analyzing if the data needed to create the output will actually be flowing readily into the AI solution in a real-world environment, or realizing that there are fragmented data systems in the customer environment that can impede the availability of the needed data, will make a huge difference. In the latter scenario, the system will often fail to work as expected and the chances of long-term adoption will significantly diminish. Or, if the medical centers or life science companies set a high bar for the amount of evidence they need to buy, you'll need to invest significant time and money to generate that evidence. That could make the investment case far less compelling and the time to an exit event much longer.

References

1. Siwicki, B. (2021, May 10). Mass General Brigham and the future of AI in radiology. Healthcare IT News. https://www.healthcareitnews.com/news/mass-general-brigham-and-future-ai-radiology
2. Perna, G. (2022, August 4). Digital health-pharma relationships face intellectual property uncertainty. Digital Health Business & Technology. https://digitalhealth.modernhealthcare.com/mergers-acquisitions-ma/digital-health-pharma-relationships-face-intellectual-property-uncertainty
3. Andrade, J. C. (2019, May 6). The AI industry series: top Healthcare AI trends to watch. Judith Chao Andrade.
4. Ross, C. (2022, September 12). Epic's AI algorithms, shielded from scrutiny by a corporate firewall, are delivering inaccurate information on seriously ill patients. STAT. https://www.statnews.com/2021/07/26/epic-hospital-algorithms-sepsis-investigation/

5. Sullivan, T. (2018, November 8). Mount Sinai finds deep learning algorithms inconsistent when applied. Healthcare IT News. https://www.healthcareitnews.com/news/mount-sinai-finds-deep-learning-algorithms-inconsistent-when-applied-outside-imaging-data-sets

6. Timsina, P., Kia, A. (2020, January 28). Machine learning platform at Mount Sinai Health System (co-presentation). [Video]. YouTube. https://www.youtube.com/watch?v=aKAvj7njGw8&ab_channel=Ai4

7. Kennedy, S. (2022, December 12). Coalition for Health AI unveils blueprint for ethical AI implementation. HealthITAnalytics. https://healthitanalytics.com/news/coalition-for-health-ai-unveils-blueprint-for-ethical-ai-implementation

8. Dreyer, K. J., & Geis, J. R. (2017b). When machines think: radiology's next frontier. Radiology, 285(3), 713–718. https://doi.org/10.1148/radiol.2017171183

9. Diagnostic informatics | Medical Software | Philips Healthcare. (2022). Philips. https://www.usa.philips.com/healthcare/solutions/clinical-informatics

10. Wilson, J., Daugherty, P. (2018, March 27). AI will change Health Care jobs for the better. Harvard Business Review https://hbr.org/2018/03/ai-will-change-health-care-jobs-for-the-better

11. Hernandez, D., & Greenwald, T. (2018, August 11). IBM has a Watson Dilemma. WSJ. https://www.wsj.com/articles/ibm-bet-billions-that-watson-could-improve-cancer-treatment-it-hasnt-worked-1533961147?mod=article_inline

12. Associated Press. (2016, March 9). Google's software beats human go champion. WSJ. https://www.wsj.com/articles/googles-software-beats-human-go-champion-1457516770?mod=article_inline

13. Copeland, R., & Olson, P. (2021, January 26). Artificial intelligence will define Google's future. For now, it's a management challenge. WSJ. https://www.wsj.com/articles/artificial-intelligence-will-define-googles-future-for-now-its-a-management-challenge-11611676945?mod=article_inline

14. Hernandez, D., & Fitch, A. (2021, February 23). IBM's retreat from Watson highlights broader AI struggles in health. WSJ. https://www.wsj.com/articles/ibms-retreat-from-watson-highlights-broader-ai-struggles-in-health-11613839579

15. RadNet scores 2 FDA clearances for AI programs in breast, prostate cancers. (2022, June 2). Biotech Insider. https://biotech-insider.com/radnet-scores-2-fda-clearances-for-ai-programs-in-breast-prostate-cancers/

16. Consumer, V. O. T., Adams, A., Shankar, M., Tecco, H., With help from: Evans, B., & McGuinness, D. (2021, July 31). 50 things we now know about digital health consumers | Rock Health. https://rockhealth.com/insights/digital-health-consumer-adoption-2016/

Index

Note: Page numbers in *italic* and **bold** refers to figures and tables, respectively.